Novel Wearable Antennas for Communication and Medical Systems

Novel Wearable Antennas for Communication and Medical Systems

By

Albert Sabban

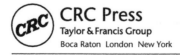

CRC Press
Taylor & Francis Group
Boca Raton London New York

CRC Press is an imprint of the
Taylor & Francis Group, an **informa** business

CRC Press
Taylor & Francis Group
6000 Broken Sound Parkway NW, Suite 300
Boca Raton, FL 33487-2742

First issued in paperback 2019

© 2018 by Taylor & Francis Group, LLC
CRC Press is an imprint of Taylor & Francis Group, an Informa business

No claim to original U.S. Government works

ISBN-13: 978-1-138-04790-7 (hbk)
ISBN-13: 978-0-367-88934-0 (pbk)

Library of Congress Cataloging-in-Publication Data

Names: Sabban, Albert, author.
Title: Novel wearable antennas for communication and medical systems / Albert Sabban.
Description: Boca Raton : Taylor & Francis, 2017. | "A CRC title, part of the Taylor & Francis imprint, a member of the Taylor & Francis Group, the academic division of T&F Informa plc." | Includes bibliographical references.
Identifiers: LCCN 2017014864 | ISBN 9781138047907 (harback : alk. paper)
Subjects: LCSH: Biomedical engineering--Instruments. | Smart materials.
Classification: LCC R856 .S23 2017 | DDC 610.28--dc23
LC record available at https://lccn.loc.gov/2017014864

Visit the Taylor & Francis Web site at
http://www.taylorandfrancis.com

and the CRC Press Web site at
http://www.crcpress.com

Dedication

This book is dedicated to the memory of my father, mother and sister. David Sabban, Dolly Sabban and Aliza Sabban

Table of Contents

Preface

The main objective of this book is to present new compact wearable antennas for communication and medical systems. Chapter 1 presents the fundamental concepts and applications of wearable communication and medical systems. Chapter 2 presents wearable communication and medical systems electromagnetics and the basic theory and fundamentals of antennas. Chapter 3 presents an introduction to the basic theory for wireless wearable communication system designers. Chapter 4 presents basic antennas for wearable communication systems. Chapter 5 presents wearable printed antennas for wireless communication systems. These chapters are written to assist electrical engineers and students in the study of basic electromagnetic, communication and antenna theory and fundamentals. There are many books on electromagnetic theory and antennas for the electromagnetic scientist. However, there are few books that help electrical engineers and undergraduate students to study and understand basic electromagnetic, communication and antenna theory and fundamentals with few integral and differential equations.

There are several 3D full-wave electromagnetics software products, such as HFSS, ADS, and CST, used to design and analyze communication systems and antennas. Communication systems and antennas developed and analyzed in this book were designed using HFSS and ADS software. For almost all antennas and devices described in this book there was good agreement between computed and measured results. Only one design and fabrication iteration was needed in the development process of the devices and antennas presented in this book.

Wideband wearable antennas for communication and medical applications are presented in Chapter 6. Several wearable antennas are presented in this chapter. Antenna electrical parameters as a function of distance from the human body is discussed in this chapter. Compact wearable radio frequency identification (RFID) antennas are presented in Section 6.8. Chapter 7 presents base station aperture antennas for communication systems. Antenna arrays for wireless communication systems are presented in Section 7.5. An integrated outdoor unit for MM wave satellite communication applications is presented in Section 7.6. A solid state power amplifier (SSPA) is presented in Section 7.7. An integrated Ku band automatic tracking system is presented in Section 7.9.

Novel wearable antennas for wireless communication systems are presented in Chapter 8. New wideband wearable meta-material antennas for communication applications are presented in Section 8.1 through 8.3. Meta-material antenna characteristics in the vicinity of the human body are discussed in Section 8.4. Wearable fractal printed antennas are presented in Sections 8.7 through 8.11. Active wearable printed antennas for medical applications are presented in Chapter 9. Wearable tunable printed antennas for medical applications are presented in Sections 9.1 through 9.8. Active wearable receiving antennas are presented in Section 9.9. An active transmitting antenna is presented in Section 9.10. New wide band passive and active wearable slot and notch antennas for wireless and medical communication systems are presented in Chapter 10.

Microwave and MM wave technologies are presented in Chapter 11. Microwave integrated circuits, monolithic microwave integrated circuits, microelectro-mechanical systems, and low temperature co-fired ceramic technologies are presented in Chapter 11. The main goal of wireless body area networks (BANs) is to continuously provide medical data to physicians.

Design considerations, computational results and measured results of wearable compact transceivers, BANs, are presented in Chapter 12. Wearable systems and antenna measurements are presented in Chapter 13.

Each chapter of the book covers sufficient details to enable students, scientists from all areas, and electrical and biomedical engineers to follow and understand the topics presented in the book. The book begins with the elementary communication, electromagnetics, and antenna topics needed for students and engineers with no background in communication, electromagnetic and antenna theory to study and understand the basic design principles and features of antennas, wearable antennas, printed antennas, and compact antennas for communication and medical applications.

Several topics and designs are presented in this book for the first time. This book may serve students and design engineers as a reference work. It presents new designs in the area of wearable antennas, meta-material antennas, fractal antennas, and active receiving and transmitting antennas. The text contains sufficient mathematical detail and explanations to enable electrical engineering and physics students to understand all topics presented in this book.

Several new wearable antennas are introduced in this book. Design considerations and computed and measured results for the new wearable systems and antennas are presented.

Acknowledgments

Acknowledgements to my family.

My wife Mazal Sabban
My daughters Dolly and Lilach
My son David Sabban
My grandchildren Nooa, Avigail, Ido, Shira, Efrat, Yael Hodaia

Acknowledgments to my engineering colleagues who helped me through the 39 years of my engineering and research career.

About the Author

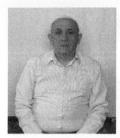 **Dr. Albert Sabban** received B.Sc and M.Sc degrees Magna Cum Laude in electrical engineering from Tel Aviv University, Israel, in 1976 and 1986, respectively. He received a Ph.D. degree in electrical engineering from University of Colorado at Boulder, USA, in 1991. He also received an MBA degree from Haifa University. His reasearch interests are microwave, antenna engineering, communication systems, biomedical and wearable systems, electromagnetics and system engineering.

From 2010 to date he has been a senior lecturer and researcher at Ort Braude College in Israel in the electrical engineering department. He also leads the communication program at Ort Braude College. Dr. Sabban was an RF and antenna specialist and project leader at hi-tech and biomedical companies. He is an expert in BAN and WBAN systems. He has designed and developed wearable medical systems and antennas for wireless communication systems.

In 1976 he joined the armament development authority, RAFAEL, in Israel. In RAFAEL he worked as a senior researcher, group leader and project leader in the electromagnetic department until 2007. He successfully passed a system engineering course in RAFAEL. During his work at RAFAEL and at other institutes and companies Dr. Sabban gained experience in project management, microwave and system engineering, sales, marketing and training. In 2007 he retired from RAFAEL. From 2008 to 2010 he worked as an RF specialist and project leader at high tech companies. At present he is a senior lecturer and researcher in academic institutes in Israel. He has published over 65 research papers and holds several patents in the antenna area. He has written three books and two chapters in books on microwave and antennas engineering.

1 Wearable Communication and Medical Systems

Wearable technology has several applications in personal wireless communication and medical devices as presented in [1–8]. The biomedical industry has been in continuous growth in the last few years. Several medical devices and systems have been developed to monitor patient health as presented in several books and papers [1–44]. Wearable technology provides a powerful new tool to medical and surgical rehabilitation services. Wearable body area networks (WBANs) can record electrocardiograms and measure body temperature, blood pressure, heartbeat rate, electro-dermal activity, and other healthcare parameters.

1.1 WEARABLE TECHNOLOGY

Accessories that can comfortably be worn on the body are called *wearable devices*. Wearable technology is a developing multidisciplinary field. Knowledge in bioengineering, electrical engineering, software engineering, and mechanical engineering is needed to design and develop wearable communication and medical system. Wearable medical systems and sensors are used to measure and monitor physiological parameters of the human body. Biomedical systems in the vicinity of human body may be wired or wireless. Many physiological parameters may be analyzed using wearable medical systems and sensors. Wearable medical systems and sensors can measure body temperature, heartbeat, blood pressure, sweat rate, and other physiological parameters of the person wearing the medical device. Wearable technology may provide scanning and sensing features that are not offered by mobile phones or laptop computers. It usually has communication capabilities and users may have access to information in real time. Several wireless technologies are used to handle data collection and processing by medical systems. The collected data may be stored or transmitted to a medical center to analyze the collected data. Wearable devices gather raw data that is fed to a database or to a software application for analysis. This analysis typically may result in a response that might alert a physician to contact a patient who is experiencing abnormal symptoms. However, a similar message may be sent to a person who achieves a fitness goal.

Examples of wearable devices include headbands, smart wristbands, belts, watches, glasses, contact lenses, e-textiles and smart fabrics, jewelry, bracelets, and hearing aid devices.

Usually wearable communication systems consist of a transmitting unit, a receiving unit, a data processing unit, and wearable antennas.

Wearable technology may influence the fields of transportation, health and medicine, fitness, aging, disabilities, education, finance, gaming, entertainment, and music. Wearable devices will be in the next decade an important part of individuals' daily lives.

1.2   WEARABLE MEDICAL SYSTEMS

One of the main goals of wearable medical systems is to increase disease prevention. By using more wearable medical devices a person can handle and be aware of his private health. Sophisticated analysis of continuously measured medical data of a large number of medical centers' patients may result in improved low-cost medical treatment.

1.2.1   APPLICATIONS OF WEARABLE MEDICAL SYSTEMS

Wearable medical devices may

- Help to monitor hospital activities
- Assist diabetes patients
- Assist asthma patients
- Help solve sleep disorders
- Help solve obesity problems
- Help solve cardiovascular diseases
- Assist epilepsy patients
- Help in treatment of Alzheimer's disease patients
- Help gather data for clinical research trials and academic research studies

1.3   WEARABLE MEDICAL SYSTEMS

Several physiological parameters can be measured using wearable medical systems and sensors. Some of this physiological data is presented in this chapter.

1.3.1   MEASUREMENT OF HUMAN BODY TEMPERATURE

The temperature of a healthy person ranges between 35°C to 38°C. Temperatures below or above this range may indicate that the person is sick. Temperatures above 40°C may cause death. A person's body temperature may be transmitted to a medical center and if needed the doctor may contact the patient for further assistance.

1.3.2   MEASUREMENT OF BLOOD PRESSURE

A blood pressure measurement indicates the arterial pressure of the blood circulating in the human body.

Some of the causes of changes in blood pressure may be stress and being over-weight. The blood pressure of a healthy person is around 80 by 120, where the systole is 120 and the diastole is 80.

Changes of ten percent above or below these values are a matter of concern and should be examined. Usually blood pressure and heartbeat are measured in the same set of measurements. The blood pressure and heartbeat may be transmitted to a medical center and if needed the doctor may contact the patient for further assistance.

1.3.3   MEASUREMENT OF HEART RATE

Measurement of the heart rate is one of the most important tests when examining the health of a patient. A change in heart rate will change the blood pressure and the amount of blood delivered to all parts of the body. The heart rate of a healthy person in 72 beats per minute. Changes in heartbeat may cause several kinds of cardiovascular disease. Traditionally heart rate is measured using a stethoscope. However, this is a manual test and is not so accurate. To measure and analyze the heartbeat a wearable medical device may be connected to a patient's chest. Medical devices that measure heartbeat can be wired or wireless.

1.3.4   MEASUREMENT OF RESPIRATION RATE

Measurement of respiration rate indicates if a person is breathing normally and if the patient is healthy. Elderly and overweight people have difficulty breathing normally. Wearable medical devices are used to measure a person's respiration rate. A wired medical device used to measure respiration rate may cause uneasiness to the patient and cause an error in measurements of respiration rate. It is better to use a wireless medical device to measure respiration rate. The measured respiration rate may be transmitted to a medical center and if needed the doctor may contact the patient for further assistance.

1.3.5   MEASUREMENT OF SWEAT RATE

Glucose is the primary energy source of human beings. Glucose is supplied to the human body usually as a monosaccharide sugar that provides energy to the human body. When a person does extensive physical activity, glucose comes out of the skin as sweat. A wearable medical device can be used to monitor and measure the sweat rate of a person during extensive physical activity. A wearable medical device can be attached to the person's clothes in proximity to the skin to monitor and measure the sweat rate. This device can also be used to measure the sweat Ph, which is important in diagnosis of diseases. Water vapor evaporated from the skin is absorbed in the medical device to determine the sweat Ph. If the amount of sweat coming out of the body is too high, the body may dehydrate. Dehydration causes tiredness and fatigue. Measurements of sweat rate and Ph may be used to monitor the physical activity of a person.

1.3.6   MEASUREMENT OF HUMAN GAIT

The movement of human limbs is called the human gait. Human gaits are the various ways in which a human can move. Different gait patterns are characterized by differences in limb movement patterns, overall velocity, forces, kinetic and potential energy cycles, and changes in contact with the ground. Walking, jogging, skipping, and sprinting are defined as natural human gaits. Gait analysis is a helpful and fundamental research tool to characterize human locomotion. Wearable devices may be attached to different parts of the body to measure and analyze human gait. The movement signal recorded by these devices can be used to analyze human gait. Temporal characteristics of gait are collected and estimated from wearable accelerometers and pressure sensors inside footwear.

In sports, gait analysis based on wearable sensors can be used for sports training and analysis and for the improvement of athletic performance. The ambulatory gait analysis results may determine whether or not a particular treatment is appropriate for a patient. Motion analysis of human limbs during gait is applied in preoperative planning for patients with cerebral palsy and can alter medical treatment decisions. Parkinson's disease is characterized by motor difficulties such as gait difficulty, slowing of movement, and limb rigidity. Gait analysis has been verified as one of the most reliable diagnostic signs of this disease. For patients with neurological problems, such as Parkinson's disease and stroke, ambulatory gait analysis is an important tool in their recovery process and can provide low-cost and convenient rehabilitation monitoring.

Gait analysis based on wearable devices can be applied in healthcare monitoring, such as in the detection of gait abnormalities, the assessment of recovery, fall risk estimation, and in sports training. In healthcare centers, gait information is used to detect walking behavior abnormalities that may predict health problems or the progression of neurodegenerative diseases. Falling is the most common type of home accident among elderly persons. It is a major threat to the health and independence among elderly people. Gait analysis using wearable devices has been used to analyze and predict falls among elderly patients.

1.3.7   WEARABLE DEVICES TRACKING AND MONITORING DOCTORS AND PATIENTS INSIDE HOSPITALS

Each patient can have a wearable device attached to the body. The wearable device is connected to several sensors. Each sensor has its own specific task to perform. For example, one sensor node may detect heart rate and body temperature while another detects blood pressure. Doctors can also carry a wearable device, which allows other hospital personnel to locate them within the hospital (Figure 1.1).

1.4   WIRELESS BODY AREA NETWORKS

The main goal of WBANs is to provide continuous biofeedback data. WBANs can record electrocardiograms, and measure body temperature, blood pressure, heartbeat rate, electro-dermal activity, and other healthcare parameters in an efficient way. For example, accelerometers can be used to sense heartbeat rate, movement, or even muscular activity. Body area networks (BANs) include applications and com-

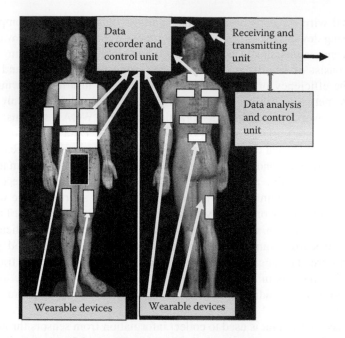

FIGURE 1.1 Wearable devices for various medical applications.

munication devices using wearable and implantable wireless networks. A sensor network that senses health parameters is called a body sensor network (BSN). A WBAN is a special-purpose wireless-sensor network that incorporates different networks and wireless devices to enable remote monitoring in various environments.

One application of WBANs is in medical centers where the condition of a large number of patients is constantly being monitored. Wireless monitoring of physiological signals of a large number of patients is needed in order to deploy a complete WSN in healthcare centers. Human health monitoring is emerging as a significant application of embedded sensor networks. A WBAN can monitor vital signs, providing real-time feedback to allow many patient diagnostic procedures using continuous monitoring of chronic conditions or progress of recovery from an illness. Recent technological advances in wireless networking promise a new generation of wireless sensor networks suitable for human body wearable network systems.

Data acquisition in WBAN devices can be point-to-point or multipoint-to-point, depending on specific applications. Detection of an athlete's health condition would require point-to-point data sharing across various on-body sensors. Human body monitoring of vital signs will require routing data from several wearable sensors, multipoint-to-point, to a sink node, which in turn can relay the information wirelessly to an out-of-body computer. Data may be transferred in real-time mode or non-real-time. Human body monitoring applications require real-time data transfer. An athlete's physiological data can be collected offline for processing and analysis purposes.

A typical wireless body area network consists of a number of compact low-power sensing devices, a control unit, and wireless transceivers. The power supply for these components should be compact, lightweight, and long lasting as well. WBANs consist of small devices with fewer opportunities for redundancy. To improve the efficiency of a WBAN it is important to minimize the number of nodes in the network. Adding more devices and path redundancy for solving node failure and network problems is not a practical option in WBAN systems. WBANs receive and transmit a large amount of data constantly. Data processing must be hierarchical and efficient to deal with the asymmetry of several resources, to maintain system efficiency, and to ensure the availability of data. WBANs in a medical area consist of wearable and implantable sensor nodes that can sense biological information from the human body and transmit it over a short distance wirelessly to a control device worn on the body or placed in an accessible location. The sensor electronics must be miniaturized, low-power, and able to detect medical signals such as electrocardiograms, electroencephalograms, pulse rate, blood pressure, and temperature. The aggregate data from the control devices is then transmitted to remote destinations in a wireless body-area network for diagnostic and therapeutic purposes by including other wireless networks for long-range transmission (Figure 1.2).

A wireless control unit is used to collect information from sensors through wires and transmits it to a remote station for monitoring (Figure 1.3).

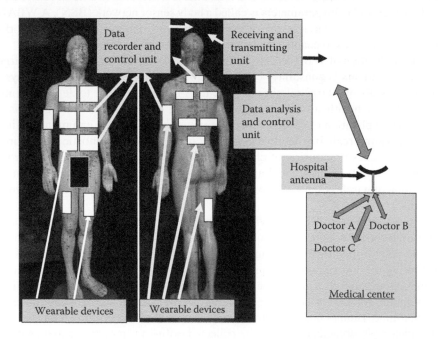

FIGURE 1.2   Wearable body area network (WBAN) for various medical applications.

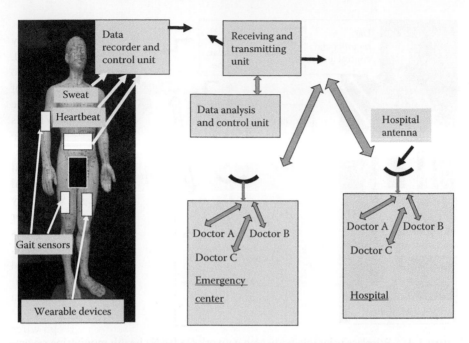

FIGURE 1.3 Wearable body area network (WBAN) health monitoring system.

1.5 WEARABLE WIRELESS BODY AREA NETWORK (WWBAN)

Wireless communication systems offer a wide range of benefits to medical centers, patients, physicians, and sports centers through continuous measuring and monitoring of medical information, early detection of abnormal conditions, supervised rehabilitation, and potential discovery of knowledge through data analysis of the collected information. Wearable health monitoring systems allow the person to follow closely changes in important health parameters and provide feedback for maintaining optimal health status. If the WWBAN is part of the telemedicine system, the medical system can alert medical personnel when life-threatening events occur, as shown in Figure 1.4. In addition, patients may benefit from continuous long-term monitoring as a part of a diagnostic procedure. We can achieve optimal maintenance of a chronic condition or monitor the recovery period after the acute event or surgical procedure. The collected medical data may be a very good indicator of the cardiac recovery of patients after heart surgery. Long-term monitoring can also confirm adherence to treatment guidelines or help monitor the effects of drug therapy. Health monitors can be used to monitor physical rehabilitation of patients during stroke rehabilitation or brain trauma rehabilitation and after hip or knee surgeries. Many people are using WBAN devices such as wearable heartrate monitors, respiration rate monitors, and pedometers for medical reasons or as part of a fitness regime. WBANs may be attached to cotton shirts to measure respiratory activity, electrocardiograms, electromyograms, and body posture.

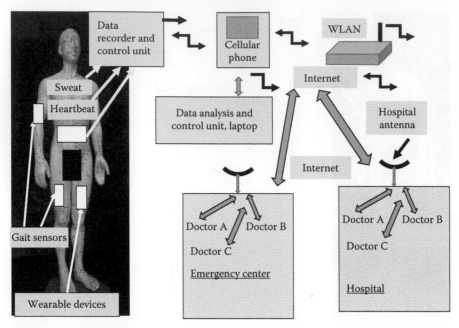

Figure 1.4: Wireless wearable body area network (WBAN) health monitoring system.

1.6 CONCLUSION

Wearable technology provides a powerful new tool to medical and surgical rehabilitation services. The WBAN is emerging as an important option for medical centers and patients. Wearable technology provides a convenient platform that may quantify the long-term context and physiological response of individuals. It will support the development of individualized treatment systems with real-time feedback to help promote the health of patients. Wearable medical systems and sensors can perform gait analysis and measure body temperature, heartbeat, blood pressure, sweat rate, and other physiological parameters of the person wearing the medical device. Gait analysis is a useful tool both in clinical practice and biomechanical research. Gait analysis using wearable sensors provides quantitative and repeatable results over extended time periods with low cost and good portability, showing better prospects and making great progress in recent years. At present, commercialized wearable sensors have been adopted in various applications of gait analysis.

REFERENCES

1. S. C. Mukhopadhyay, ed., *Wearable Electronics Sensors*, Switzerland: Springer, 2015.
2. A. Sabban, *Wideband RF Technologies and Antennas in Microwave Frequencies*, Hoboken, NJ: John Wiley & Sons, July 2016.
3. A. Sabban, *Low Visibility Antennas for Communication Systems*, Boca Raton, FL: Taylor & Francis, 2015.
4. A. Sabban, Small wearable meta materials antennas for medical systems, *The Applied Computational Electromagnetics Society Journal*, vol. 31, no. 4, April 2016.

5. A. Sabban, Microstrip Antenna Arrays, *Microstrip Antennas*, N. Nasimuddin (Ed.), pp. 361–384, Croatia: InTech, 2011, ISBN: 978-953-307-247-0, http://www.intechopen.com/articles/show/title/microstrip-antenna-arrays.
6. A. Sabban, New Wideband printed antennas for medical applications, *IEEE Journal, Transactions on Antennas and Propagation*, vol. 61, no. 1, 84–91, January 2013.
7. U.S Patent, Inventors: Albert Sabban. Dual polarized dipole wearable antenna, U.S Patent number: 8203497, June 19, 2012, USA.
8. A. Bonfiglio and D. De Rossi, eds., *Wearable Monitoring Systems*, New York, NY: Springer, 2011
9. T. Gao, D. Greenspan, M. Welsh, R. R. Juang and A. Alm, Vital signs monitoring and patient tracking over a wireless network. Proceedings of IEEE-EMBS 27th Annual International Conference of the Engineering in Medicine and Biology, Shanghai, China, 1–5 September 2005, pp. 102–105.
10. C. A. Otto, E. Jovanov and E. A. Milenkovic, WBAN-based system for health monitoring at home. Proceedings of IEEE/EMBS International Summer School, Medical Devices and Biosensors, Boston, MA, 4–6 September 2006, pp. 20–23.
11. G. H. Zhang, C. C. Y. Poon, Y. Li and Y. T. Zhang, A biometric method to secure telemedicine systems. Proceedings of the 31st Annual International Conference of the IEEE Engineering in Medicine and Biology Society, Minneapolis, MN, September 2009, pp. 701–704.
12. S. Bao, Y. Zhang and L. Shen, Physiological signal based entity authentication for body area sensor networks and mobile healthcare systems. Proceedings of the 27th Annual International Conference of the IEEE EMBS, Shanghai, China, 1–4 September 2005, pp. 2455–2458.
13. V. Ikonen and E. Kaasinen, Ethical assessment in the design of ambient assisted living. Proceedings of Assisted Living Systems—Models, Architectures and Engineering Approaches, Schloss Dagstuhl, Germany, November 2008, pp. 14–17.
14. V. Srinivasan, J. Stankovic and K. Whitehouse, Protecting your daily in home activity information from a wireless snooping attack. Proceedings of the 10th International Conference on Ubiquitous Computing, Seoul, Korea, 21–24 September 2008, pp. 202–211.
15. R. Casas, M. R. Blasco, A. Robinet, A. R. Delgado, A. R. Yarza, J. McGinn, R. Picking, and V. Grout, User modelling in ambient intelligence for elderly and disabled people. Proceedings of the 11th International Conference on Computers Helping People with Special Needs, Linz, Austria, July 2008, pp. 114–122.
16. Y. Jasemian, Elderly comfort and compliance to modern telemedicine system at home. Proceedings of the Second International Conference on Pervasive Computing Technologies for Healthcare, Tampere, Finland, 30 January–1 February 2008, pp. 60–63.
17. L. Atallah, B. Lo, G. Z. Yang and F. Siegemund, Wirelessly accessible sensor populations (WASP) for elderly care monitoring. Proceedings of the Second International Conference on Pervasive Computing Technologies for Healthcare, Tampere, Finland, 30 January–1 February 2008, pp. 2–7.
18. T. Hori, Y. Nishida, T. Suehiro and S. Hirai, SELF-Network: Design and implementation of network for distributed embedded sensors. Proceedings of IEEE/RSJ International Conference on Intelligent Robots and Systems, Takamatsu, Japan, 30 October–5 November 2000, pp. 1373–1378.
19. Y. Mori, M. Yamauchi and K. Kaneko, Design and implementation of the Vital Sign Box for home healthcare. Proceedings of IEEE EMBS International Conference on Information Technology Applications in Biomedicine, Arlington, VA, November 2000, pp. 104–109.

20. C. Lauterbach, M. Strasser, S. Jung and W. Weber, Smart clothes self-powered by body heat. Proceedings of Avantex Symposium, Frankfurt, Germany, May 2002, pp. 5259–5263.

21. S. Marinkovic and E. Popovici, Network coding for efficient error recovery in wireless sensor networks for medical applications. Proceedings of International Conference on Emerging Network Intelligence, Sliema, Malta, 11–16 October 2009, pp. 15–20.

22. T. Schoellhammer, E. Osterweil, B. Greenstein, M. Wimbrow and D. Estrin, Lightweight temporal compression of microclimate datasets. Proceedings of the 29th Annual IEEE International Conference on Local Computer Networks, Tampa, FL, 16–18 November 2004, pp. 516–524.

23. A. T. Barth, M. A. Hanson, H .C. Powell, Jr and J. Lach, Tempo 3.1: A body area sensor network platform for continuous movement assessment. Proceedings of the 6th International Workshop on Wearable and Implantable Body Sensor Networks, Berkeley, CA, June 2009, pp. 71–76.

24. M. Gietzelt, K. H. Wolf, M. Marschollek and R. Haux, Automatic self-calibration of body worn triaxial-accelerometers for application in healthcare. Proceedings of the Second International Conference on Pervasive Computing Technologies for Healthcare, Tampere, Finland, January 2008, pp. 177–180.

25. T. Gao, D. Greenspan, M. Welsh, R. R. Juang, and A. Alm. Vital signs monitoring and patient tracking over a wireless network. Proceedings of the 27th Annual International Conference of the IEEE EMBS, Shanghai, China, 1–4 September 2005; pp. 102–105.

26. A. Purwar, D. U. Jeong and W. Y. Chung, Activity monitoring from realtime triaxial accelerometer data using sensor network. Proceedings of International Conference on Control, Automation and Systems, Hong Kong, 21–23 March 2007, pp. 2402–2406.

27. C. Baker, K. Armijo, S. Belka, M. Benhabib, V. Bhargava, N. Burkhart, et al., Wireless sensor networks for home health care. Proceedings of the 21st International Conference on Advanced Information Networking and Applications Workshops, Niagara Falls, Canada, 21–23 May 2007, pp. 832–837.

28. L. Schwiebert, S. K. S. Gupta and J. Weinmann, Research challenges in wireless networks of biomedical sensors. Proceedings of the 7th Annual International Conference on Mobile Computing and Networking, Rome, Italy, 16–21 July 2001, pp. 151–165.

29. O. Aziz, B. Lo, R. King, A. Darzi and G. Z. Yang, Pervasive body sensor network: An approach to monitoring the postoperative surgical patient. Proceedings of International Workshop on Wearable and implantable Body Sensor Networks (BSN 2006), Cambridge, MA, 2006, pp. 13–18.

30. J. M. Kahn, R. H. Katz and K. S. J. Pister, Next century challenges: Mobile networking for smart dust. Proceedings of the ACM MobiCom'99, Washington, DC, August 1999, pp. 271–278.

31. N. Noury, T. Herve, V. Rialle, G. Virone, E. Mercier, G. Morey, et al., Monitoring behavior in home using a smart fall sensor. Proceedings of IEEE-EMBS Special Topic Conference on Micro-technologies in Medicine and Biology, Lyon, France, 12–14 October 2000, pp. 607–610.

32. D. Y. Kwon and M. Gross, Combining body sensors and visual sensors for motion training. Proceedings of the 2005 ACM SIGCHI International Conference on Advances in Computer Entertainment Technology, Valencia, Spain, 15–17 June 2005, pp. 94–101.

33. N. K. Boulgouris, D. Hatzinakos and K. N. Plataniotis, Gait recognition: A challenging signal processing technology for biometric identification. *IEEE Signal Processing Magazine*, vol. 22, 78–90, 2005.

34. S. Kimmeskamp and E. M. Hennig, Heel to toe motion characteristics in Parkinson patients during free walking. *Clinical Biomechanics*, vol. 16, 806–812, 2001.

35. K. Turcot, R. Aissaoui, K. Boivin, M. Pelletier, N. Hagemeister and J. A. de Guise, New accelerometric method to discriminate between asymptomatic subjects and patients with medial knee osteoarthritis during 3-D gait. *IEEE Transactions Biomedical Engineering*, vol. 55, 1415–1422.

36. H. Furnée, Real-time motion capture systems, *Three-Dimensional Analysis of Human Locomotion*. In P. Allard, A. Cappozzo, A. Lundberg and C.L. Vaughan, eds., Chichester: John Wiley & Sons, 1997. pp. 85–108.

37. S. J.M. Bamberg, A. Y. Benbasat, D. M. Scarborough, D. E. Krebs and J. A. Paradiso, Gait analysis using a shoe-integrated wireless sensor system. *IEEE Transactions on Information Technology in Biomedicine*, vol. 12, 413–423, 2008.

38. J.H. Choi, J. Cho, J.H. Park, J.M. Eun and M.S. Kim, An efficient gait phase detection device based on magnetic sensor array. Proceedings of the 4th Kuala Lumpur International Conference on Biomedical Engineering, Kuala Lumpur, Malaysia, 25–28 June 2008; 21, pp. 778–781.

39. J. Hidler, Robotic assessment of walking in individuals with gait disorders. Proceedings of the 26th Annual International Conference of the IEEE Engineering in Medicine and Biology Society, San Francisco, CA, 1–5 September 2004; 7, pp. 4829–4831.

40. Y. Wahab and N.A. Bakar, Gait analysis measurement for sport application based on ultrasonic system. Proceedings of the 2011 IEEE 15th International Symposium on Consumer Electronics, Singapore, 14–17 June 2011, pp. 20–24.

41. B. De Silva, A.N. Jan, M. Motani and K.C. Chua, A real-time feedback utility with body sensor networks. Proceedings of the 5th International Workshop on Wearable and Implantable Body Sensor Networks (BSN 08), Hong Kong, 1–3 June 2008, pp. 49–53.

42. A. Salarian, H. Russmann, F.J.G. Vingerhoets, C. Dehollain, Y. Blanc, P.R. Burkhard and K. Aminian, Gait assessment in Parkinson's disease: Toward an ambulatory system for long-term monitoring. *IEEE Transactions on Biomedical Engineering*, vol. 51, 1434–1443, 2004.

43. L. Atallah, G.G. Jones, R. Ali, J.J.H. Leong, B. Lo and G.Z. Yang, Observing recovery from knee-replacement surgery by using wearable sensors. Proceedings of the 2011 International Conference on Body Sensor Networks, Dallas, TX, 23–25 May 2011, pp. 29–34.

44. M. ElSayed, A. Alsebai, A. Salaheldin, N. El Gayar and M. ElHelw, Ambient and wearable sensing for gait classification in pervasive healthcare environments. Proceedings of the 12th IEEE International Conference on e-Health Networking Applications and Services (Healthcom), Lyon, France, 1–3 July 2010, pp. 240–245.

2 Electromagnetic Waves and Transmission Lines for Wearable Communication Systems Designers

Data transfer from point to point in communication systems can be done by transmitting electromagnetic waves or by connecting the points via transmission lines. Time-varying currents and charges create electromagnetic waves. Propagation of electromagnetic waves in space and in materials obeys Maxwell's equations [1–8]. Electromagnetic fields may be viewed as a combination of electric and magnetic fields. Stationary charges produce electric fields. Moving charges and currents produce magnetic fields. The electromagnetic spectrum and basic definitions of electromagnetic wave propagation are presented in this chapter. Transmitting and receiving information in microwave frequencies is based on electromagnetic wave propagation.

2.1 ELECTROMAGNETIC SPECTRUM

The electromagnetic spectrum corresponds to electromagnetic waves from the meter range to the mm wave range. The characteristic feature of these phenomena is the short wavelength involved. The wavelength is of the same order of magnitude as the circuit devices used. The propagation time from one point of the circuit to another point of the circuit is comparable to the period of the oscillating voltages and currents in the circuit. Conventional low-circuit analysis based on Kirchhoff's and Ohm's laws can not analyze and describe the variation of fields, voltages, and currents along the length of the components. Components whose dimensions are lower than a tenth of a wavelength are called lumped elements. Components whose dimensions are higher than a tenth of a wavelength are called distributed elements. Kirchhoff's and Ohm's laws may be applied to lumped elements. However, Kirchhoff's and Ohm's laws cannot be applied to distributed elements.

To prevent interference and to provide efficient use of the radio spectrum, similar services are allocated in bands, see [11–14]. Bands are divided at wavelengths of 10^n meters, or frequencies of 3×10^n hertz. Each of these bands has a basic band plan which dictates how it is to be used and shared to avoid interference and to set protocol for the compatibility of transmitters and receivers. In Table 2.1 the electromagnetic spectrum and applications are listed. In Table 2.2 the IEEE standard for radar

TABLE 2.1

Electromagnetic Spectrum and Applications

Band Name	Abbreviation	ITU	Frequency\$\lambda 0$	Applications
Tremendously low frequency	TLF		< 3 Hz> 100,000 km	Natural and artificial EM noise
Extremely low frequency	ELF		3–30 Hz 100,000 km–10,000 km	Communication with submarines
Super low frequency	SLF		30–300 Hz 10,000 km–1000 km	Communication with submarines
Ultra low Frequency	ULF		300–3000 Hz 1000 km–100 km	Submarine communication, communication within mines
Very low frequency	VLF	4	3–30 kHz 100 km–10 km	Navigation, time signals, submarine communication, wireless heart rate monitors, geophysics
Low frequency	LF	5	30–300 kHz 10 km–1 km	Navigation, clock time signals, AM longwave broadcasting (Europe and parts of Asia), RFID, amateur radio
Medium frequency	MF	6	300–3000 kHz 1 km–100 m	AM (medium-wave) broadcasts, amateur radio, avalanche beacons
High frequency	HF	7	3–30 MHz 100 m–10 m	Shortwave broadcasts, radio, amateur radio and aviation, communications, RFID, radar, near-vertical incidence sky wave (NVIS) radio communications, marine and mobile radio telephony
Very high frequency	VHF	8	30–300 MHz 10 m–1 m	FM, television broadcasts and line-of-sight ground-to-aircraft and aircraft-to-aircraft communications, land mobile and maritime mobile communications, amateur radio, weather radio
Ultra high frequency	UHF	9	300–3000 MHz 1 m–100 mm	Television broadcasts, microwave oven, radio astronomy, mobile phones, wireless LAN, Bluetooth, ZigBee, GPS and two-way radios such as land mobile, FRS and GMRS radios
Super high frequency	SHF	10	3–30 GHz 100 mm–10 mm	Radio astronomy, wireless LAN, modern radars, communications satellites, satellite television broadcasting, DBS

(Continued)

TABLE 2.1 (*Continued*)
Electromagnetic Spectrum and Applications

Band Name	Abbreviation	ITU	Frequency\λ0	Applications
Extremely high frequency	EHF	11	30–300 GHz 10 mm–1 mm	Radio astronomy, microwave radio relay, microwave remote sensing, directed-energy weapons, scanners
Terahertz or Tremendously high frequency	THz or THF	12	300–3,000 GHz 1 mm–100 μm	Terahertz imaging, ultrafast molecular dynamics, condensed-matter physics, terahertz time-domain spectroscopy, terahertz computing/communications

TABLE 2.2
IEEE Standard Radar Frequency Bands

Microwave Frequency Bands-IEEE Standard

Designation	Frequency Range
L band	1 to 2 GHz
S band	2 to 4 GHz
C band	4 to 8 GHz
X band	8 to 12 GHz
K_u band	12 to 18 GHz
K band	18 to 26.5 GHz
K_a band	26.5 to 40 GHz
Q band	30 to 50 GHz
U band	40 to 60 GHz
V band	50 to 75 GHz
E band	60 to 90 GHz
W band	75 to 110 GHz
F band	90 to 140 GHz
D band	110 to 170 GHz

frequency bands is listed. In Table 2.3 the International Tel-communication Union (ITU) bands are given. In Table 2.4 radar-frequency bands as defined by NATO for ECM systems are listed, see [13].

2.2 BASIC ELECTROMAGNETIC WAVE DEFINITIONS

Field: A field is a physical quantity that has a value for each point in space and time.

Wavelength: The wavelength is the distance between two sequential equivalent points. Wavelength, λ, is measured in meters.

Wave period: The period is the time, *T*, for one complete cycle of an oscillation of a wave. The period is measured in seconds.

Frequency: The frequency, *f*, is the number of periods per unit time (second) and is measured in hertz.

TABLE 2.3
The International Tel-Communication Union Bands

Band Number	Symbols	Frequency Range	Wavelength Range
4	VLF	3 to 30 kHz	10 to 100 km
5	LF	30 to 300 kHz	1 to 10 km
6	MF	300 to 3000 kHz	100 to 1000 m
7	HF	3 to 30 MHz	10 to 100 m
8	VHF	30 to 300 MHz	1 to 10 m
9	UHF	300 to 3000 MHz	10 to 100 cm
10	SHF	3 to 30 GHz	1 to 10 cm
11	EHF	30 to 300 GHz	1 to 10 mm
12	THF	300 to 3000 GHz	0.1 to 1 mm

TABLE 2.4
Radar-Frequency Bands as Defined by NATO for ECM Systems

Band	Frequency Range
A band	0 to 0.25 GHz
B band	0.25 to 0.5 GHz
C band	0.5 to 1.0 GHz
D band	1 to 2 GHz
E band	2 to 3 GHz
F band	3 to 4 GHz
G band	4 to 6 GHz
H band	6 to 8 GHz
I band	8 to 10 GHz
J band	10 to 20 GHz
K band	20 to 40 GHz
L band	40 to 60 GHz
M band	60 to 100 GHz

Source: AFR 55-44/AR 105-86/OPNAVINST 3430.9A/MCO 3430.1, 27 October 1964 superseded by AFR 55-44/AR 105-86/OPNAVINST 3430.1A/MCO 3430.1A, 6 December 1978: Performing Electronic Countermeasures in the United States and Canada, Attachment 1, ECM Frequency Authorizations.

Phase velocity: The phase velocity, v, of a wave is the rate at which the phase of the wave propagates in space. Phase velocity measured in $\frac{m}{s}$.

$$\lambda = v * T$$

$$T = 1/f \qquad (2.1)$$

$$\lambda = v/f$$

Electromagnetic waves propagate in free space at the phase velocity of light.

$$v = 3 \cdot 10^8 \quad \frac{m}{s} \tag{2.2}$$

Wavenumber: A wavenumber, k, is the spatial frequency of the wave in radians per unit distance (per meter). $k = 2\pi/\lambda$.

Angular frequency: The angular frequency, ω, represents the frequency in radians per second. $\omega = v*k = 2\pi f$.

Polarization: A wave is polarized if it oscillates in one direction or plane. The polarization of a transverse wave describes the direction of oscillation in the plane perpendicular to the direction of propagation.

Antenna: An antenna is used to efficiently radiate electromagnetic energy in desired directions. Antennas match radio frequency systems to space. All antennas may be used to receive or radiate energy. They transmit or receive electromagnetic waves, and convert electromagnetic radiation into electric current, or vice versa. Antennas transmit and receive electromagnetic radiation at radio frequencies. They are a necessary part of all communication links and radio equipment. Antennas are used in systems such as radio and television broadcasting, point-to-point radio communication, wireless LAN, cell phones, radar, medical systems, and spacecraft communication. Antennas are most commonly employed in air or outer space, but can also be operated underwater, on and inside the human body, or even through soil and rock at low frequencies for short distances.

2.3 ELECTROMAGNETIC WAVE THEORY

2.3.1 MAXWELL'S EQUATIONS

Maxwell's equations are presented in several books [1–10]. Maxwell's equations describe how electric and magnetic fields are generated and altered by each other. They are a classical approximation to the more accurate and fundamental theory of quantum electrodynamics. Quantum deviations from Maxwell's equations are usually small. Inaccuracies occur when the particle nature of light is important or when electric fields are strong. Symbols and abbreviations of physical parameters and electromagnetic fields are listed in Tables 2.5 and 2.6.

2.3.2 GAUSS'S LAW FOR ELECTRIC FIELDS

Gauss's law for electric fields states that the electric flux via any closed surface S is equal to the net charge q divided by the free space dielectric constant.

$$\oint_S E \cdot ds = \frac{1}{\varepsilon_0} \int_V \rho \, dv = \frac{1}{\varepsilon_0} q$$

$$D = \varepsilon E \tag{2.3}$$

$$\nabla \cdot D = \rho_v$$

TABLE 2.5

Symbols and Abbreviations of Physical Parameters

Dimensions	Parameter	Symbol
Wb/m	Magnetic potential	A
m/s^2	Acceleration	a
tesla	Magnetic field	B
F	Capacitance	C
V/m	Electric field displacement	D
V/m	Electric field	E
N	Force	F
A/m	Magnetic field strength	H
A	Current	I
A/m^2	Current density	J
H	Self-inductance	L
m	Length	l
H	Mutual inductance	M
C	Charge	q
W/m^2	Poynting vector	$\mathbf{P}$
W	Power	P
Ω	Resistance	R
m^3	Volume	V
m/s	Velocity	v
F/m	Dielectric constant	ε
–	Relative dielectric constant	ε_r
H/m	Permeability	μ
1/$\Omega \cdot$m	Conductivity	σ
Wb	Magnetic flux	ψ

2.3.3 Gauss's Law for Magnetic Fields

Gauss's law for magnetic fields states that the magnetic flux via any closed surface S is equal to zero. There is no magnetic charge in nature.

$$\oint_S B \cdot ds = 0$$

$$B = \mu H$$

$$\psi_m = \int_S B \cdot ds \tag{2.4}$$

$$\nabla \bullet B = 0$$

TABLE 2.6
Symbols and Abbreviations of Electromagnetic Fields

Parameter	Symbol	Dimensions
Electric field displacement	D	V/m
Electric field	E	V/m
Magnetic field strength	H	A/m
Dielectric constant in space	ε_0	$8.854 \cdot 10^{-12}$ F/m
Permeability in space	μ_0	$\mu_0 = 4\pi \cdot 10^{-7}$ H/m
Volume charge density	ρ_V	C/m^3
Magnetic field	B	Tesla, Wb/m^2
Conductivity	σ	$1 / \Omega \cdot m$
Magnetic flux	ψ	Wb
Skin depth	δ_s	m

2.3.4 Ampère's Law

The original "Ampère's law" stated that magnetic fields can be generated by electrical current. Ampère's law has been corrected by Maxwell who stated that magnetic fields can also be generated by time variant electric fields. The corrected "Ampère's law" shows that a changing magnetic field induces an electric field and also that a time-variant electric field induces a magnetic field.

$$\oint_C \frac{B}{\mu_0} \cdot dl = \int_S J \cdot ds + \frac{d}{dt} \int_s \varepsilon_0 E \cdot ds$$

$$\nabla X H = J + \frac{\partial D}{\partial t} \tag{2.5}$$

$$J = \sigma E$$

$$i = \int_S J \cdot ds$$

2.3.5 Faraday's Law

Faraday's law describes how a propagating time-varying magnetic field through a surface S creates an electric field, as shown in Figure 2.1.

$$\oint_C E \cdot dl = -\frac{d}{dt} \int_s B \cdot ds$$

$$\nabla X E = -\frac{\partial B}{\partial t} \tag{2.6}$$

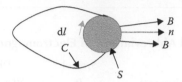

FIGURE 2.1   Faraday's law.

2.3.6 Wave Equations

The variation of electromagnetic waves as a function of time may be written as $e^{j\omega t}$. The derivative as a function of time is $j\omega e^{j\omega t}$. Maxwell's equations may be written as:

$$\nabla X E = -j\omega\mu H$$
$$\nabla X H = (\sigma + j\omega\varepsilon)E \tag{2.7}$$

A ∇X (curl) operation on the electric field E results in:

$$\nabla X \nabla X E = -j\omega\mu \nabla X H \tag{2.8}$$

By substituting the expression of $\nabla X H$ in this equation we get:

$$\nabla X \nabla X E = -j\omega\mu(\sigma + j\omega\varepsilon)E \tag{2.9}$$

$$\nabla X \nabla X E = -\nabla^2 E + \nabla(\nabla \bullet E) \tag{2.10}$$

In free space there is no charge so $\nabla \bullet E = 0$. Equation 2.11 presents the wave equation for electric fields, where γ is the complex propagation constant, α represents losses in the medium, and β represents the wave phase constant in radians per meter.

$$\nabla^2 E = j\omega\mu(\sigma + j\omega\varepsilon)E = \gamma^2 E$$
$$\gamma = \sqrt{j\omega\mu(\sigma + j\omega\varepsilon)} = \alpha + j\beta \tag{2.11}$$

If we follow the same procedure on the magnetic field we will get the wave equation for magnetic field.

$$\nabla^2 H = j\omega\mu(\sigma + j\omega\varepsilon)H = \gamma^2 H \tag{2.12}$$

The law of conservation of energy imposes boundary conditions on electric and magnetic fields. When an electromagnetic wave travels from medium 1 to medium 2 the electric and magnetic fields should be continuous as presented in Figure 2.2.

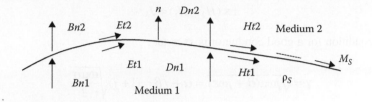

FIGURE 2.2 Fields between two media.

2.3.7 GENERAL BOUNDARY CONDITIONS

$$n \cdot (D_2 - D_1) = \rho_S \qquad (2.13)$$

$$n \cdot (B_2 - B_1) = 0 \qquad (2.14)$$

$$(E_2 - E_1) \times n = M_S \qquad (2.15)$$

$$n \times (H_2 - H_1) = J_S \qquad (2.16)$$

2.3.8 BOUNDARY CONDITIONS FOR DIELECTRIC MEDIUM

$$n \cdot (D_2 - D_1) = 0 \qquad (2.17)$$

$$n \cdot (B_2 - B_1) = 0 \qquad (2.18)$$

$$(E_2 - E_1) \times n = 0 \qquad (2.19)$$

$$n \times (H_2 - H_1) = 0 \qquad (2.20)$$

2.3.9 BOUNDARY CONDITIONS FOR CONDUCTOR

$$n \cdot (D_2 - D_1) = \rho_S \qquad (2.21)$$

$$n \cdot (B_2 - B_1) = 0 \qquad (2.22)$$

$$(E_2 - E_1) \times n = 0 \qquad (2.23)$$

$$n \times (H_2 - H_1) = J_S \qquad (2.24)$$

The condition for a good conductor is $\sigma \gg \omega\epsilon$.

$$\gamma = \sqrt{j\omega\mu(\sigma + j\omega\varepsilon)} = \alpha + j\beta \approx (1+j)\sqrt{\frac{\omega\mu\sigma}{2}} \qquad (2.25)$$

$$\delta_s = \sqrt{\frac{2}{\omega\mu\sigma}} = \frac{1}{\alpha} \qquad (2.26)$$

The conductor skin depth is given as δ_s. The wave attenuation is α.

2.4   WAVE PROPAGATION THROUGH HUMAN BODY

The electrical properties of human body tissues should be considered in the design of wearable communication and medical systems. The conductivity and dielectric constants of human body tissues are listed in Table 2.7; see [15–16]. The complex propagation constant γ, given in Equation 2.11, can be calculated as a function of frequency by using the conductivity and dielectric constant values listed in Table 2.7. The major issue in the design of wearable antennas is the interaction between RF transmission and the human body. Electrical properties of human body tissues should be considered in the design of wearable antennas. The attenuation, α, of RF transmission through the human body is the real value of the propagation constant γ, where $\alpha = \text{Real}(\gamma)$. For example, stomach tissue attenuation is around 1.67 dB/cm at 500 MHz and 2.2 dB/cm at 1000 MHz. Blood attenuation is around 3.38 dB/cm at

TABLE 2.7
Properties of Human Body Tissues

Tissue	Property	434 MHz	800 MHz	1000 MHz
Prostate	σ	0.75	0.90	1.02
	ε	50.53	47.4	46.65
Stomach	σ	0.67	0.79	0.97
	ε	42.9	40.40	39.06
Colon, Heart	σ	0.98	1.15	1.28
	ε	63.6	60.74	59.96
Kidney	σ	0.88	0.88	0.88
	ε	117.43	117.43	117.43
Nerve	σ	0.49	0.58	0.63
	ε	35.71	33.68	33.15
Fat	σ	0.045	0.056	0.06
	ε	5.02	4.58	4.52
Lung	σ	0.27	0.27	0.27
	ε	38.4	38.4	38.4

500 MHz and 4.02 dB/cm at 1000 MHz. The attenuation of stomach tissues, skin, and pancreas at frequencies from 150 MHz to 1000 MHz is listed in Table 2.8. The attenuation of fat, small-intestine tissues, and blood at frequencies from 150 MHz to 1000 MHz is listed in Table 2.9.

2.5   MATERIALS

In Table 2.10, hard materials are presented. Alumina is the most popular hard substrate in microwave integrated circuits (MIC). Gallium arsenide is the most popular hard substrate in monolithic microwave integrated circuits (MIMIC) technology at microwave frequencies.

In Table 2.11, soft materials are presented. Duroid is the most popular soft substrate in MIC circuits and in the printed antennas industry. Dielectric losses in Duroid are significantly lower than dielectric losses in FR-4 substrate. However, the cost of FR-4 substrate is significantly lower than the cost of Duroid. Commercial MIC devices use usually FR-4 substrate. Duroid is the most popular soft substrate used in the development of printed antennas with high efficiency at microwave frequencies.

2.6   TRANSMISSION LINES THEORY

Transmission lines are used to transfer electromagnetic energy from one point to another with minimum losses over a wide band of frequencies. There are three major

TABLE 2.8
Attenuation of Stomach Tissues, Skin, and Pancreas

Frequency MHz	Attenuation Stomach dB/cm	Attenuation Skin dB/cm	Attenuation Pancreas dB/cm
150	1.09643156	0.99356488	1.15470908
200	1.20939308	1.08475696	1.2702312
250	1.31292812	1.16787664	1.37479916
300	1.41391992	1.24912144	1.4755566
350	1.48670172	1.30428284	1.54858144
400	1.55709652	1.35728292	1.61897624
450	1.62247428	1.40642908	1.68601188
500	1.67844292	1.44867464	1.74763988
550	1.73350016	1.49011296	1.80851272
600	1.78806264	1.53108256	1.86901232
650	1.83840664	1.57730356	1.9296508
700	1.88836872	1.62329888	1.99015908
750	1.93809644	1.669164	2.05065868
800	1.98771132	1.71496836	2.11124508
850	2.0487404	1.7427704	2.15668488
900	2.1098476	1.77030336	2.20203788
950	2.17106764	1.79764536	2.2473822
1000	2.23242656	1.82481376	.29276992

TABLE 2.9
Attenuation of Fat, Small Intestine, and Blood

Frequency MHz	Attenuation Fat dB/cm	Attenuation Small Intestine dB/cm	Attenuation Blood dB/cm
150	0.16276736	1.45260668	2.30187524
200	0.199694684	1.86289292	2.55900288
250	0.224987336	2.08283544	2.7694842
300	0.247448572	2.21293128	2.95151248
350	0.269270092	2.29457536	3.08230272
400	0.291230492	2.34826984	3.19356296
450	0.303265312	2.38501228	3.29175112
500	0.315080528	2.41105228	3.38202312
550	0.327376616	2.4300528	3.46402308
600	0.340818464	2.444288	3.53959984
650	0.354259444	2.45519876	3.607191
700	0.367729068	2.4637312	3.67058972
750	0.371782628	2.4705016	3.73061192
800	0.375756332	2.47597868	3.7879086
850	0.37967188	2.48044888	3.84912864
900	0.383546632	2.48415524	3.90854324
950	0.38876852	2.487254	3.9664562
1000	0.393995616	2.48986668	4.02311056

TABLE 2.10
Hard Materials—Ceramics

Material	Symbol or Formula	Dielectric Constant	Dissipation Factor (tan δ)	Coefficient of Thermal Expansion ppm/Â°C	Thermal Cond. (W/mÂ°C)	Mass Density (gr/cc)
Alumina 99.5%	Al_2O_3	9.8	0.0001	8.2	35	3.97
Alumina 96%	Al_2O_3	9.0	0.0002	8.2	24	3.8
Aluminum Nitride	AlN	8.9	0.0005	7.6	290	3.26
Beryllium Oxide	BeO	6.7	0.003	6.05	250	
Gallium Arsenide	GaAs	12.88	0.0004	6.86	46	5.32
Indium Phosphide	InP	12.4	–	–	–	–
Quartz	–	3.8	0.0001	0.6	5	
Sapphire	–	9.3, 11.5	–	–	–	–
Silicon (high resistivity)	Si (HRS)	4	–	2.5	138	2.33
Silicon Carbide	SiC	10.8	0.002	4.8	350	3.2

TABLE 2.11

Soft Materials

Manufacturer and Material	Symbol or Formula	Relative Dielectric Constant ε_r	Tolerance on Dielectric Constant	tan δ	Mass Density(gr/cc)	Thermal Conductivity (W/mÅ°C)	Coefficient of Thermal Expansion PPM/Å°C x/y/z
Rogers Duroid 5870	PTFE/Random glass	2.33	0.02	0.0012	2.2	0.26	22/28/173
Rogers Duroid 5880	PTFE/Random glass	2.2	0.02	0.0012	2.2	0.26	31/48/237
Rogers Duroid 6002	PTFE/Random glass	2.94	0.04	0.0012	2.1	0.44	16/16/24
Rogers Duroid 6006	PTFE/Random glass	6	0.15	0.0027	2.7	0.48	38/42/24
Rogers Duroid 6010	PTFE/Random glass	10.2–10.8	0.25	0.0023	2.9	0.41	24/24/24
FR-4	Glass/epoxy	4.8	–	0.022	–	0.16	–
Polyethylene	–	2.25	–	–	–	–	–
Polyflon CuFlon	PTFE	2.1	–	0.00045	–	–	12.9
Polyflon PolyGuide	Polyolefin	2.32	–	0.0005	–	–	108
Polyflon Norclad	Thermoplastic	2.55	–	0.0011	–	–	53
Polyflon Clad Ultem	Thermoplastic	3.05	–	0.003	1.27	–	56
PTFE	PTFE	2.1	–	0.0002	2.1	0.2	–
Rogers R/flex 3700	Thermally stable thermoplastic	2.0	–	0.002	–	–	8
Rogers RO3006	PTFE ceramic	6.15	0.15	0.0025	2.6	0.61	17/17/24
Rogers RO3010	PTFE ceramic	10.2	0.3	0.0035	3	0.66	17/17/24
Rogers RO3203	PTFE ceramic	3.02	–	–	–	–	–
Rogers RO3210	PTFE ceramic	10.2	–	–	–	–	–
Rogers RO4003	Thermoset plastic ceramic glass	3.38	0.05	0.0027	1.79	0.64	11/14/46
Rogers RO4350B	Thermoset plastic ceramic glass	3.48	0.05	0.004	1.86	0.62	14/16/50
Rogers TMM 3	Ceramic/thermos	3.27	0.032	0.002	1.78	0.7	15/15/23
Rogers TMM 10	Ceramic/thermoset	9.2	0.23	0.0022	2.77	0.76	21/21/20

types of transmission lines [1–10]: transmission lines whose cross section is very small compared to wavelengths on which the dominant mode of propagation is transverse electromagnetic (TEM) mode; closed rectangular and cylindrical conducting tubes on which the dominant modes of propagation are tranverse electric (TE) and transverse magnetic (TM) modes; open boundary structures whose cross section is greater than 0.1 λ that may support the surface wave mode of propagation.

For TEM modes $Ez = Hz = 0$, for TE modes $Ez = 0$, and for TM modes $Hz = 0$.

Voltage and currents in transmission lines are derived using the transmission lines equations. Transmission line equations are derived using the Maxwell equations and the boundary conditions on the transmission line section shown in Figure 2.3. Equation 2.27 is the first lossless transmission line equation. l_e is the self-inductance per length.

$$\frac{\partial V}{\partial Z} = -\frac{\partial}{\partial t} l_e I = -l_e \frac{\partial I}{\partial t} \tag{2.27}$$

$$\frac{\partial I}{\partial Z} = -c \frac{\partial V}{\partial t} - gV \tag{2.28}$$

Equation 2.28 is the second lossless transmission line equation. $c = \dfrac{\Delta C}{\Delta Z} \quad \dfrac{F}{m}$

$$g = \frac{\Delta G}{\Delta Z} \quad \frac{m}{\Omega}$$

Equation 2.29 is the first transmission line equation with losses.

$$-\frac{\partial v}{\partial z} = Ri + L \frac{\partial i}{\partial t} \tag{2.29}$$

Equation 2.30 is the second transmission line equation with losses.

$$-\frac{\partial i}{\partial z} = Gv + C \frac{\partial v}{\partial t} \tag{2.30}$$

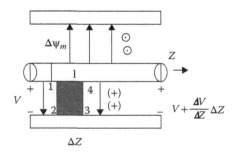 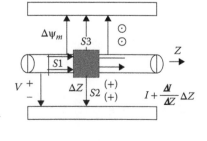

FIGURE 2.3 Transmission line geometry.

where $\qquad C = \dfrac{\Delta C(z)}{\Delta Z} \qquad \dfrac{F}{m} \qquad L = \dfrac{\Delta L(z)}{\Delta Z} \qquad \dfrac{H}{m}$

By differentiating Equation 2.29 with respect to z and by differentiating Equation 2.30 with respect to t and adding the result we get:

$$-\frac{\partial^2 v}{\partial z^2} = RGv + (RC + LG)\frac{\partial v}{\partial t} + LC\frac{\partial^2 v}{\partial t^2} \qquad (2.31)$$

By differentiating Equation 2.30 with respect to z and by differentiating Equation 2.29 with respect to t and adding the result we get:

$$-\frac{\partial^2 i}{\partial z^2} = RGi + (RC + LG)\frac{\partial i}{\partial t} + LC\frac{\partial^2 i}{\partial t^2} \qquad (2.32)$$

Equations 2.31 and 2.32 are analogs to the wave equations. The solution of these equations is a superposition of a forward wave, $+z$, and backward wave, $-z$.

$$V(z,t) = V_+\left(t - \frac{z}{v}\right) + V_-\left(t + \frac{z}{v}\right)$$

$$I(z,t) = Y_0\left\{V_+\left(t - \frac{z}{v}\right) - V_-\left(t + \frac{z}{v}\right)\right\} \qquad (2.33)$$

Y_0 is the characteristic admittance of the transmission line $Y_0 = \dfrac{1}{Z_0}$.

The variation of electromagnetic waves as a function of time may be written as $e^{j\omega t}$. The derivative as a function of time is $j\omega e^{j\omega t}$. By using these relations we write the phazor transmission line equations.

$$\frac{dV}{dZ} = -ZI$$

$$\frac{dI}{dZ} = -YV$$

$$\frac{d^2 V}{dz^2} = \gamma^2 V \qquad (2.34)$$

$$\frac{d^2 I}{dz^2} = \gamma^2 I$$

where

$$Z = R + j\omega L$$

$$(2.35)$$

$$Y = G + j\omega C$$

The solution of the transmission line equations in harmonic steady state is:

$$v(z,t) = \mathrm{Re}\, V(z)e^{j\omega t} \qquad (2.36)$$

$$i(z,t) = \mathrm{Re}\, I(z)e^{j\omega t}$$

$$V(z) = V_+ e^{-\gamma z} + V_- e^{\gamma z}$$

$$(2.37)$$

$$I(z) = I_+ e^{-\gamma z} + I_- e^{\gamma z}$$

For a lossless transmission line we write:

$$\frac{dV}{dZ} = -j\omega L I$$

$$\frac{dI}{dZ} = --j\omega C V$$

$$2.38)$$

$$\frac{d^2 V}{dz^2} = -\omega^2 L C V$$

$$\frac{d^2 I}{dz^2} = -\omega^2 L C I$$

The solution of the lossless transmission line equations is:

$$V(z) = e^{j\omega t}(V^+ e^{-j\beta z} + V^- e^{j\beta z}) \qquad (2.39)$$

$$I(z) = Y_0 (e^{j\omega t}(V^+ e^{-j\beta z} - V^- e^{j\beta z}))$$

$$v_{\mathrm{p}} = \frac{\omega}{\beta} = \frac{1}{\sqrt{LC}} = \frac{1}{\sqrt{\mu\varepsilon}}$$

where v_{p} represents phase velocity.

Z_0 is the characteristic impedance of the transmission line.

$$Z_0 = \frac{V_+}{I_+} = \frac{V_-}{I_-} = \sqrt{\frac{(R+j\omega L)}{(G+j\omega C)}}$$

$$\text{for} \quad R = 0 \quad G = 0 \qquad (2.40)$$

$$Z_0 = \frac{V_+}{I_+} = \frac{V_-}{I_-} = \sqrt{\frac{L}{C}}$$

Waves in transmission lines

A load Z_L is connected, at $z = 0$, to a transmission line with impedance Z. The voltage on the load is V_L. The current on the load is I_L (Figure 2.4).

$$V(0) = V_L = I(0) \cdot Z_L$$
$$I(0) = I_L$$

(2.41)

For $z = 0$ we write:

$$V(0) = I(0) \cdot Z_L = V_+ + V_-$$
$$I(0) = Y_0(V_+ - V_-)$$

(2.42)

By substituting $I(0)$ in $V(0)$ we get:

$$Z_L = Z_0 \frac{V_+ + V_-}{V_+ - V_-}$$

$$Z_L = Z_0 \frac{1 + \dfrac{V_-}{V_+}}{1 - \dfrac{V_-}{V_+}}$$

(2.43)

The ratio $\dfrac{V_-}{V_+}$ is defined as the reflection coefficient: $\Gamma_L = \dfrac{V_-}{V_+}$.

$$Z_L = Z_0 \frac{1 + \Gamma_L}{1 - \Gamma_L}$$

(2.44)

$$\Gamma_L = \frac{\dfrac{Z_L}{Z_0} - 1}{\dfrac{Z_L}{Z_0} + 1}$$

(2.45)

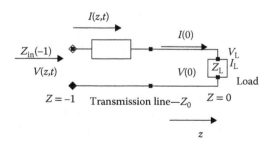

FIGURE 2.4 Transmission line with load.

The reflection coefficient as a function of z is written as:

$$\Gamma(Z) = \frac{V_-}{V_+} = \frac{V_- e^{j\beta z}}{V_+ e^{-j\beta z}} = \Gamma_L e^{2j\beta z} \tag{2.46}$$

The input impedance as a function of z is written as:

$$Z_{in}(z) = \frac{V(z)}{I(z)} = \frac{V_+ e^{-j\beta z} + V_- e^{j\beta z}}{(V_+ e^{-j\beta z} - V_- e^{j\beta z})Y_0}$$

$$= Z_0 \frac{1 + \Gamma_L e^{2j\beta z}}{1 - \Gamma_L e^{2j\beta z}} \tag{2.47}$$

$$Z_{in}(-l) = Z_L \frac{\cos\beta l + j\dfrac{Z_0}{Z_L}\sin\beta l}{\cos\beta l + j\dfrac{Z_L}{Z_0}\sin\beta l} \tag{2.48}$$

The voltage and current as a function of z may be written as:

$$V(z) = V_+ e^{-j\beta z}(1 + \Gamma(z))$$

$$I(z) = Y_0 V_+ e^{-j\beta z}(1 - \Gamma(z)) \tag{2.49}$$

The ratio between the maximum and minimum voltage along a transmission line is called the voltage standing wave ratio (VSWR), represented by S.

$$S = \left|\frac{V(z)\max}{V(z)\min}\right| = \frac{1 + |\Gamma(z)|}{1 - |\Gamma(z)|} \tag{2.50}$$

2.7   MATCHING TECHNIQUES

Usually in communication systems the load impedance is not the same as the impedance of commercial transmission lines. We get maximum power transfer from source to load if impedances are matched [1–10]. A perfect impedance match corresponds to a VSWR 1:1. A reflection coefficient magnitude of zero is a perfect match; a value of one is perfect reflection. The reflection coefficient (Γ) of a short circuit has a value of –1 (1 at an angle of 180°). The reflection coefficient of an open circuit is one at an angle of 0°. The return loss of a load is merely the magnitude of the reflection coefficient expressed in decibels. The correct equation for return loss is:

$$\text{Return loss} = -20 \times \log\,[\text{mag}(\Gamma)]$$

For a maximum voltage V_m in a transmission line the maximum power is:

$$P_{max} = \frac{V_m^2}{Z_0} \tag{2.51}$$

For a unmatched transmission line the maximum power is:

$$P_{max} = \frac{(1-|\Gamma|^2)V_+^2}{Z_0}$$

$$V_{max} = (1+|\Gamma|)V_+ \tag{2.52}$$

$$V_+^2 = \frac{V_{max}^2}{(1+|\Gamma|)^2}$$

$$P_{max} = \frac{1-|\Gamma|}{1+|\Gamma|} \cdot \frac{V_{max}^2}{Z_0} = \frac{V_{max}^2}{VSWR \cdot Z_0} \tag{2.53}$$

A 2:1 VSWR will result in half of the maximum power being transferred to the load. The reflected power may cause damage to the source.

Equation 2.47 indicates that there is a one-to-one correspondence between the reflection coefficient and input impedance. A movement of distance z along a transmission line corresponds to a change of $e^{-2j\beta}z$, which represents a rotation via an angle of $2\beta z$. In the reflection coefficient plane we may represent any normalized impedance by contours of constant resistance, r, and contours of constant reactance, x. The corresponding impedance moves on a constant radius circle via an angle of $2\beta z$ to a new impedance value. Those relations may be presented by a graphic aid called a Smith chart. They may be also presented by the following set of equations:

$$\Gamma_L = \frac{\dfrac{Z_L}{Z_0} - 1}{\dfrac{Z_L}{Z_0} + 1}$$

$$z(l) = \frac{Z_L}{Z_0} = r + jx \tag{2.54}$$

$$\Gamma_L = \frac{r + jx - 1}{r + jx + 1} = p + jq$$

$$\frac{Z(z)}{Z_0} = \frac{1+\Gamma(z)}{1-\Gamma(z)} = r + jx$$

$$\Gamma(z) = u + jv \tag{2.55}$$

$$\frac{1+u+jv}{1-u-jv} = r + jx$$

$$\left(u - \frac{r}{1+r}\right) + v^2 = \frac{1}{(1+r)^2}$$

$$(u-1)^2 + \left(v - \frac{1}{x}\right) = \frac{1}{x^2}$$

(2.56)

Equation 2.56 presents two families of circles in the reflection coefficient plane. The first family are contours of constant resistance, r, and the second family are contours of constant reactance, x. The center of the Smith chart is $r = 1$. Moving away from the load corresponds to mowing around the chart in a clockwise direction. Moving away from the generator toward the load corresponds to moving around the chart in a counterclockwise direction (Figure 2.5).

A complete revolution around the chart in a clockwise direction corresponds to a movement of half a wavelength away from the load. The Smith chart can be employed to calculate the reflection coefficient and the input impedance for a given transmission line and load impedance. If we are at a matched impedance condition at the center of the Smith chart, any length of transmission line with impedance Z_0 does nothing to the input match. But if the reflection coefficient of the network (S_{11}) is at some non-ideal impedance, adding a transmission line between the network and the reference plane rotates the observed reflection coefficient clockwise about the center of the Smith chart. Further, the rotation occurs at a fixed radius (and VSWR magnitude) if the transmission line has the same characteristic impedance as the source impedance Z_0. Adding a quarter wavelength means a 180° phase rotation. Adding one quarter wavelength from a short circuit moves us 180° to the right side of the chart, to an open circuit.

2.7.1 SMITH CHART GUIDELINES

The Smith chart contains almost all possible complex impedances within one circle.

- The smith chart horizontal center line represents resistance/conductance.
- Zero resistance is located on the left end of the horizontal center line.
- Infinite resistance is located on the right end of the horizontal center line.
- The horizontal centerline represents the resistive conductive horizontal scale of the chart.
- Impedances in the Smith chart are normalized to the characteristic impedance of the transmission line and are independent of the characteristic impedance of the transmission.
- The center of the line and also of the chart is the 1.0 point, where $R = Z_0$ or $G = Y_0$.

At point $r = 1.0$, $Z = Z_0$ and no reflection will occur.

2.7.2 QUARTER-WAVE TRANSFORMERS

A quarter-wave transformer may be used to match a device with impedance Z_L to a system with impedance Z_0, as shown in Figure 2.6. A quarter-wave transformer is a matching network with bandwidth somewhat inversely proportional to the relative

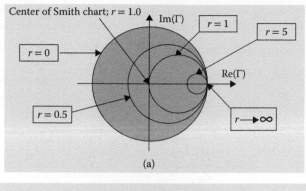

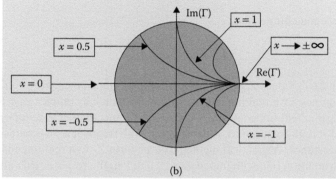

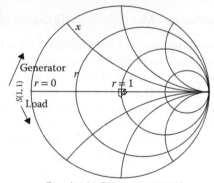

FIGURE 2.5 (a) r circles. (b) x circles. (c) Smith chart.

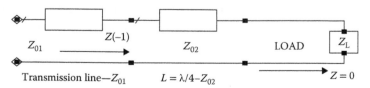

FIGURE 2.6 Quarter-wave transformer.

mismatch we are trying to match. For a single-stage quarter-wave transformer, the correct transformer impedance is the geometric mean between the impedances of the load and the source. Substituting $l = \dfrac{\lambda}{4}$, $\beta = \dfrac{2\pi}{\lambda}$ in Equation 2.47 we get:

$$\bar{Z}(-l) = \frac{\dfrac{Z_L}{Z_{02}}\cos\beta\dfrac{\lambda}{4} + j\sin\beta\dfrac{\lambda}{4}}{\cos\beta\dfrac{\lambda}{4} + j\dfrac{Z_L}{Z_{00}}\sin\beta\dfrac{\lambda}{4}} = \frac{Z_{02}}{Z_L} \tag{2.57}$$

$$\bar{Z}(-l) = \frac{Z_{01}}{Z_{02}} = \frac{Z_{02}}{Z_L}$$

We achieve matching when

$$Z_{02} = \sqrt{Z_L Z_{01}} \tag{2.58}$$

For complex Z_L values Z_{02} also will be complex impedance. However, standard transmission lines have real impedance values. To match a complex $Z_L = R + jX$ we transform Z_L to a real impedance $Z_{L1} - jX$ to Z_L. Connecting a capacitor $-jX$ to Z_L is not practical at high frequencies. A capacitor at high frequencies has parasitic inductance and resistance. A practical method to transform Z_L to a real impedance Z_{L1} is to add a transmission line with impedance Z_0 and length l to get a real value Z_{L1}.

2.7.3 WIDEBAND MATCHING—MULTI-SECTION TRANSFORMERS

Multi-section quarter-wave transformers are employed for wideband applications. Responses such as Chebyshev (equi-ripple) and maximally flat are possible for multi-section transformers. Each section brings us to intermediate impedance. In four section transformers from 25 Ω to 50 Ω intermediate impedances are chosen by using an arithmetic series. For an arithmetic series the steps are equal, $\Delta Z = 6.25\,\Omega$, so the impedances are 31.25 Ω, 37.5 Ω, 43.75 Ω. Solving for the transformers yields Z1 = 27.951, Z2 = 34.233, Z3 = 40.505 and Z4 = 46.771 Ω. A second solution to multi-section transformers involves a geometric series from impedance Z_L to impedance Z_S. Here the impedance from one section to the next adjacent section is a constant ratio.

2.7.4 SINGLE STUB MATCHING

A device with admittance Y_L can be matched to a system with admittance Y_0 by using a shunt or series single stub. At a distance l from the load we can get a normalized admittance $\bar{Y}$ in $= 1 + j\bar{B}$. By solving Equation 2.58 we can calculate l.

$$\bar{Y}(l) = \frac{1 + j\dfrac{Z_L}{Z_0}\tan\beta l}{\dfrac{Z_L}{Z_0} + j\tan\beta l} = 1 + j\bar{B} \tag{2.59}$$

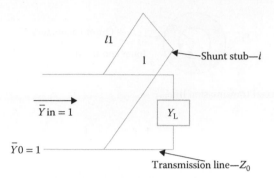

FIGURE 2.7 Single stub matching.

At this location we can add a shunt stub with normalized input susceptance, $-j\bar{B}$ to yield $\bar{Y}$ in $= 1$ as presented in Equation 2.60. $\bar{Y}$ in $= 1$ represents a matched load. The stub can be short-circuited line or open-circuited line. The susceptance $\bar{B}$ is given in Equation 2.60.

$$\bar{Y} \text{ in} = 1 + j\bar{B}$$

$$\bar{Y}_{1\text{in}} = -j\bar{B} \tag{2.60}$$

$$\bar{B} = ctg\beta l_1$$

The length l_1 of the short-circuited line may be calculated by solving Equation 2.61 (Figure 2.7).

$$\text{Im}\left\{ \frac{1 + j\dfrac{Z_L}{Z_0}\tan\beta l}{\dfrac{Z_L}{Z_0} + j\tan\beta l} \right\} = ctg\beta l_1 \tag{2.61}$$

2.8 COAXIAL TRANSMISSION LINE

A coax transmission line consists of two round conductors, one of which completely surrounds the other, with the two separated by a continuous solid dielectric [1–9]. The desired propagation mode is TEM. The major advantage of coax over a microstrip line is that the transmission line does not radiate. The disadvantages are that coax lines are more expensive. Coax lines are usually employed up to 18 GHz. They are highly expensive at frequencies higher than 18 GHz. To obtain good performance at higher frequencies, a small-diameter cable is required to stay below the cutoff frequency. Maxwell's laws are employed to compute the electric and magnetic fields in the coax transmission line. A cross section of the coaxial transmission line is shown in Figure 2.8.

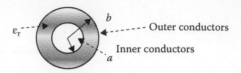

FIGURE 2.8   Coaxial transmission line.

$$\oint_S E \cdot ds = \frac{1}{\varepsilon_0} \int_V \rho \, dv = \frac{1}{\varepsilon_0} q$$

(2.62)

$$E_r = \frac{\rho_L}{2\pi r \varepsilon}$$

$$V = \int_a^b E \cdot dr = \int_a^b \frac{\rho_L}{2\pi r \varepsilon} \cdot dr = \frac{\rho_L}{2\pi \varepsilon} \ln \frac{b}{a}$$

(2.63)

Ampere's law is employed to calculate the magnetic field.

$$\oint H \cdot dl = 2\pi r H_\varphi = I$$

(2.64)

$$H_\varphi = \frac{I}{2\pi r}$$

$$V = \int_a^b E_r \cdot dr = -\int_a^b \eta H_\varphi \cdot dr = \frac{I\eta}{2\pi} \ln \frac{b}{a}$$

(2.65)

$$Z_0 = \frac{V}{I} = \frac{\eta}{2\pi} \ln \frac{b}{a} \quad \eta = \sqrt{\mu/\varepsilon}$$

The power flow in the coaxial transmission line may be calculated by calculating the Poynting vector.

$$P = (E \times H) \cdot n = EH$$

$$P = \frac{VI}{2\pi r^2 \ln(b/a)}$$

(2.66)

$$W = \int_S P \cdot ds = \int_a^b \frac{VI}{2\pi r^2 \ln(b/a)} 2\pi r \, dr = VI$$

Table 2.12 presents several industry-standard coax cables. The cable dimensions, cable impedance, and cable cutoff frequency are given in Table 2.12. RG cables are flexible cables. SR cables are semi-rigid cables.

TABLE 2.12
Industry-Standard Coax Cables

Cable Type	Outer Diameter (in.)	2b (in.)	2a (in.)	Z_0 (Ω)	f_c (GHz)
RG-8A	0.405	0.285	0.089	50	14.0
RG-58A	0.195	0.116	0.031	50	35.3
RG-174	0.100	0.060	0.019	50	65.6
RG-196	0.080	0.034	0.012	50	112
RG-214	0.360	0.285	0.087	50	13.9
RG-223	0.216	0.113	0.037	50	34.6
SR-085	0.085	0.066	.0201	50	60.2
SR-141	0.141	0.1175	0.0359	50	33.8
SR-250	0.250	0.210	0.0641	50	18.9

2.8.1 CUTOFF FREQUENCY AND WAVELENGTH OF COAX CABLES

f_c Cutoff frequency

The criterion for cutoff frequency is that the circumference at the midpoint inside the dielectric must be less than a wavelength. Therefore the cutoff wavelength for the TE01 mode is $\lambda_c = \pi(a+b)\sqrt{\mu_r \varepsilon_r}$.

2.9 MICROSTRIP LINE

Microstrip is a planar printed transmission line. It has been the most popular RF transmission line over the last twenty years [3–10]. Microstrip transmission lines consist of a conductive strip of width "W" and thickness "t" and a wider ground plane, separated by a dielectric layer of thickness "H." In practice, microstrip line is usually made by etching circuitry on a substrate that has a ground plane on the opposite face. A cross section of the microstrip line is shown in Figure 2.9. The major advantage of microstrip over stripline is that all components can be mounted on top of the board. The disadvantage is that when high isolation is required such as in a filter or switch, some external shielding is needed. Microstrip circuits may radiate, causing unintended circuit response. Microstrip is dispersive; signals of different frequencies travel at slightly different speeds. Other microstrip line configurations are offset strip line and suspended air microstrip line. For microstrip lines, not all the fields are constrained to the same dielectric. At the line edges the fields pass via air and dielectric substrate. The effective dielectric constant should be calculated.

2.9.1 EFFECTIVE DIELECTRIC CONSTANT

Part of the field in the microstrip line structure exists in air and the other part of the field exists in the dielectric substrate. The effective dielectric constant is somewhat less than the substrate's dielectric constant.

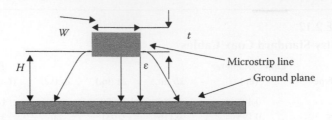

FIGURE 2.9 Microstrip line cross section.

The effective dielectric constant of the microstrip line is calculated by:
For

$$\left(\frac{W}{H}\right) < 1 \tag{2.67}$$

$$\varepsilon_e = \frac{\varepsilon_r + 1}{2} + \frac{\varepsilon_r - 1}{2}\left[\left(1 + 12\left(\frac{H}{W}\right)\right)^{-0.5} + 0.04\left(1 - \left(\frac{W}{H}\right)\right)^2\right]$$

For

$$\left(\frac{W}{H}\right) \geq 1 \tag{2.68}$$

$$\varepsilon_e = \frac{\varepsilon_r + 1}{2} + \frac{\varepsilon_r - 1}{2}\left[\left(1 + 12\left(\frac{H}{W}\right)\right)^{-0.5}\right]$$

This calculation ignores strip thickness and frequency dispersion, but their effects are negligible.

2.9.2 Characteristic Impedance

The characteristic impedance Z_0 is a function of the ratio of the height to the width W/H of the transmission line, and also has separate solutions depending on the value of W/H. The characteristic impedance Z_0 of microstrip is calculated by:

For

$$\left(\frac{W}{H}\right) < 1 \tag{2.69}$$

$$Z_0 = \frac{60}{\sqrt{\varepsilon_e}} \ln\left[8\left(\frac{H}{W}\right) + 0.25\left(\frac{H}{W}\right)\right] \Omega$$

For $$\left(\frac{W}{H}\right) \geq 1 \qquad (2.70)$$

$$Z_0 = \frac{120\pi}{\sqrt{\varepsilon_e}\left[\left(\frac{H}{W}\right)+1.393+0.66*\ln\left(\frac{H}{W}+1.444\right)\right]} \ \Omega$$

We can calculate Z_0 by using Equations 2.69 and 2.70 for a given $\left(\frac{W}{H}\right)$. However, to calculate $\left(\frac{W}{H}\right)$ for a given Z_0 we first should calculate ε_e. However, to calculate ε_e we should know $\left(\frac{W}{H}\right)$. We first assume that $\varepsilon_e = \varepsilon_r$ and compute $\left(\frac{W}{H}\right)$. For this value of $\left(\frac{W}{H}\right)$ we compute ε_e. Then we compute a new value of $\left(\frac{W}{H}\right)$. Two to three iterations are needed to calculate accurate values of $\left(\frac{W}{H}\right)$ and ε_e. *We may calculate* $\left(\frac{W}{H}\right)$ with around 10% accuracy by using Equation 2.71. Table 2.13 presents examples of microstrip line parameters.

$$\frac{W}{H} = 8\frac{\sqrt{[e^{\frac{Z_0}{42.4}\sqrt{(\varepsilon_r+1)}}-1]\left[\frac{7+\frac{4}{\varepsilon_r}}{11}\right]+\left[\frac{1+\frac{1}{\varepsilon_r}}{0.81}\right]}}{[e^{\frac{Z_0}{42.4}\sqrt{(\varepsilon_r+1)}}-1]} \qquad (2.71)$$

2.9.3 Higher-Order Transmission Modes in Microstrip Line

In order to prevent higher-order transmission modes we should limit the thickness of the microstrip substrate to 10% of a wavelength. The cutoff frequency of the higher-order transmission mode is given as $-f_c = \frac{c}{4H\sqrt{\varepsilon-1}}$.

Examples: Higher order modes will not propagate in microstrip lines printed on alumina substrate 15 mil thick up to 18 GHz. Higher order modes will not propagate in microstrip lines printed on GaAs substrate 4 mil thick up to 80 GHz. Higher order

---

TABLE 2.13

Examples of Microstrip Line Parameters

Substrate	W/H	Impedance Ω
Alumina ($\varepsilon_r = 9.8$)	0.95	50
GaAs ($\varepsilon_r = 12.9$)	0.75	50
$\varepsilon_r = 2.2$	3	50

modes will not propagate in a microstrip lines printed on quartz substrate 5 mil thick up to 120 GHz.

Losses in microstrip line:

Losses in microstrip line are due to conductor loss, radiation loss, and dielectric loss.

2.9.4 CONDUCTOR LOSS

Conductor loss may be calculated by using Equation 2.72.

$$\alpha_c = 8.686 \log(R_S/(2WZ_0)) \quad \text{dB/cm}$$

$$R_S = \sqrt{\pi f \mu \rho} \quad \text{Skin Resistance}$$

(2.72)

Conductor losses may also be calculated by defining an equivalent loss tangent δc, given by $\delta c = \delta s / h$, where $\delta s = \sqrt{2/\omega \mu \sigma}$, where σ is the strip conductivity, h is the substrate height, and μ is the free space permeability.

2.9.5 DIELECTRIC LOSS

Dielectric loss may be calculated by using Equation 2.73.

$$\alpha_d = 27.3 \frac{\varepsilon_r}{\sqrt{\varepsilon_{eff}}} \frac{\varepsilon_{eff} - 1}{\varepsilon_r - 1} \frac{tg\delta}{\lambda_0} \quad \text{dB/cm}$$

(2.73)

$$tg\delta = \text{dielectric loss coefficent}$$

Losses in microstrip lines are presented in Tables 2.14 through 2.16 for several microstrip line structures. For example, the total loss of a microstrip line presented in Table 2.15 at 40 GHz is 0.5 dB/cm. The total loss of a microstrip line presented in Table 2.16 at 40 GHz is 1.42 dB/cm. We may conclude that losses in microstrip lines limit the applications of microstrip technology at mm wave frequencies.

TABLE 2.14

Microstrip Line Losses for Alumina Substrate 10-mil Thick

Frequency (GHz)	Loss Tangent Loss (dB/cm)	Metal Loss (dB/cm)	Total Loss (dB/cm)
10	−0.005	−0.12	−0.124
20	−0.009	−0.175	−0.184
30	−0.014	−0.22	−0.23
40	−0.02	−0.25	−0.27

Alumina, $H = 254$ μ (10 mils), $W = 247$ μ, $E_r = 9.9$, Tan$\delta = 0.0002$, 3 μ gold, conductivity 3.5 E7 mhos/m

---

TABLE 2.15
Microstrip Line Losses for Alumina Substrate 5-mil Thick

Frequency (GHz)	Loss Tangent Loss (dB/cm)	Metal Loss (dB/cm)	Total Loss (dB/cm)
10	−0.004	−0.23	−0.23
20	−0.009	−0.333	−0.34
30	−0.013	−0.415	−0.43
40	−0.018	−0.483	−0.5

Alumina, H = 127 μ (5 mils), W = 120 μ, ER = 9.9, Tanδ = 0.0002, 3 μ gold, conductivity 3.5E7 mhos/m

TABLE 2.16
Microstrip Line Losses for GaAs Substrate 2-mil Thick

Frequency (GHz)	Tangent Loss (dB/cm)	Metal Loss (dB/cm)	Total Loss (dB/cm)
10	−0.010	−0.66	−0.67
20	−0.02	−0.96	−0.98
30	−0.03	−1.19	−1.22
40	−0.04	−1.38	−1.42

GaAs, H = 50 μ (2 mils), W = 34 μ, ER = 12.88, Tanδ = 0.0004, 3 μ gold, conductivity 3.5E7 mhos/m

2.10 WAVEGUIDES

Waveguides are low loss transmission lines. They may be rectangular or circular. A rectangular waveguide structure is presented in Figure 2.10. A waveguide structure is uniform in the z direction. Fields in waveguides are evaluated by solving the Helmolz equation. The wave equation is given in Equation 2.74. The wave equation in a rectangular coordinate system is given in Equation 2.75.

$$\nabla^2 E = \omega^2 \mu \varepsilon E = -k^2 E$$

$$\nabla^2 H = \omega^2 \mu \varepsilon H = -k^2 H \tag{2.74}$$

$$k = \omega\sqrt{\mu\varepsilon} = \frac{\omega}{v} = \frac{2\pi}{\lambda}$$

$$\nabla^2 E = \frac{\partial^2 E_i}{\partial x^2} + \frac{\partial^2 E_i}{\partial y^2} + \frac{\partial^2 E_i}{\partial z^2} + k^2 E_i = 0 \quad i = x, y, z$$

$$\tag{2.75}$$

$$\nabla^2 H = \frac{\partial^2 H_i}{\partial x^2} + \frac{\partial^2 H_i}{\partial y^2} + \frac{\partial^2 H_i}{\partial z^2} + k^2 H_i = 0$$

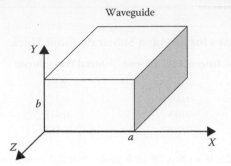

FIGURE 2.10 Rectangular waveguide structure.

The wave equation solution may be written as $E = f(z)g(x,y)$. Field variation in the z direction may be written as $e^{-j\beta z}$. The derivative of this expression in the z direction may be written as $-j\beta e^{j\beta z}$. Maxwell's equations may be presented as written in Equations 2.76 and 2.77. A field may be represented as a superposition of waves in the transverse and longitudinal directions.

$$E(x,y,z) = e(x,y)e^{-j\beta z} + e_z(x,y)e^{-j\beta z}$$

$$H(x,y,z) = h(x,y)e^{-j\beta z} + h_z(x,y)e^{-j\beta z}$$

$$\nabla XE = (\nabla_t - j\beta a_z) \times (e + e_z)e^{-j\beta z} = -j\omega\mu(h + h_z)e^{-j\beta z}$$

$$\nabla_t \times e - j\beta a_z \times e + \nabla_t \times e_z - j\beta a_z \times e_z = -j\omega\mu(h + h_z) \qquad (2.76)$$

$$a_z \times e_z = 0$$

$$\nabla_t \times e = -j\omega\mu h_z$$

$$-j\beta a_z \times e + \nabla_t \times e_z = -a_z \times \nabla_t e_z - j\beta a_z \times e = -j\omega\mu h$$

$$\nabla_t \times h = -j\omega\varepsilon e_z$$

$$a_z \times \nabla_t h_z + j\beta a_z \times h = -j\omega\varepsilon e \qquad (2.77)$$

$$\nabla \cdot \mu H = (\nabla_t - j\beta a_z) \cdot (h + h_z)\mu e^{-j\beta z} = 0$$

$$\nabla_t \cdot h - j\beta a_z \cdot h_z = 0 \qquad (2.78)$$

$$\nabla \cdot \varepsilon E = 0 \quad \nabla_t \cdot e - j\beta a_z \cdot e_z = 0$$

Waves are characterized as TEM, TE, or TM waves. In TEM waves $e_z = h_z = 0$. In TE waves $e_z = 0$. In TM waves $h_z = 0$.

2.10.1 TE WAVES

In TE waves $e_z = 0$. h_z is as solution of Equation 2.79. The solution to Equation 2.79 is written as $h_z = f(x)g(y)$.

$$\nabla_t^2 h_z = \frac{\partial^2 h_z}{\partial x^2} + \frac{\partial^2 h_z}{\partial y^2} + k_c^2 h_z = 0 \tag{2.79}$$

By applying $h_z = f(x)g(y)$ to Equation 2.79 and dividing by fg we get Equation 2.80.

$$\frac{f''}{f} + \frac{g''}{g} + k_c^2 = 0 \tag{2.80}$$

f is a function that varies in the x direction and g is a function that varies in the y direction. The sum of f and g may be equal to zero only if they are equal to a constant. These facts are written in Equation 2.81.

$$\frac{f''}{f} = -k_x^2; \frac{g''}{g} = -k_y^2 \tag{2.81}$$

$$k_x^2 + k_y^2 = k_c^2$$

The solutions for f and g are given in Equation 2.82. A_1, A_2, B_1, and B_2 are derived by applying the h_z boundary conditions to Equation 2.80.

$$f = A_1 \cos k_x x + A_2 \sin k_x x$$
$$g = B_1 \cos k_y y + B_2 \sin k_y y \tag{2.82}$$

The h_z boundary conditions are written in Equation 2.83.

$$\frac{\partial h_z}{\partial x} = 0 \quad @ \quad x = 0, a$$

$$\frac{\partial h_z}{\partial y} = 0 \quad @ \quad y = 0, b \tag{2.83}$$

By applying the h_z boundary conditions to Equation 2.82 we get the relations written in Equation 2.84.

$$-k_x A_1 \sin k_x x + k_x A_2 \cos k_x x = 0$$

$$-k_y B_1 \sin k_y y + k_y B_2 \cos k_y y = 0$$

$$A_2 = 0 \qquad k_x a = 0 \qquad k_x = \frac{n\pi}{a} \qquad n = 0,1,2 \tag{2.84}$$

$$B_2 = 0 \qquad k_y b = 0 \qquad k_y = \frac{m\pi}{b} \qquad m = 0,1,2$$

The solution for h_z is given in Equation 2.85.

$$h_z = A_{nm} \cos \frac{n\pi x}{a} \cos \frac{m\pi y}{b}$$

$$n = m \neq 0 \qquad n = 0,1,2 \qquad m = 0,1,2 \qquad\qquad (2.85)$$

$$k_{c,nm} = \left[\left(\frac{n\pi}{a} \right)^2 + \left(\frac{m\pi}{b} \right)^2 \right]^{1/2}$$

Both n and m cannot be zero. The wavenumber at cutoff is $k_{c,nm}$ and depends on the waveguide dimensions. The propagation constant γ_{nm} is given in Equation 2.86.

$$\gamma_{nm} = j\beta_{nm} = j(k_0^2 - k_c^2)^{1/2} =$$

$$= j \left[\left(\frac{2\pi}{\lambda_0} \right)^2 - \left(\frac{n\pi}{a} \right)^2 - \left(\frac{m\pi}{b} \right)^2 \right]^{1/2} \qquad\qquad (2.86)$$

For $k_0 \rangle k_{c,nm}$, β is real and the wave will propagate. For $k_0 \langle k_{c,nm}$, β is imaginary and the wave will decay rapidly. Frequencies that define propagating and decaying waves are called cutoff frequencies. We calculate cutoff frequencies using Equation 2.87.

$$f_{c,nm} = \frac{c}{2\pi} k_{c,nm} = \frac{c}{2\pi} \left[\left(\frac{n\pi}{a} \right)^2 + \left(\frac{m\pi}{b} \right)^2 \right]^{1/2} \qquad\qquad (2.87)$$

For $a = 2$, the cutoff wavelength is computed by using Equation 2.88.

$$\lambda_{c,nm} = \frac{2ab}{\left[n^2 b^2 + m^2 a^2 \right]^{1/2}} = \frac{2a}{\left[n^2 + 4m^2 \right]^{1/2}}$$

$$\lambda_{c,10} = 2a \qquad \lambda_{c,01} = a \qquad \lambda_{c,11} = 2a/\sqrt{5} \qquad\qquad (2.88)$$

$$\frac{c}{2a} \langle f_{01} \rangle \frac{c}{a}$$

For $\frac{c}{2a} \langle f_{01} \rangle \frac{c}{a}$ the dominant is TE10.

We use Equations 2.76 through 2.78 to derive the electromagnetic fields that propagate in the waveguide as given in Equation 2.89.

$$H_z = A_{nm} \cos\frac{n\pi x}{a} \cos\frac{m\pi y}{b} e^{\pm j\beta_{nm}z}$$

$$H_x = \pm j\frac{n\pi\beta_{nm}}{ak_{c,nm}^2} A_{nm} \sin\frac{n\pi x}{a} \cos\frac{m\pi y}{b} e^{\pm j\beta_{nm}z}$$

$$H_y = \pm j\frac{m\pi\beta_{nm}}{bk_{c,nm}^2} A_{nm} \cos\frac{n\pi x}{a} \sin\frac{m\pi y}{b} e^{\pm j\beta_{nm}z} \tag{2.89}$$

$$E_X = Z_{h,nm} j\frac{m\pi\beta_{nm}}{bk_{c,nm}^2} A_{nm} \cos\frac{n\pi x}{a} \sin\frac{m\pi y}{b} e^{\pm j\beta_{nm}z}$$

$$E_Y = -jZ_{h,nm} \frac{n\pi\beta_{nm}}{ak_{c,nm}^2} A_{nm} \sin\frac{n\pi x}{a} \cos\frac{m\pi y}{b} e^{\pm j\beta_{nm}z}$$

The impedance of the nm modes is given as $Z_{h,nm} = \dfrac{e_x}{h_y} = \dfrac{k_0}{\beta_{nm}}\sqrt{\dfrac{\mu_0}{\varepsilon_0}}$.

The power of the nm mode is computed by using Poynting vector calculation as shown in Equation 2.90.

$$P_{nm} = 0.5\,\mathrm{Re} \int_0^a\int_0^b E \times H^* \cdot a_z\,dx\,dy = 0.5\,\mathrm{Re}\,Z_{h,nm} \int_0^a\int_0^b (H_y H_Y^* + H_x H_x^*)\,dx\,dy$$

$$\int_0^a\int_0^b \cos^2\frac{n\pi x}{a}\sin^2\frac{m\pi y}{b}\,dx\,dy = \frac{ab}{4} \qquad n \neq 0 \qquad m \neq 0$$

$$\tag{2.90}$$

$$\text{or} \quad \frac{ab}{2} \qquad n \quad \text{or} \quad m = 0$$

$$P_{nm} = \frac{|A_{nm}|^2}{2\varepsilon_{0n}\varepsilon_{0m}}\left(\frac{\beta_{nm}}{k_{c,nm}}\right)^2 Z_{h,nm} \qquad \varepsilon_{0n} = 1, \quad n = 0 \qquad \varepsilon_{0n} = 2, \quad n \succ 0$$

The TE mode with the lowest cutoff frequency in a rectangular waveguide is TE10. TE10 fields in a rectangular waveguide are shown in Figure 2.11.

2.10.2 TM WAVES

In TM waves, $h_z = 0$. e_z is a solution of Equation 2.91. The solution to Equation 2.13 may be written as $e_z = f(x)g(y)$. e_z should be zero at the metallic walls. The e_z boundary conditions are written in Equation 2.92. The solution for e_z is given in Equation 2.93.

$$\nabla_t^2 e_z = \frac{\partial^2 e_z}{\partial x^2} + \frac{\partial^2 e_z}{\partial y^2} + k_c^2 e_z = 0 \tag{2.91}$$

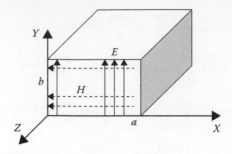

FIGURE 2.11 TE10 mode.

$$e_z = 0 \quad @ \quad x = 0, a$$

$$e_z = 0 \quad @ \quad y = 0, b \tag{2.92}$$

$$e_z = A_{nm} \sin \frac{n\pi x}{a} \sin \frac{m\pi y}{b}$$

$$n = m \neq 0 \qquad n = 0, 1, 2 \qquad m = 0, 1, 2 \tag{2.93}$$

$$k_{c,nm} = \left[\left(\frac{n\pi}{a} \right)^2 + \left(\frac{m\pi}{b} \right)^2 \right]^{1/2}$$

The first propagating TM mode is TM11, $n = m = 1$. By using Equations 2.76 through 2.78 and 2.91 we can derive the electromagnetic fields that propagate in the waveguide as given in Equation 2.94.

$$E_z = \sin \frac{n\pi x}{a} \sin \frac{m\pi y}{b} e^{\pm j\beta_{nm}z}$$

$$E_x = -j \frac{n\pi \beta_{nm}}{ak_{c,nm}^2} \cos \frac{n\pi x}{a} \sin \frac{m\pi y}{b} e^{\pm j\beta_{nm}z}$$

$$E_y = -j \frac{m\pi \beta_{nm}}{bk_{c,nm}^2} A_{nm} \sin \frac{n\pi x}{a} \cos \frac{m\pi y}{b} e^{\pm j\beta_{nm}z} \tag{2.94}$$

$$H_X = \frac{-E_y}{Z_{e,nm}}$$

$$H_Y = \frac{E_x}{Z_{e,nm}}$$

The impedance of the nm modes $\quad Z_{e,nm} = \frac{\beta_{nm}}{k_0} \sqrt{\frac{\mu_0}{\varepsilon_0}}$.

The TM mode with the lowest cutoff frequency in the rectangular waveguide is TM11. TM11 fields in the rectangular waveguide are shown in Figure 2.12.

2.11 CIRCULAR WAVEGUIDE

A circular waveguide is used to transmit electromagnetic waves in circular polarization. At high frequencies attenuation of several modes in a circular waveguide is lower than in a rectangular waveguide. The circular waveguide structure is uniform in the z direction. Fields in waveguides are evaluated by solving the Helmolz equation in cylindrical coordinate system. A circular waveguide in a cylindrical coordinate system is presented in Figure 2.13. The wave equation is given in Equation 2.95. The wave equation in a cylindrical coordinate system is given in Equation 2.96.

$$\nabla^2 E = \omega^2 \mu\varepsilon E = -k^2 E$$

$$\nabla^2 H = \omega^2 \mu\varepsilon H = -k^2 H \tag{2.95}$$

$$k = \omega\sqrt{\mu\varepsilon} = \frac{\omega}{v} = \frac{2\pi}{\lambda}$$

$$\nabla^2 E = \frac{1}{r}\frac{\partial}{\partial r}\left(r\frac{\partial E_i}{\partial r}\right) + \frac{1}{r^2}\frac{\partial^2 E_i}{\partial \varphi^2} + \frac{\partial^2 E_i}{\partial z^2} - \gamma^2 E_i = 0 \qquad i = r, \varphi, z$$

$$\nabla^2 H = \frac{1}{r}\frac{\partial}{\partial r}\left(r\frac{\partial H_i}{\partial r}\right) + \frac{1}{r^2}\frac{\partial^2 H_i}{\partial \varphi^2} + \frac{\partial^2 H_i}{\partial z^2} - \gamma^2 H_i = 0 \tag{2.96}$$

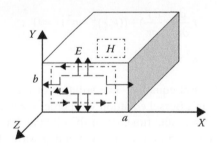

FIGURE 2.12 TM11 mode.

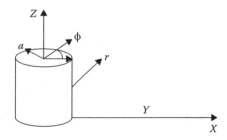

FIGURE 2.13 Circular waveguide structure.

The solution to Equation 2.96 is written as $E = f(r)g(\varphi)h(z)$. By applying E to Equation 2.96 and dividing by $f(r)g(\varphi)h(z)$ we get Equation 2.97.

$$\nabla^2 E = \frac{1}{rf}\frac{\partial}{\partial r}(r\frac{\partial f}{\partial r}) + \frac{1}{r^2 g}\frac{\partial^2 g}{\partial \varphi^2} + \frac{\partial^2 h}{h\partial z^2} - \gamma^2 = 0 \qquad (2.97)$$

f is a function that varies in the r direction, g is a function that varies in the φ direction, and h is function that varies in the z direction. The sum of f, g, and h may be equal to zero only if they equal to a constant. The solution for h is written in Equation 2.98. The propagation constant is γ_g.

$$\frac{\partial^2 h}{h\partial z^2} - \gamma_g^2 = 0 \qquad (2.98)$$

$$h = Ae^{-\gamma_g z} + Be^{\gamma_g z}$$

$$\frac{r}{f}\frac{\partial}{\partial r}(r\frac{\partial f}{\partial r}) + \frac{1}{g}\frac{\partial^2 g}{\partial \varphi^2} - (\gamma^2 - \gamma_g^2) = 0 \qquad (2.99)$$

The solution for g is written in Equation 2.100.

$$\frac{\partial^2 g}{g\partial \varphi^2} + n^2 = 0 \qquad (2.100)$$

$$g = A_n \sin n\varphi + B_n \cos n\varphi$$

$$r\frac{\partial}{\partial r}(r\frac{\partial f}{\partial r}) + ((k_c r)^2 - n^2)f = 0 \qquad (2.101)$$

$$k_c^2 + \gamma^2 = \gamma_g^2$$

Equation 2.101 is a Bessel equation. The solution of this equation is written in Equation 2.102. $J_n(k_c r)$ is a Bessel equation with order n and represents a standing wave. The wave varies as a cosine function in the circular waveguide. $N_n(k_c r)$ is a Bessel equation with order n and represents a standing wave. The wave varies as a sine function in the circular waveguide.

$$f = C_n J_n(k_c r) + D_n N_n(k_c r) \qquad (2.102)$$

The general solution for the electric fields in a circular waveguide is given in Equation 2.103. For $r = 0$, $N_n(k_c r)$ goes to infinity, so $D_n = 0$.

$$E(r,\varphi,z) = (C_n J_n(k_c r) + D_n N_n(k_c r))(A_n \sin n\varphi + B_n \cos n\varphi)e^{\pm\gamma_g z} \qquad (2.103)$$

$$A_n \sin n\varphi + B_n \cos n\varphi = \sqrt{A_n^2 + B_n^2}\cos\left(n\varphi + \tan^{-1}\left(\frac{A_n}{B_n}\right)\right) = F_n \cos n\varphi \qquad (2.104)$$

The general solution for the electric fields in a circular waveguide is given in Equation 2.105.

$$E(r,\varphi,z) = E_0(J_n(k_c r))(\cos n\varphi)e^{\pm\gamma_g z} \quad \text{If} \quad \alpha = 0$$

$$E(r,\varphi,z) = E_0(J_n(k_c r))(\cos n\varphi)e^{\pm\beta_g z} \quad (2.105)$$

$$\beta_g = \pm\sqrt{\omega^2\mu\varepsilon - k_c^2}$$

2.11.1 TE Waves in a Circular Waveguide

In TE waves, $e_z = 0$. H_z is as solution of Equation 2.106. The solution to Equation 2.106 may be written as given in Equation 2.107.

$$\nabla^2 H_z = \gamma^2 H_z \quad (2.106)$$

$$H_z = H_{0z}(J_n(k_c r))(\cos n\varphi)e^{\pm j\beta_g z} \quad (2.107)$$

The electric and magnetic fields are solutions of Maxwell's equations as written in Equations 2.108 and 2.109.

$$\nabla X E = -j\omega\mu H \quad (2.108)$$

$$\nabla \times H = j\omega\varepsilon E \quad (2.109)$$

Field variation in the z direction may be written as $e^{-j\beta z}$. The derivative of this expression in the z direction may be written as $-j\beta e^{j\beta z}$. The electric and magnetic field components are solutions of Equations 2.110 and 2.111.

$$E_r = -\frac{j\omega\mu}{k_c^2}\frac{1}{r}\left(\frac{\partial H_z}{\partial\varphi}\right)$$

$$(2.110)$$

$$E_\varphi = \frac{j\omega\mu}{k_c^2}\left(\frac{\partial H_z}{\partial r}\right)$$

$$H_\varphi = -\frac{-j\beta_g}{k_c^2}\frac{1}{r}\left(\frac{\partial H_z}{\partial\varphi}\right)$$

$$(2.111)$$

$$H_r = \frac{-j\beta_g}{k_c^2}\left(\frac{\partial H_z}{\partial r}\right)$$

The H_z, H_r, and E_φ boundary conditions are written in Equation 2.112.

$$\frac{\partial H_z}{\partial r} = 0 \quad @ \quad r = a$$

$$H_r = 0 \quad @ \quad r = a \tag{2.112}$$

$$E_\varphi = 0 \quad @ \quad r = a$$

By applying the boundary conditions to Equation 2.107 we get the relations written in Equation 2.113. The solutions of Equation 2.113 are listed in Table 2.17.

$$\frac{\partial H_z}{\partial r}\Big|r = a = H_{0z}(J_n'(k_c a))(\cos n\varphi)e^{-\beta_g z} = 0 \tag{2.113}$$

$$J_n'(k_c a) = 0$$

The wavenumber at the cutoff is $k_{c,np}$. $k_{c,np}$ depends on the waveguide dimensions. The propagation constant $\gamma_{g,np}$ is given in Equation 2.114.

$$\gamma_{g,np} = j\beta_{g,np} = j(k_0^2 - k_c^2)^{1/2}$$

$$= j\left[\left(\frac{2\pi}{\lambda_0}\right)^2 - \left(\frac{X_{np}'}{a}\right)^2\right]^{1/2} \tag{2.114}$$

For $k_0 \rangle k_{c,nm}$, β is real and the wave will propagate. For $k_0 \langle k_{c,nm}$, β is imaginary and the wave will decay rapidly. Frequencies that define propagating and decaying waves are called cutoff frequencies. We may calculate cutoff frequencies by using Equation 2.115.

$$f_{c,nm} = \frac{cX_{np}'}{2\pi a} \tag{2.115}$$

We get the field components by solving Equations 2.110 and 2.111. The field components are written in Equation 2.116.

TABLE 2.17

Circular Waveguide TE Modes

p	$(n = 0)$ X_{np}'	$(n = 1)$ X_{np}'	$(n = 2)$ X_{np}'	$(n = 3)$ X_{np}'	$(n = 4)$ X_{np}'	$(n = 5)$ X_{np}'
1	3.832	1.841	3.054	4.201	5.317	6.416
2	7.016	5.331	6.706	8.015	9.282	10.52
3	10.173	8.536	9.969	11.346	12.682	13.987
4	13.324	11.706	13.170	–	–	–

$$H_z = H_{0z}\left(J_n\left(\frac{X'_{np}r}{a}\right)\right)(\cos n\varphi)e^{-j\beta_g z}$$

$$H_\varphi = \frac{E_{0r}}{Z_g}\left(J_n\left(\frac{X'_{np}r}{a}\right)\right)(\sin n\varphi)e^{-j\beta_g z}$$

$$H_r = \frac{E_{0\varphi}}{Z_g}\left(J'_n\left(\frac{X'_{np}r}{a}\right)\right)(\cos n\varphi)e^{-j\beta_g z} \qquad (2.116)$$

$$E_\varphi = E_{0\varphi}\left(J'_n\left(\frac{X'_{np}r}{a}\right)\right)(\cos\varphi)e^{-j\beta_g z}$$

$$E_r = E_{0r}\left(J_n\left(\frac{X'_{np}r}{a}\right)\right)(\sin\varphi)e^{-j\beta_g z}$$

The impedance of the np modes is written in Equation 2.117.

$$Z_{g,np} = \frac{E_r}{H_\varphi} = \frac{\omega\mu}{\beta_{g,np}} = \frac{\eta}{\sqrt{1-\left(\frac{f_c}{f}\right)^2}} \qquad (2.117)$$

2.11.2 TM Waves in a Circular Waveguide

In TM waves, $h_z = 0$. e_z is as solution of Equation 2.118. The solution to Equation 2.118 is written in Equation 2.119.

$$\nabla^2 E_z = \gamma^2 E_z \qquad (2.118)$$

$$E_z = E_{0z}(J_n(k_c r))(\cos n\varphi)e^{+j\beta_g z} \qquad (2.119)$$

The electric and magnetic fields are solutions of Maxwell's equations as written in Equations 2.120 and 2.121.

$$\nabla X E = -j\omega\mu H \qquad (2.120)$$

$$\nabla \times H = j\omega\varepsilon E \qquad (2.121)$$

Field variation in the z direction is written as $e^{-j\beta z}$. The derivative of this expression in the z direction may be written as $-j\beta e^{j\beta z}$. The electric and magnetic fields components are the solutions of Equations 2.122 and 2.123.

$$H_r = \frac{j\omega\varepsilon}{k_c^2}\frac{1}{r}\left(\frac{\partial H_z}{\partial\varphi}\right)$$

$$H_\varphi = \frac{-j\omega\varepsilon}{k_c^2}\left(\frac{\partial H_z}{\partial r}\right)$$

(2.122)

$$E_\varphi = -\frac{-j\beta_g}{k_c^2}\frac{1}{r}\left(\frac{\partial E_z}{\partial\varphi}\right)$$

$$E_r = \frac{-j\beta_g}{k_c^2}\left(\frac{\partial E_z}{\partial r}\right)$$

(2.123)

The E_r boundary condition is written in Equation 2.124.

$$E_z = 0 \quad @ \quad r = a$$

(2.124)

By applying the boundary conditions to Equation 2.119 we get the relations written in Equation 2.125. The solutions of Equation 2.125 are listed in Table 2.18.

$$E_z|(r = a) = H_{0z}(J_n(k_c a))(\cos n\varphi)e^{-j\beta_g z} = 0$$

$$J_n(k_c a) = 0$$

(2.125)

The wavenumber at the cutoff is $k_{c,np}$. $k_{c,np}$ depends on the waveguide dimensions. The propagation constant $\gamma_{g,np}$ is given in Equation 2.126.

$$\gamma_{g,np} = j\beta_{g,np} = j(k_0^2 - k_c^2)^{1/2}$$

$$= j\left[\left(\frac{2\pi}{\lambda_0}\right)^2 - \left(\frac{X_{np}}{a}\right)^2\right]^{1/2}$$

(2.126)

For $k_0 \rangle k_{c,nm}$, β is real and the wave will propagate. For $k_0 \langle k_{c,nm}$, β is imaginary and the wave will decay rapidly. Frequencies that define propagating and decaying

TABLE 2.18

Circular Waveguide TM Modes

P	$n=0$, X_{np}	$n=1$, X_{np}	$n=2$, X_{np}	$n=3$, X_{np}	$n=4$, X_{np}	$n=5$, X_{np}
1	2.405	3.832	5.136	6.38	7.588	8.771
2	5.52	7.106	8.417	9.761	11.065	12.339
3	8.645	10.173	11.62	13.015	14.372	
4	11.792	13.324	14.796	–	–	–

waves are called cutoff frequencies. We calculate the cutoff frequencies by using Equation 2.127.

$$f_{c,nm} = \frac{cX_{np}}{2\pi a} \tag{2.127}$$

We get the field components by solving Equations 2.122 and 2.123. The field components are written in Equation 2.128.

$$E_z = E_{0z}\left(J_n\left(\frac{X_{np}r}{a}\right) \right)(\cos n\varphi)e^{-j\beta_g z}$$

$$H_\varphi = \frac{E_{0r}}{Z_g}\left(J_n'\left(\frac{X_{np}r}{a}\right) \right)(\cos n\varphi)e^{-j\beta_g z}$$

$$H_r = \frac{E_{0\varphi}}{Z_g}\left(J_n\left(\frac{X_{np}r}{a}\right) \right)(\sin n\varphi)e^{-j\beta_g z} \tag{2.128}$$

$$E_\varphi = E_{0\varphi}\left(J_n\left(\frac{X_{np}r}{a}\right) \right)(\sin \varphi)e^{-j\beta_g z}$$

$$E_r = E_{0r}\left(J_n'\left(\frac{X_{np}r}{a}\right) \right)(\cos \varphi)e^{-j\beta_g z}$$

The impedance of the np modes is written in Equation 2.129.

$$Z_{g,np} = \frac{E_r}{H_\varphi} = \frac{\beta_{g,np}}{\omega\varepsilon} = \eta\sqrt{1-\left(\frac{f_c}{f}\right)^2} \tag{2.129}$$

The mode with the lowest cutoff frequency in a circular waveguide is TE11. TE11 fields in a circular waveguide are shown in Figure 2.14.

REFERENCES

1. W. Ramo and T. Van Duzer, *Fields and Waves in Communication Electronics*. 3rd Edition, Hoboken, NJ: John Wiley & Sons, 1994.

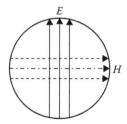

2.14 TE11 fields in a circular waveguide.

2. R. E. Collin, *Foundation for Microwave Engineering*, Tokyo, Japan: McGraw-Hill, 1966.
3. C. A. Balanis, *Antenna Theory: Analysis and Design*, 2nd Edition. Hoboken, NJ: John Wiley & Sons, 1996
4. A. Sabban, *Low Visibility Antennas for Communication Systems*, Boca Raton, FL: Taylor & Francis, 2015.
5. A. Sabban, *Wideband RF Technologies and Antenna in Microwave Frequencies*, Hoboken, NJ: John Wiley & Sons, July 2016.
6. L. C. Godara, Editor, *Handbook of Antennas in Wireless Communications*, Boca Raton, FL: CRC Press, 2002
7. J. D. Kraus and R. J. Marhefka, *Antennas for All Applications*, 3rd Edition, New Delhi, India: McGraw Hill, 2002.
8. F. T. Ulaby, *Electromagnetics for Engineers*, Upper Sadddle River, NJ: Pearson Education, 2005.
9. J. R. James, P. S. Hall and C. Wood, *Microstrip Antenna Theory and Design*, London, 1981.
10. A. Sabban, *RF Engineering, Microwave and Antennas*, Israel: Saar Publication, 2014.
11. ITU-R Recommendation V.431: Nomenclature of the frequency and wavelength bands used in telecommunications. International Telecommunication Union, Geneva, 2015.
12. IEEE Standard 521–2002: Standard Letter Designations for Radar-Frequency Bands. E-ISBN: 0–7381–335–6. USA, 2003.
13. AFR 55-44/AR 105-86/OPNAVINST 3430.9A/MCO 3430.1, 27 October 1964 superseded by AFR 55-44/AR 105–86/OPNAVINST 3430.1A/MCO 3430.1A, 6 December 1978: Performing Electronic Countermeasures in the United States and Canada, Attachment 1, ECM Frequency Authorizations.
14. L. A. Belov, S. M. Smolskiy and V. N. Kochemasov, *Handbook of RF, Microwave, and Millimeter-Wave Components*, pp. 27–28, Norwood, MA: Artech House. ISBN 978-1-60807-209-5.
15. L.C. Chirwa, P. A. Hammond, S. Roy and D. R. S. Cumming, Electromagnetic radiation from ingested sources in the human intestine between 150 MHz and 1.2 GHz, *IEEE Transaction on Biomedical Engineering*, vol. 50, no. 4, 484–492, April 2003.
16. D. Werber, A. Schwentner and E. M. Biebl, Investigation of RF transmission properties of human tissues, *Advances in Radio Science*, vol. 4, 357–360, 2006.

3 Introduction to Basic Theory for Wireless Wearable Communication System Designers

This chapter provides a short introduction to wireless wearable communication systems. Transmitting and receiving information in microwave frequencies is based on electromagnetic wave propagation. Wireless wearable communication systems operate in the vicinity of the human body.

3.1 WIRELESS WEARABLE COMMUNICATION SYSTEM FREQUENCY RANGE

The electromagnetic spectrum of wireless wearable communication systems corresponds to electromagnetic waves from the meter range to the centimeter wave range to date. However, there are some new designs in the mm wave rage. The characteristic feature of this phenomena is the short wavelength involved. The wavelength is of the same order of magnitude as the circuit device used. The propagation time from one point of the circuit to another point of the circuit is comparable to the period of the oscillating voltages and currents in the circuit. Conventional low circuit analysis based on Kirchhoff's and Ohm's laws can not analyze and describe the variation of fields, voltages, and currents along the length of the components. Components whose dimensions are lower than a tenth of a wavelength are called lumped elements. Components whose dimensions are higher than a tenth of a wavelength are called distributed elements. Kirchhoff's and Ohm's laws may be applied to lumped elements. However, Kirchhoff's and Ohm's laws cannot be applied to distributed elements.

To prevent interference and to provide efficient use of the frequency spectrum, similar services are allocated in frequency bands, see [1–4]. Bands are divided at wavelengths of 10^n meters or frequencies of 3×10^n hertz. Each band has a basic band plan which dictates how it is to be used and shared, to avoid interference and to set the protocol for the compatibility of transmitters and receivers. Table 3.1 lists the electromagnetic spectrum and applications of wireless wearable communication systems. Table 3.2 gives the International Tel-communication Union (ITU) Bands. Table 3.3 lists IEEE standard frequency bands for wireless wearable communication systems.

TABLE 3.1

Electromagnetic Spectrum and Applications of Wireless Wearable Communication Systems

Band Name	Abbreviation	ITU	Frequency\λ0	Applications
Low frequency	LF	5	30–300 kHz 10 km–1 km	Wearable RFID
Medium frequency	MF	6	300–3000 kHz 1 km–100 m	Wearable RFID
High frequency	HF	7	3–30 MHz 100 m–10 m	Shortwave broadcasts, wearable RFID communications, mobile radio telephony
Very high frequency	VHF	8	30–300 MHz 10 m–1 m	FM, television broadcasts, land mobile communications, weather radio,
Ultra high frequency	UHF	9	300–3000 MHz 1 m–100 mm	Mobile phones, wireless LAN, Bluetooth, Zig Bee, GPS and two-way radios such as land mobile, wireless wearable communication systems
Super high frequency	SHF	10	3–30 GHz 100 mm–10 mm	Wireless LAN, wireless wearable communication systems, DBS

TABLE 3.2

The International Tel-Communication Union Bands for Wireless Wearable Communication Systems

Band Number	Symbols	Frequency Range	Wavelength Range
4	VLF	3 to 30 kHz	10 to 100 km
5	LF	30 to 300 kHz	1 to 10 km
6	MF	300 to 3000 kHz	100 to 1000 m
7	HF	3 to 30 MHz	10 to 100 m
8	VHF	30 to 300 MHz	1 to 10 m
9	UHF	300 to 3000 MHz	10 to 100 cm
10	SHF	3 to 30 GHz	1 to 10 cm

TABLE 3.3

IEEE Standard Frequency Bands for Wireless Wearable Communication Systems

Symbols	Frequency Range
L band	1 to 2 GHz
S band	2 to 4 GHz
C band	4 to 8 GHz

3.2   FREE SPACE PROPAGATION

The fundamentals of wireless communication systems are presented in several papers and books [5–7].

Flux density at distance R of an isotropic source radiating P_t watts uniformly into free space is given by Equation 3.1. At distance R, the area of the spherical shell with center at the source is $4\pi R^2$.

$$F = \frac{P_t}{4\pi R^2} \text{ W/m}^2 \qquad (3.1)$$

$$G(\theta) = \frac{P(\theta)}{P_0/4\pi} \qquad (3.2)$$

$P(\theta)$ is variation of power with angle.

$G(\theta)$ is gain at the direction θ.

P_0 is total power transmitted.

Sphere = 4π solid radians.

Gain is a usually expressed in **decibels** (dB). G [dB] = $10 \log_{10} G$. Gain is realized by focusing power. An isotropic radiator is an antenna which radiates in all directions equally. Effective isotropic radiated power (EIRP) is the amount of power the transmitter would have to produce if it was radiating to all directions equally. The EIRP may vary as a function of direction because of changes in the antenna gain versus angle. We now want to find the power density at the receiver. We know that power is conserved in a lossless medium. The power radiated from a transmitter must pass through a spherical shell on the surface of which is the receiver.

The area of this spherical shell is $4\pi R^2$. Therefore spherical spreading loss is $1/4\pi R^2$.

We can rewrite the power flux density, as given in Equation 3.3, now considering the transmit antenna gain:

$$F = \frac{\text{EIRP}}{4\pi R^2} = \frac{P_t G_t}{4\pi R^2} \text{ W/m}^2 \qquad (3.3)$$

The power available to a receiving antenna of area A_r is given in Equation 3.4:

$$P_r = F \times A_r = \frac{P_t G_t A_r}{4\pi R^2} \qquad (3.4)$$

Real antennas have effective flux collecting areas which are less than the physical aperture area. A_e is defined as the antenna effective aperture area, where $A_e = A_{phy} \times \eta$ where η = aperture efficiency.

Antennas have maximum gain G related to the effective aperture area as f as given in Equation 3.5, where A_e is effective aperture area.

$$G = \text{Gain} = \frac{4\pi A_e}{\lambda^2} \qquad (3.5)$$

Aperture antennas (horns and reflectors) have a physical collecting area that can be easily calculated from their dimensions:

$$A_{\text{phy}} = \pi r^2 = \pi \frac{D^2}{4} \qquad (3.6)$$

Therefore, using Equation 3.5 and Equation 3.6 we can obtain the formula for aperture antenna gain as given in Equations 3.7 and 3.8.

$$\text{Gain} = \frac{4\pi A_e}{\lambda^2} = \frac{4\pi A_{\text{phy}}}{\lambda^2} \times \eta \qquad (3.7)$$

$$\text{Gain} = \left(\frac{\pi D}{\lambda}\right)^2 \times \eta \qquad (3.8)$$

$$\text{Gain} \cong \eta \left(\frac{75\pi}{\theta_{3\,dB}}\right)^2 = \eta \frac{(75\pi)^2}{\theta_{3\,dBH}\theta_{3\,dBE}} \qquad (3.9)$$

where $\theta_{3\,dB} \cong \dfrac{75\lambda}{D}$.

$\theta_{3\,dB}$ is the antenna half power beam width. Assuming for instance a typical aperture efficiency of 0.55 gives:

$$\text{Gain} \cong \frac{30,000}{(\theta_{3\,dB})^2} = \frac{30,000}{\theta_{3\,dBH}\theta_{3\,dBE}} \qquad (3.10)$$

3.3   FRIIS TRANSMISSION FORMULA

The Friis transmission formula is presented in Equation 3.11.

$$P_r = P_t G_t G_r \left(\frac{\lambda}{4\pi R}\right)^2 \qquad (3.11)$$

Free space loss (L_p) represents propagation loss in free space. Losses due to attenuation in atmosphere, L_a, should also be accounted for in the transmission equation. $L_p = \left(\dfrac{4\pi R}{\lambda}\right)$. The received power may be given as $P_r = \dfrac{P_t G_t G_r}{L_p}$

Losses due to polarization mismatch, L_{pol}, should also be accounted. Losses associated with the receiving antenna, L_{ra}, and with the receiver, L_r, cannot be neglected in computation of a transmission budget. Losses associated with the transmitting antenna are written as L_{ta}.

$$P_r = \frac{P_t G_t G_r}{L_p L_a L_{ta} L_{ra} L_{pol} L_o L_r} \tag{3.12}$$

$P_t = P_{out}/L_t$
EIRP $= P_t G_t$
where
P_t = transmitting antenna power
L_t = loss between power source and antenna
EIRP = effective isotropic radiated power

$$P_r = \frac{P_t G_t G_r}{L_p L_a L_{ta} L_{ra} L_{pol} L_{other} L_r}$$

$$= \frac{EIRP \times G_r}{L_p L_a L_{ta} L_{ra} L_{pol} L_{other} L_r} \tag{3.13}$$

$$= \frac{P_{out} G_t G_r}{L_t L_p L_a L_{ta} L_{ra} L_{pol} L_{other} L_r}$$

where

$$G = 10 \log\left(\frac{P_{out}}{P_{in}}\right) \text{ dB gain in dB}$$

$$L = 10 \log\left(\frac{P_{in}}{P_{out}}\right) \text{ dB loss in dB}$$

Gain may be derived as given in Equation 3.14.

$$P_{in} = \frac{V_{in}^2}{R_{in}} \qquad P_{out} = \frac{V_{out}^2}{R_{out}}$$

$$G = 10\log\left(\frac{P_{out}}{P_{in}}\right) = 10\log\left(\frac{\dfrac{V_{out}^2}{R_{out}}}{\dfrac{V_{in}^2}{R_{in}}}\right) \tag{3.14}$$

$$G = 10\log\left(\frac{V_{out}^2}{V_{in}^2}\right) + 10\log\left(\frac{R_{in}}{R_{out}}\right) = 20\log\left(\frac{V_{out}}{V_{in}}\right) + 10\log\left(\frac{R_{in}}{R_{out}}\right)$$

3.3.1 LOGARITHMIC RELATIONS

Important logarithmic operations are listed in Equations 3.15 through 3.18.

$$10\log_{10}(A \times B)$$
$$= 10\log_{10}(A) + 10\log_{10}(B)$$
$$= A\ \text{dB} + B\ \text{dB} \tag{3.15}$$
$$= (A + B)\ \text{dB}$$

$$10\log_{10}(A/B)$$
$$= 10\log_{10}(A) - 10\log_{10}(B)$$
$$= A\ \text{dB} - B\ \text{dB} \tag{3.16}$$
$$= (A - B)\ \text{dB}$$

$$10\log_{10}(A^2)$$
$$= 2 \times 10\log_{10}(A) \tag{3.17}$$
$$= 20\log_{10}(A)$$
$$= 2 \times (A\ \text{in dB})$$

$$10\log_{10}(\sqrt{A})$$
$$= \frac{10}{2}\log_{10}(A) \tag{3.18}$$
$$= \frac{1}{2} \times (A\ \text{in dB})$$

In Table 3.4 the linear ratio versus logarithmic ratio is listed.

TABLE 3.4
Linear Ratio versus Logarithmic Ratio

Linear Ratio	dB	Linear Ratio	dB
0.001	−30.0	2.000	3.0
0.010	−20.0	3.000	4.8
0.100	−10.0	4.000	6.0
0.200	−7.0	5.000	7.0
0.300	−5.2	6.000	7.8
0.400	−4.0	7.000	8.5
0.500	−3.0	8.000	9.0
0.600	−2.2	9.000	9.5
0.700	−1.5	10.000	10.0
0.800	−1.0	100.000	20.0
0.900	−0.5	1000.000	30.0
1.000	0.0	18.000	12.6

The received power P_r in dBm is given in Equation 3.19. The received power P_r is commonly referred to as "Carrier Power," C.

$$P_r = \text{EIRP} - L_{ta} - L_p - L_a - L_{pol} - L_{ra} - L_{other} + G_r - L_r \qquad (3.19)$$

The surface area of a sphere of radius d is $4\pi d^2$, so that the power flow per unit area W (power flux in W/m²) at distance d from a transmitter antenna with input power P_T and antenna gain G_T is given in Equation 3.20.

$$W = \frac{P_r G_r}{4\pi d^2} \qquad (3.20)$$

The received signal strength depends on the "size" or aperture of the receiving antenna. If the antenna has an effective area A, then the received signal strength is given in Equation 3.21.

$$P_R = P_T G_T (A/(4\pi d^2)) \qquad (3.21)$$

Define the receiver antenna gain G_R as $4\pi A/\lambda^2$, where $\lambda = c/f$.

3.4   LINK BUDGET EXAMPLES

$F = 2.4$ GHz $\Rightarrow \lambda = 3e8\text{m/s}/2.4e9\text{/s} = 12.5$ cm
At 933 MHz $\Rightarrow \lambda = 32$ cm
Receiver signal strength: $P_R = P_T G_T G_R (\lambda/4\pi d)^2$
P_R (dBm) $= P_T$ (dBm) $+ G_T$ (dBi) $+ G_R$ (dBi) $+ 10\log_{10}((\lambda/4\pi)^2) - 10\log_{10}(d^2)$

For $F = 2.4$ GHz => $10 \log_{10} ((\lambda/4\pi)^2) = -40$ dB
For $F = 933$ MHz => $10 \log_{10} ((\lambda/4\pi)^2) = -32$ dB

Mobile phone downlink

$\lambda = 12.5$ cm
$f = 2.4$ GHz
P_R (dBm) $= (P_T\, G_T\, G_R L)$ (dBm) $- 40$ dB $+ 10 \log_{10} (1/d^2)$
$P_R - (P_T + G_T + G_R + L) - 40$ dB $= 10 \log_{10} (1/d^2)$
Or $155 - 40 = 10 \log_{10} (1/d^2)$
Or $(155 - 40)/20 = \log_{10} (1/d)$
$d = 10\wedge ((155 - 40)/20) = 562$ km

Mobile phone uplink

$d = 10\wedge ((153 - 40)/20) = 446$ km
For standard 802.11
- $P_R - P_T = -113.2$ dBm
- 6 Mbps
  - $d = 10^{(113.2 - 40)/20} = 4500$ m
  - $d = 10^{(113.2 - 40 - 3)/20} = 3235$ m with 3 dB gain margin
  - $d = 10^{(113.2 - 40 - 3 - 9)/20} = 1148$ m with 3 dB gain margin and neglecting antenna gains
- 54 Mbps needs -85 dBm
  - $d = 10^{(99.2 - 40)/20} = 912$ m
  - $d = 10^{(99.2 - 40 - 3)/20} = 646$ m with 3 dB gain margin
  - $d = 10^{(99.2 - 40 - 3 - 9)/20} = 230$ m with 3 dB gain margin and neglecting antenna gains

Signal strength

- Measure signal strength in
  - dBW $= 10*\log$ (power in watts)
  - dBm $= 10*\log$ (power in mW)
- 802.11 can legally transmit at 30 dBm.
- Most 802.11 PCMCIA cards transmit at 10–20 dBm.
- Mobile phone base station: 20 W, but 60 users, so 0.3W/user, but antenna has gain $= 18$ dBi.
- Mobile phone handset: 21 dBm.

3.5 NOISE

Noise limits a system's ability to process weak signals. System dynamic range is defined as the system's capability to detect weak signals in the presence of large-amplitude signals.

Noise sources:

1. Random noise in resistors and transistors
2. Mixer noise

3. Undesired cross-coupling noise from other transmitters and equipment
4. Power supply noise
5. Thermal noise present in all electronics and transmission media due to thermal agitation of electrons

Thermal noise = kTB(W) where k is Boltzmann's constant = 1.38×10^{-23}, T is temperature in Kelvin (C + 273), and B is bandwidth.

Examples

For temperature = 293°C => –203dB, –173 dBm/Hz
For temperature = 293°C and 22 MHz => –130 dB, –100 dBm

Random noise

- External noise
- Atmospheric noise
- Interstellar noise

Receiver internal noise

- Thermal noise
- Flicker noise (low frequency)
- Shot noise

SNR is defined as signal-to-noise ratio. It varies with frequency.
SNR = signal power / noise power, and is given in Equation 3.22.

$$\text{SNR} = \frac{S(f)}{N(f)} = \frac{\text{Average signal power}}{\text{Average noise power}} \tag{3.22}$$

- SNR (dB) = 10*log10 (signal power / noise power)

Noise factor, F, is a measure of the degradation of SNR due to the noise added as we process the signal. F is given in Equations 3.23 and 3.24.

$$F = \frac{\text{Available output noise power}}{\text{Available output noise due to source}} \tag{3.23}$$

Noise figure = NF = $10\log(F)$.
The multistage noise figure is given by Equation 3.24:

$$F = F_1 + \frac{F_2 - 1}{G_1} + \frac{F_3 - 1}{G_1 G_2} + \cdots + \frac{F_n - 1}{G_1 G_2 \cdots G_{n-1}} \tag{3.24}$$

Signal strength is the transmitted power multiplied by a gain minus losses.

Loss sources

- Distance between the transmitter and the receiver.
- The signal passes through rain or fog at high frequencies.
- The signal passes through an object.
- Part of the signal is reflected from an object.
- Signal interferes, multi-path fading.
- An object not directly in the way impairs the transmission.

The received signal must have a strength that is larger than the receiver sensitivity. An SNR of 20 dB or larger would be good. Sensitivity is defined as minimum detectable input signal level for a given output SNR; this is also called the noise floor.

3.6   COMMUNICATION SYSTEMS LINK BUDGET

The link budget determines if the received signal is larger than the receiver sensitivity.

A link budget analysis determines if there is enough power at the receiver to recover the information. The link budget must account for effective transmission power. It takes into account the following parameters. The transmitting channel power budget is presented in Table 3.5.

Transmitter

- Transmission power
- Antenna gain
- Losses in cable and connectors

Path losses

- Attenuation
- Ground reflection
- Fading (self-interference)

Receiver

- Receiver sensitivity
- Losses in cable and connectors

A transmitter block diagram for a wireless wearable communication system is shown in Figure 3.1. A receiver block diagram is shown in Figure 3.2.

3.7   PATH LOSS

Path loss is a reduction in the signal's power, which is a direct result of the distance between the transmitter and the receiver in the communication path.

There are many models used in the industry today to estimate the path loss. The most common are the free space and Hata models. Each model has its own requirements that need to be met in order to be utilized correctly. The free space path loss is the reference point other models use.

Free space path loss

Free space path loss (dB) $= 20\log_{10} f + 20\log_{10} d - 147.56$ where F is frequency in Hz, and d is the distance in meters.

The free Space model typically underestimates the path loss experienced for mobile communications. It predicts a point-to-point fixed path loss.

Hata model

The Hata model is used extensively in cellular communications. The basic model is for urban areas, with extensions for suburbs and rural areas.

TABLE 3.5

Transmitting Channel Power Budget for Wireless Wearable Communication System

Component	Gain (dB)/Loss (dB)	Power (dBm)	Remarks
Input power	–	–10	–
Transmitter gain	40	–	–
Power amplifier output power	–	30	–
Filter loss	1	29	–
Line loss	1	28	–
Matching loss	1	27	–
Radiated power	–	27	–

TABLE 3.6

Receiving Channel Power Budget for Wireless Wearable Communication System

Component	Gain (dB)/Loss (dB)	Power (dBm)	Remarks
Input power	–	–20	–
Receiver gain	23	–	–
Line losses	1	–21	–
Filter loss	1	–22	–
Matching loss	1	–23	–
LNA amplifier output power	–	0	–

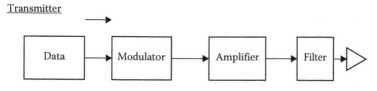

FIGURE 3.1   Transmitter block diagram for wireless wearable communication system.

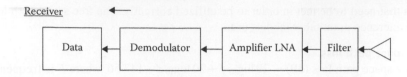

FIGURE 3.2   Receiver block diagram for wireless wearable communication system.

The Hata model is valid only for these ranges:

- Distance 1–20 km
- Base height 30–200 m
- Mobile height 1–10 m
- 150 MHz to 1500 MHz

Hata formula for urban areas

$$L_\mathrm{H} = 69.55 + 26.16\log_{10}f_\mathrm{c} - 13.82\log_{10}h_\mathrm{b} - \mathrm{env}(h_\mathrm{m}) + (44.9 - 6.55\log_{10}h_\mathrm{b})\log_{10}R$$

- h_b is the base station antenna height in meters.
- h_m is the mobile antenna height, also measured in meters.
- R is the distance from the cell site to the mobile in km.
- f_c is the transmit frequency in MHz.
- $\mathrm{env}(h_\mathrm{m})$ is an adjustment factor for the type of environment and the height of the mobile. $\mathrm{env}(h_\mathrm{m}) = 0$ for urban environments with a mobile height of 1.5 m.

3.8   RECEIVER SENSITIVITY

Sensitivity describes the weakest signal power level that the receiver is able to detect and decode. Sensitivity is determined by the lowest signal-to-noise ratio at which the signal can be recovered. Different modulation and coding schemes have different minimum SNRs. Sensitivity is determined by adding the required SNR to the noise present at the receiver.

Noise sources

- Thermal noise
- Noise introduced by the receiver's amplifier

Thermal noise $= N = kTB$ (watts)

- $k = 1.3803 \times 10^{-23}$ J/K
- $T =$ temperature in Kelvin
- $B =$ receiver bandwidth

N (dBm) $= 10\log_{10}(kTB) + 30$
Thermal noise is usually very small for reasonable bandwidths.

Basic receiver sensitivity calculation

Sensitivity (W) = kTB * NF(linear) * minimum SNR required (linear)
Sensitivity (dBm) = $10\log_{10}(kTB*1000)$ + NF (dB) + minimum SNR required (dB)
Sensitivity (dBm) = $10\log_{10}(kTB)$ + 30 + NF (dB) + minimum SNR required (dB)

Sensitivity decreases in communication systems when:

- Bandwidth increases
- Temperature increases
- Amplifier introduces more noise
- Losses in space, rain, and snow

3.9 RECEIVER DEFINITIONS AND FEATURES

Figure 3.3 presents a basic receiver block diagram.

3.9.1 RECEIVER DEFINITIONS

RF, IF, and LO frequencies
When a receiver uses a mixer we refer to the input frequency as the RF frequency. The system must provide a signal to mix down the RF; this is called the local oscillator. The resulting lower frequency is called the intermediate frequency (IF), because it is somewhere between the RF frequency and the base band frequency.
Base band frequency
The base band is the frequency where the information you want to process is.
Preselector filter
A preselector filter is used to keep undesired radiation from saturating a receiver. For example, we don't want our cell phone to pick up air-traffic control radar.
Amplitude and phase matching versus tracking
In a multi-channel receiver (more than one receiver), it is important for the channels to match and track each other over a frequency. Amplitude and phase *matching* means that the relative magnitude and phase of signals that pass through the two paths must be almost equal.
Tunable bandwidth versus instantaneous bandwidth
Instantaneous bandwidth is what we get with a receiver when we keep the LO at a fixed frequency, and sweep the input frequency to measure the response. The result-

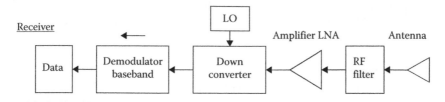

FIGURE 3.3 Basic receiver block diagram for wearable communication system.

ing bandwidth is a function of the frequency responses of everything in the chain. Their instantaneous bandwidth has a direct effect on the minimum detectable signal. Tunable bandwidth implies that we change the frequency of the LO to track the RF frequency. The bandwidth in this case is only a function of the preselector filter, the LNA, and the mixer. Tunable bandwidth is often many times greater than instantaneous bandwidth.

Gain

The gain of a receiver is the ratio of input signal power to output signal power.

Noise figure

The figure of a receiver is a measure of how much the receiver degrades the ratio of signal to noise of the incoming signal. It is related to the minimum detectable signal. If the LO signal has a high AM and/or FM noise, it could degrade the receiver noise figure because, far from the carrier, the AM and FM noise originates from thermal noise. Remember that the effect of LO AM noise is reduced by the balance of the balanced mixer.

1 dB compression point

The 1 dB compression point is the power level where the gain of the receiver is reduced by 1 dB due to compression.

Linearity

A receiver operates linearly if a 1 dB increase in input signal power results in a 1 dB increase in IF output signal strength.

Dynamic range

The dynamic range of a receiver is a measurement of the range from minimum detectable signal to the maximum signal that will start to compress the receiver.

Signal to noise ratio (*S/N*) (SNR)

SNR is a measure of how far a signal is above the noise floor.

Noise factor, noise figure, and noise temperature

- Noise factor is a measure of how the signal to noise ratio is degraded by a device:
  - F = noise factor = $(S_{in}/N_{in})/(S_{out}/N_{out})$.
  - S_{in} is the signal level at the input>
  - N_{in} is the noise level at the input.
  - S_{out} is the signal level at the output.
  - N_{out} is the noise level at the output.

- The noise factor of a device is specified with noise from a noise source at room temperature (N_{in} = KT), where K is Boltzmann's constant and T is approximately room temperature in Kelvin. KT is somewhere around −174 dBm/Hz. The noise figure is the noise factor, expressed in decibels:

  - NF (dB) = noise figure = $10*\log (F)$.
  - T = noise temperature = $290*(F-1)$.
  - 1 dB NF is about 75° K, and 3 dB is 288 K.
  - The noise factor contributions of each stage in a four-stage system are given in Equation 3.25.

$$F = F1 + \frac{F2-1}{G1} + \frac{F3-1}{G1G2} + \frac{F4-1}{G1G2G3} \qquad (3.25)$$

3.10 TYPES OF RADARS

- In **monostatic radars** the transmitting and receiving antennas are co-located. Most radars are monostatic.
- In **bistatic radars,** the transmitting and receiving antennas are not co-located.
- **Doppler radar** is used to measure the velocity of a target, due to its Doppler shift. Police radar is a classic example of Doppler radar.
- **Frequency modulated/continuous wave** (FMCW) radar implies that the radar signal is "chirped," or its frequency is varied in time. By varying the frequency in this manner, you can gather both range and velocity information.
- **Synthetic aperture radar (SAR)** uses a moving platform to "scan" the radar in one or two dimensions. Satellite radar images are mostly done using SAR.

3.11 TRANSMITTER DEFINITIONS AND FEATURES

Figure 3.4 presents a basic transmitter block diagram.

3.11.1 AMPLIFIERS

- **Class A:** The amplifier is biased at close to half of its saturated current. The output conducts during the entire 360° phase of the input signal sine wave. Class A does not give maximum efficiency, but provides the best linearity. Drain efficiencies of 50% are possible in Class A.
- **Class B:** The power amplifier is biased at a point where it draws nearly zero DC current; for a FET, this means that it is biased at pinch-off. During one half of the input signal sine wave it conducts, but not the other half. A Class B amplifier can be very efficient, with theoretical efficiency of 80%–85%. However, we are giving up 6 dB of gain when we move from Class A to Class B.

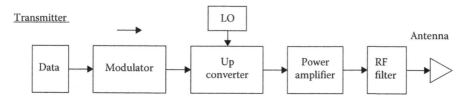

FIGURE 3.4 Basic transmitter block diagram for a wearable communication system.

- **Class C:** Class C occurs when the device is biased so that the output conducts for even less than 180° of the input signal. The output power and gain decrease.
- **Power density:** This is a measure of power divided by transistor size. In the case of FETs it is expressed in W/mm. GaN transistors have more than 10 W/mm power density.
- **Saturated output power: PSAT** is the output power where the Pin/Pout curve slope goes to zero.
- **Load pull:** The process of varying the impedance seen by the *output* of an active device to other than 50 Ω in order to measure performance parameters, in the simplest case, gain. In the case of a power device, a load pull power bench is used to evaluate large signal parameters such as compression characteristics, saturated power, efficiency, and linearity as the output load is varied across the Smith chart.
- **Harmonic load pull:** The process of varying the impedance at the output of a device, with separate control of the impedances at F0, 2F0, 3F0, etc.
- **Source pull:** The process of varying the impedance seen by the input of an active device to other than 50 Ω in order to measure performance parameters. In the case of a low noise device, source pull is used in a noise parameter extraction setup to evaluate how signal-to-noise ratio (noise figure) varies with source impedance.

3.11.2 Amplifier Temperature Considerations

In the case of an FET amplifier, the gain drops and the noise figure increases. The gain drop is around −0.006 dB/stage/°C.

The noise figure of an LNA increases by +0.006 dB/°C. In an LNA, the first stage will dominate the temperature effect.

3.11.3 Power Amplifiers

Power amplifiers are used to boost a small signal to a large signal. Solid-state amplifiers and tube amplifiers are usually employed as power amplifiers.

The output power capabilities of power amplifiers are listed in Table 3.7.

TABLE 3.7
Power Amplifiers Output Power Capabilities

Frequency Band	Solid State	Tube Type
L-band through C-band	200 watts (LDMOS) GaN	
X-band	50 watts (GaN HEMT device)	3000 watts (TWT)
Ka-band	6 watts (GaAs PHEMT device)	1000 watts (klystron)
Q-band	4 watts (GaAs PHEMT device)	

3.12 SATELLITE COMMUNICATION TRANSCEIVER

This section presents an example of a satellite communication transceiver, describing the design, performance, and fabrication of a compact and low-cost MIC RF-Head for satellite communication applications. Surface mount MIC technology is employed to fabricate the RF-Head.

3.12.1 INTRODUCTION

The mobile telecommunication industry is currently in continuous growth [8–15]. Moreover, the great public demand for cellular and cordless telephones has stimulated a wide interest in new mobile services such as portable satellite communication terminals. For example, the Inmarsat-M system provides digital communications between the public switched terrestrial networks and mobile users.

Communication links to and from mobile installations are established via the Inmarsat geostationary satellite and the associated ground station.

The RF-Head includes receiving and transmitting channels, an RF controller, synthesizers, a modem, and a DC supply unit. The size of the RF-Head is $30 \times 20 \times 2.5$ cm and it weighs 1 kg. The transmitting channel may be operated in high power mode to transmit 10 W or in low power mode to transmit 4 W. The transmitted power level is controlled by an automatic leveling control unit to ensure low power consumption over the entire frequency and temperature range. The RF-Head vent is set to on and off automatically by the RF controller. The gain of the receiving channel is 76 dB and is temperature compensated using a temperature sensor and a voltage-controlled attenuator. Surface mount technology (SMT) is employed to fabricate the RF-Head.

3.12.2 DESCRIPTION OF THE RECEIVING CHANNEL

Figure 3.5 shows a block diagram of the receiving channel. The receiving channel consists of low noise amplifier, filters, an active mixer, a saw filter, a temperature sensor, a voltage-controlled attenuator, and IF amplifiers.

The low noise amplifier has 10 dB gain and a 0.9 dB noise figure for frequencies ranging from 1.525 to 1.559 GHz. The total gain of the receiving channel is 76 dB.

The low noise amplifier employs a $1.8 (GaAS) Fet.

Table 3.8 gives the noise figure and power budget calculation. The channel gain is temperature compensated by connecting the output port of a temperature sensor to the reference voltage port of a voltage-controlled attenuator. The variation of the sensor output voltage as a function of temperature varies the attenuation level of the attenuator. Gain stability as a function of temperature is less than 1 dB. The receiving channel noise figure is less than 2.2 dB, including 1 dB diplexer losses. The receiving channel rejects out of band signals with power level lower than –20 dBm.

Receiving channel specifications
- Frequency range: 1525–1559 MHz
- Local oscillator frequency: 1355–1389 MHz

- IF frequency: 170 MHz
- Channel 1 dB bandwidth: 50 kHz
- Noise figure: 3 dB
- Input signals: −105 to −135 dBm
- Output signals: −30 to −60 dBm
- Receiving sensitivity: C/N = 41 dB/Hz for −130 dBm input signal

3.12.3 RECEIVING CHANNEL DESIGN AND FABRICATION

A major parameter in the receiving channel design was to achieve a very low target price in manufacturing hundreds of units. The components were selected to meet the electrical requirements for a given low target price assigned to each component. The low production cost of the RF-Head is achieved by using SMT to manufacture the RF-Head. Trimming is not required in the fabrication procedure of the receiving channel. The gain and noise-figure values of the receiving channel are measured in each RF-Head. Around 300 receiving channels have been manufactured to date.

3.12.4 DESCRIPTION OF THE TRANSMITTING CHANNEL

A block diagram of the transmitting channel is shown in Figure 3.6. The transmitting channel consists of low power amplifiers, pass band filters, voltage-controlled attenuator, an active mixer, medium power and high power amplifiers, a high power isolator, a coupler, a power detector, and a DC supply unit.

The power budget of the transmitting channel is given in Table 3.9.

Five stages of power amplifiers amplify the input signal from 0 dBm to 40 dBm. The fifth stage is a 10 W power amplifier with high efficiency. The amplifier may transmit 10 W in high power mode or 4 W in low power mode. The DC bias voltage

---

TABLE 3.8

Noise Figure and Gain Calculations

Component	Noise Figure (dB)	Gain (dB)	Pout (dBm)
Diplexer	1	−1	−131
LNA	0.95	20	−111
VCA	3.5	−3.5	−114.5
Filter	2	−2	−116.5
Matched LNA unit	1.45	14	−102.5
Filter	2	−2	−104.5
LNA	0.9	10	−94.5
VCA	3.5	−3.5	−98
Filter	2	−2	−100
Mixer	20	15	−85
Saw filter	8	−8	−93
IF amplifiers	2.5	42.5	−50.5
Transmission line losses	2.5	−2.5	−53
Total	2.35	77	−53

System1

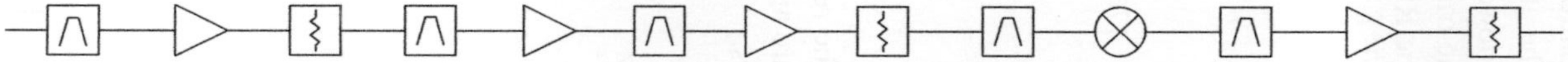

	Diplexer	LNA	VCA	Matched LNA	Filter	LNA	VCA	Filter	Mixer magnum	Saw filter	IF AMP	Losses	Total
Gain (dB)	-1.00	20.00	-3.50	14.00	-2.00	10.00	-3.50	-2.00	15.00	-8.00	42.00	-2.50	76.33*
NF (dB)	1.00	0.95	3.50	1.45	2.00	0.90	3.50	2.00	20.00	8.00	2.50	2.50	2.35
IP1dB (dBm)	20.00	-2.00	20.00	4.00	20.00	7.00	20.00	20.00	8.00	20.00	10.00	20.00	-59.50
NF+ (dB)	0.71	0.86	0.04	0.04	0.00	0.00	0.00	0.00	0.26	0.00	0.00	0.00	

Input Pwr (dBm) -60.00
System Temp (K) 290.00

Modulation: FM
System BW (MHz) 0.03
S/N (dB, Actual) 66.18
Srce Temp (K) 290.00
Te Eff. (K) 208.30
SFDR3 (dB) N/A

MDS (dBm) -126.86
S/N (dB, Req'd) 6.00
Sens. Loss (dB) 0.00
Sensitivity (dBm) -120.86
G/T (dB/K) -16.97

Input IP3 (dBm) N/A
Output IP3 (dBm) N/A
OIM3 (dBm) N/A
ORR3 (dB) N/A
IRR3 (dB) N/A

FIGURE 3.5 Block diagram and gain budget of the receiving channel.

of the power amplifier is automatically controlled by the RF-Controller to set the power amplifier to the required mode and power level. A −30 dB coupler and a power detector are used to measure the output power level. The measured power level is transferred via an A/D converter to the RF-Controller to monitor the output power level of the transmitting channel by varying the attenuation of the voltage-controlled attenuator. This feature ensures low DC power consumption and high efficiency of the RF-Head. The RF-Controller sets the transmitting channel to ON and OFF. A temperature sensor is used to measure the RF-Head temperature. The RF-Controller sets the RF-Head vent to ON and OFF according to the measured RF-Head temperature.

3.12.4.1   Transmitting Channel Specifications

- Frequency range: 1626.5–1660.5 MHz
- IF frequency range: 99.5–133.5 MHz
- LO f   requency: 1760 MHz
- Input power: 0 dBm
- Output power (High Mode): 38–40 dBm
- Output power (Low Mode): 34–36 dBm
- Power consumption: 42 W

3.12.4.2   Diplexer Specifications

A very compact and lightweight diplexer connects the receiving and transmitting channels to the antenna. The diplexer's simple structure and easy manufacturability ensure lower costs in production than similar diplexers.

Transmit filter
- Pass band frequency range: 1626.5–1660.5 MHz
- Pass band insertion loss: 0.7 dB
- Pass band VSWR < 1.3:1
- Rejection > 54 dB at 1525–1559 Mhz

Receive filter
- Pass band frequency range: 1525–1559 MHz
- Pass band insertion loss < 1.3 dB
- Pass band VSWR <1.3:1
- Rejection > 65 dB at 1626.5–1660.5 MHz
- Size: 86 × 36 × 25 mm

3.12.5   Transmitting Channel Fabrication

Figure 3.7 shows a photo of the RF-Head prototype for the Inmarsat-M ground terminal. A major parameter in the transmitting channel design was to achieve a low target price in the fabrication of hundreds of units. The components were selected to meet the target price given to each component and the electrical requirements. Low production cost is achieved by using SMT technology to manufacture the transmitting channel. A quick trimming procedure is required in the fabrication of the trans-

TABLE 3.9
Transmitting Channel Power Budget

Component	Gain/Loss (dB)	Pout (dBm)
Input	0	0
VCA	−4	−4
Tr. line loss	−0.5	−4.5
Mixer	2	−2.5
Filter	−2	−4.5
Low power amplifiers	20.5	16
Filter	−2	14
Medium power amplifier	16	30
Power amplifier	11.5	41.5
Isolator	−0.5	41
Diplexer	−1	40
Total	40.0	40

System1

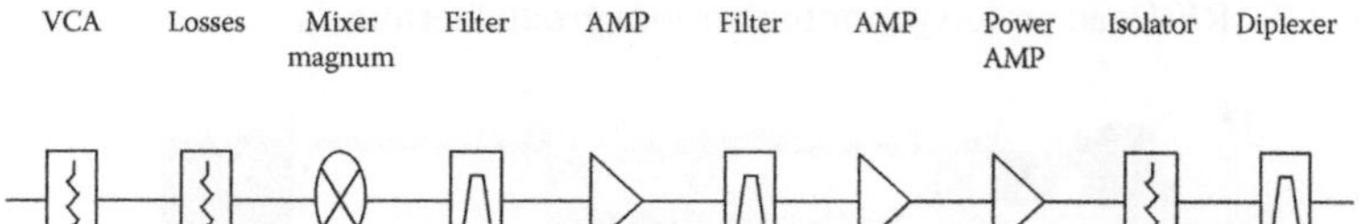

	VCA	Losses	Mixer magnum	Filter	AMP	Filter	AMP	Power AMP	Isolator	Diplexer	Total
Gain (dB)	−4.00	−0.50	2.00	−2.00	20.50	−2.00	16.00	11.50	−0.50	−1.00	40.00
NF (dB)	4.00	0.50	2.00	2.00	3.00	2.00	3.00	5.00	0.50	1.00	9.23
IP1dB (dBm)	20.00	20.00	10.00	20.00	10.00	20.00	10.00	20.00	20.00	20.00	−21.67
NF+ (dB)	0.87	0.16	0.95	0.58	1.77	0.01	0.02	0.00	0.00	0.00	

Input Pwr (dBm) −60.00 System Temp (K) 290.00

Modulation: FM

System BW (MHz)	0.03	MDS (dBm)	−119.98	Input IP3 (dBm) N/A
S/N (dB, Actual)	59.98	S/N (dB, Req'd)	6.00	Output IP3 (dBm) N/A
Srce Temp (K)	290.00	Sens. Loss (dB)	0.00	OIM3 (dBm) N/A
Te E . (K)	2136.86	Sensitivity (dBm)	−113.98	ORR3 (dB) N/A
SFDR3 (dB)	N/A	G/T (dB/K)	−23.85	IRR3 (dB) N/A

FIGURE 3.6 Block diagram and gain budget of the transmitting channel.

mitting channel to achieve the required output power and efficiency. The output power and spurious level of the transmitting channel are tested in the fabrication procedure of each RF-Head. Around 300 transmitting channels have been manufactured during the first production cycle.

Figure 3.8 shows the RF-Head modules for the Inmarsat-M ground terminal. The RF-Head is separated into five sections: receiving and transmitting channels, diplexer, synthesizers, RF controller, and a DC supply unit. A metallic fence and cover separate the transmitting and receiving channels.

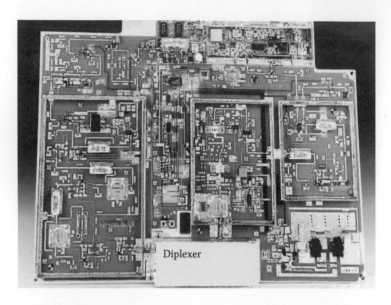

FIGURE 3.7   RF-Head prototype for Inmarsat-m ground terminal.

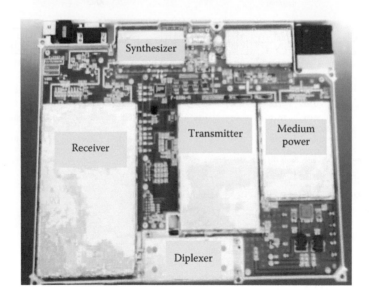

FIGURE 3.8   RF-Head modules for Inmarsat-M ground terminal.

3.12.6   RF Controller

The RF controller is based on an 87c51 microcontroller. The RF controller communicates with the system controller via a full duplex serial bus. The communication is based on message transfer. The RF controller sets the transmitting channel to on and off by controlling the DC voltage switching unit. The RF controller monitors the output power level of the transmitting channel by varying the attenuation of the voltage-controlled attenuator in the transmitting channel. It sets the transmitting channel to burst or SCPC modes with high or low power level. The RF controller produces the clock data and enables signals for the Rx and Tx synthesizers.

3.12.7 CONCLUDING REMARKS

This section presents a compact and low-cost RF-Head for Inmarsat-M applications. The RF-Head is part of a portable satellite communication ground terminal, "Caryphone," which supplies phone and fax services to the customer.

The RF controller automatically monitors the output power level to ensure low DC power consumption. A DC-to-DC converter supplies to the power amplifier a controlled DC bias voltage to set the power amplifier to high power level mode, 10 W, or 4 W.

The receiving channel noise figure is less than 2.2 dB. The total gain of the receiving channel is 76 dB with gain stability of 1 dB as a function of temperature.

The RF-Head size is 30 × 20 × 2.5 cm and weighs less than 1 kg.

REFERENCES

1. ITU-R Recommendation V.431: Nomenclature of the frequency and wavelength bands used in telecommunications. Geneva: International Telecommunication Union, Geneva, 2015.
2. IEEE Standard 521–2002: Standard Letter Designations for Radar-Frequency Bands. E-ISBN: 0-7381-3356-6. USA, 2003.
3. AFR 55-44/AR 105-86/OPNAVINST 3430.9A/MCO 3430.1, 27 October 1964 superseded by AFR 55-44/AR 105-86/OPNAVINST 3430.1A/MCO 3430.1A, 6 December 1978: Performing Electronic Countermeasures in the United States and Canada, Attachment 1, ECM Frequency Authorizations.
4. L. A. Belov, S. M. Smolskiy and V. N. Kochemasov, Handbook of RF, Microwave, and Millimeter-Wave Components. Boston, MA: Artech House, pp. 27–28, 2012, ISBN 978-1-60807-209-5.
5. W. C. Y. Lee, *Mobile Communication Engineering*, New York, NY: McGraw Hill, 1982.
6. K. Fujimoto and J. R. James, Ed., *Mobile Antenna Systems Handbook*, Boston, MA: Artech House, 1994.
7. M. L. Skolnik, *Introduction to Radar Systems*, New York, NY: McGraw Hill, 1980.
8. A. Sabban, *Wideband RF Technologies and Antenna in Microwave Frequencies*, Hoboken, NJ: Wiley Sons, July 2016.
9. A. Sabban, Ultra-wideband RF modules for communication systems, PARIPEX, *Indian Journal of Research*, vol. 5, no. 1, 91–95, January 2016.
10. A. Sabban, Wideband RF modules and antennas at microwave and MM wave frequencies for communication applications, *Journal of Modern Communication Technologies & Research*, vol. 3, 89–97, March 2015.
11. A. Sabban, J. Cabiri and E. Carmeli, 18 to 40 GHz integrated compact switched filter bank module, ISSSE 2007 Conference, Montreal, Canada, pp. 347–350, August 2007.

12. A. Sabban., Applications of MM wave microstrip antenna arrays, ISSSE 2007 Conference, Montreal, Canada, pp. 119–122, August 2007.
13. A. Sabban, A. Britebard and Y. Shemesh, Development and fabrication of a compact integrated RF-head for Inmarsat-M ground terminal, European Microwave Conference 1997, Jerusalem, Israel, pp. 1186–1191. September 1997.
14. A. Madjar, D. Behar, A. Sabban and I. Shapir, RF front end prototype for a millimeter wave (Ka/K) band VSAT satellite communication earth terminal, European Microwave Conference 1996, Prague, pp. 953–955. September 1996.
15. A. Sabban and Y. Shemesh, A compact low power consumption integrated RF-head for Inmarsat-M ground terminal, European Microwave Conference, Bologna, Italy, pp. 81–82, September 1995.

4 Basic Antennas for Wearable Communication Systems

4.1 INTRODUCTION TO ANTENNAS

Antennas are a major component in communication systems [1–16]. Mobile antenna systems are presented in [12]. An antenna is used to efficiently radiate electromagnetic energy in desired directions. Antennas match radio frequency systems, sources of electromagnetic energy, to space. All antennas can be used to receive or radiate energy. They transmit or receive electromagnetic waves, and can convert electromagnetic radiation into electric current, or vice versa. Antennas transmit and receive electromagnetic radiation at radio frequencies, and are a necessary part of all communication links and radio equipment. They are used in systems such as radio and television broadcasting, point-to-point radio communication, wireless LAN, cell phones, radar, medical systems, and spacecraft communication. Antennas are most commonly employed in air or outer space, but can also be operated underwater, on and inside the human body, or even through soil and rock at low frequencies for short distances. Physically, an antenna is an arrangement of one or more conductors. In transmitting mode, an alternating current is created in the elements by applying a voltage at the antenna terminals, causing the elements to radiate an electromagnetic field. In receiving mode, an electromagnetic field from another source induces an alternating current in the elements and a corresponding voltage at the antenna's terminals. Some receiving antennas (such as parabolic and horn) incorporate shaped reflective surfaces to receive the radio waves striking them and direct or focus them onto the actual conductive elements.

4.2 ANTENNA DEFINITIONS

Radiation pattern: A radiation pattern is the antenna-radiated field as a function of the direction in space. It is a way of plotting the radiated power from an antenna. This power is measured at various angles at a constant distance from the antenna.

Radiator: This is the basic element of an antenna. An antenna can be made up of multiple radiators.

Bore sight: The direction in space to which the antenna radiates maximum electromagnetic energy.

Range: Antenna range is the radial range from an antenna to an object in space.

Azimuth (AZ): The angle from left to right from a reference point, from 0° to 360°.

Elevation (EL): The EL angle is the angle from the horizontal (x, y) plane, from $-90°$ (down) to $+90°$ (up).

Main beam: The region around the direction of maximum radiation, usually the region that is within 3 dB of the peak of the main lobe.

Beam Width: The beam width is the angular range of the antenna pattern in which at least half of the maximum power is emitted. This angular range, of the major lobe, is defined as the points at which the field strength falls around 3 dB in relation to the maximum field strength.

Side lobes: Side lobes are smaller beams that are away from the main beam. They present radiation in undesired directions. The side-lobe level is a parameter used to characterize the antenna radiation pattern. It is the maximum value of the side lobes away from the main beam and is usually expressed usually in decibels.

Radiated power: Total radiated power when the antenna is excited by a current or voltage of known intensity.

Isotropic radiator: Theoretical lossless radiator that radiates, or receives, equal electromagnetic energy in free space to all directions.

Wearable antenna: Antenna worn on human body.

Directivity: The ratio between the amounts of energy propagating in a certain direction compared to the average energy radiated to all directions over a sphere.

$$D = \frac{P(\theta,\phi)\text{maximal}}{P(\theta,\phi)\text{average}} = 4\pi \frac{P(\theta,\phi)\text{maximal}}{P\,\text{rad}} \tag{4.1}$$

$$P(\theta,\phi)\text{average} = \frac{1}{4}\iint P(\theta,\phi)\sin\theta\,d\theta\,d\phi = \frac{P\,\text{rad}}{4\pi} \tag{4.2}$$

$$D \sim \frac{4\pi}{\theta E \times \theta H} \tag{4.3}$$

θE—Beam width in radian in EL plane

θH—Beam width in radian in AZ plane

Antenna effective area (A_{eff}): The antenna area which contributes to the antenna directivity.

$$D = \frac{4\pi A_{\text{eff}}}{\lambda^2} \tag{4.4}$$

Antenna gain (G): The ratio between the amounts of energy propagating in a certain direction compared to the energy that would be propagated in the same direction if the antenna were a non-directional, isotropic radiator is known as its gain.

Radiation efficiency (α): Radiation efficiency is the ratio of power radiated to the total input power. The efficiency of an antenna takes into account losses, and is equal to the total radiated power divided by the radiated power of an ideal lossless antenna.

$$G = \alpha D \tag{4.5}$$

4.2.1 TYPES OF ANTENNA

4.2.1.1 Wire-Type Antennas

Dipoles
Monopoles
Bi-conical antennas
Loop antennas
Helical antennas

4.2.1.2 Aperture-Type Antennas

Horn and open waveguide
Reflector antennas
Arrays
Microstrip and printed antennas
Slot antennas

A comparison of directivity and gain values for several antennas is given in Table 4.1.

$$\text{For small antennas} \left(l < \frac{\lambda}{2} \right) \quad G \cong \frac{41,000}{\theta E^\circ \times \theta H^\circ} \tag{4.6}$$

$$\text{For medium size antennas} \left(\lambda < l < 8\lambda \right) \quad G \cong \frac{31,000}{\theta E^\circ \times \theta H^\circ} \tag{4.7}$$

TABLE 4.1
Antenna Directivity versus Antenna Gain

Antenna Type	Directivity (dBi)	Gain (dBi)
Isotropic radiator	0	0
Dipole $\lambda/2$	2	2
Dipole above ground plane	6–4	6–4
Microstrip antenna	7–8	6–7
Yagi antenna	6–18	5–16
Helix antenna	7–20	6–18
Horn antenna	10–30	9–29
Reflector antenna	15–60	14–58

$$\text{For big antennas}\left(8\lambda < l\right) \quad G \cong \frac{27{,}000}{\theta E^\circ \times \theta H^\circ} \tag{4.8}$$

Antenna impedance: Antenna impedance is the ratio of the voltage at any given point along the antenna to the current at that point. It depends upon the height of the antenna above the ground and the influence of surrounding objects. The impedance of a quarter-wave monopole near perfect ground is approximately 36 Ω. The impedance of a half-wave dipole is approximately 75 Ω.

Antenna array: An array of antenna elements is a set of antennas used for transmitting or receiving electromagnetic waves.

Active antenna: An antenna consists of a radiating element and active elements such as amplifiers.

Phased arrays: Phased array antennas are electrically steerable. The physical antenna can be stationary. Phased arrays, smart antennas, incorporate active components for beam steering.

4.2.1.3   Steerable Antennas

- Arrays with switchable elements and partially mechanically and electronically steerable arrays.
- Hybrid antenna systems: fully electronically steerable arrays. Such systems can be equipped with phase and amplitude shifters for each element or the design can be based on digital beam forming (DBF).
- This technique, in which the steering is performed directly on a digital level, allows the most flexible and powerful control of the antenna beam.

4.3   DIPOLE ANTENNA

A dipole antenna is a small wire antenna consisting of two straight conductors excited by a voltage fed via a transmission line as shown in Figure 4.1. Each side of the transmission line is connected to one of the conductors. The most common dipole is the half-wave dipole, in which each of the two conductors is approximately a quarter wavelength long, so the length of the antenna is half of a wavelength.

We can calculate the fields radiated from the dipole by using a potential function. The electric potential function is φ_l. The electric potential function is A. The potential function is given in Equation 4.9.

$$\varphi_l = \frac{1}{4\pi\varepsilon_0} \int_c \frac{\rho_l e^{j(\omega t - \beta R)}}{R} \, \mathrm{d}l$$

$$A_l = \frac{\mu_0}{4\pi} \int_c \frac{i e^{j(\omega t - \beta R)}}{R} \, \mathrm{d}l \tag{4.9}$$

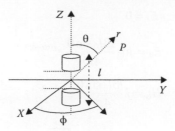

FIGURE 4.1 Dipole antenna.

4.3.1 RADIATION FROM SMALL DIPOLE

The length of a small dipole is small compared to wavelength and is called an elementary dipole. We can assume that the current along the elementary dipole is uniform. We can solve the wave equation in spherical coordinates by using the potential function given in Equation 4.9. The electromagnetic fields in a point $P(r, \theta, \varphi)$ are given in Equation 4.10. The electromagnetic fields in Equation 4.2 vary as $\dfrac{1}{r}, \dfrac{1}{r^2}, \dfrac{1}{r^3}$. For $r \ll 1$, the dominant component of the field varies as $\dfrac{1}{(r)^3}$ and is given in Equation 4.11. These fields are the dipole near fields. In this case the waves are standing waves and the energy oscillates in the antenna near zone and is not radiated to open space. The real part of the poynting vector is equal to zero. For $r \gg 1$, the dominant component of the field varies as $1/r$ as given in Equation 4.12. These fields are the dipole far fields.

$$E_r = \eta_0 \frac{ll_0 \cos\theta}{2\pi r^2}\left(1 - \frac{j}{\beta r}\right)e^{j(\omega t - \beta r)}$$

$$E_\theta = j\eta_0 \frac{\beta ll_0 \sin\theta}{4\pi r}\left(1 - \frac{j}{\beta r} - \frac{1}{(\beta r)^2}\right)e^{j(\omega t - \beta r)}$$

$$H_\varphi = j\frac{\beta ll_0 \sin\theta}{4\pi r}\left(1 - \frac{j}{\beta r}\right)e^{j(\omega t - \beta r)} \tag{4.10}$$

$$H_r = 0 \qquad H_\theta = 0 \qquad E_\phi = 0$$

$$I = I_0 \cos\omega t$$

$$E_r = -j\eta_0 \frac{ll_0 \cos\theta}{2\pi\beta r^3}e^{j(\omega t - \beta r)}$$

$$E_\theta = -j\eta_0 \frac{ll_0 \sin\theta}{4\pi\beta r^3}e^{j(\omega t - \beta r)} \tag{4.11}$$

$$H_\varphi = \frac{ll_0 \sin\theta}{4\pi r^2}e^{j(\omega t - \beta r)}$$

$$E_r = 0$$

$$E_\theta = j\eta_0 \frac{l\beta I_0 \sin\theta}{4\pi r} e^{j(\omega t - \beta r)} \tag{4.12}$$

$$H_\varphi = j \frac{l\beta I_0 \sin\theta}{4\pi r} e^{j(\omega t - \beta r)}$$

$$\frac{E_\theta}{H_\varphi} = \eta_0 = \sqrt{\frac{\mu_0}{\varepsilon_0}} \tag{4.13}$$

In the far fields the electromagnetic fields vary as $1/r$ and $\sin\theta$. Equation 4.13 gives wave impedance in free space.

4.3.1.1 Dipole Radiation Pattern

The antenna radiation pattern represents the radiated fields in space at a point $P(r, \theta, \varphi)$ as a function of θ, φ. The antenna radiation pattern is three dimensional. When φ is constant and θ varies we get the E plane radiation pattern. When φ varies and θ is constant, usually $\theta = \pi/2$, we get the H plane radiation pattern.

4.3.1.2 Dipole E Plane Radiation Pattern

The dipole E plane radiation pattern is given in Equation 4.14 and presented in Figure 4.2.

$$|E_\theta| = \eta_0 \frac{l\beta I_0 |\sin\theta|}{4\pi r} \tag{4.14}$$

At a given point $P(r, \theta, \varphi)$ the dipole E plane radiation pattern is given in Equation 4.15.

$$|E_\theta| = \eta_0 \frac{l\beta I_0 |\sin\theta|}{4\pi r} = A|\sin\theta|$$

$$\text{Choose} \quad A = 1 \tag{4.15}$$

$$|E_\theta| = |\sin\theta|$$

The dipole E plane radiation pattern in a spherical coordinate system is shown in Figure 4.3.

4.3.1.3 Dipole *H* Plane Radiation Pattern

For $\theta = \pi/2$ the dipole *H* plane radiation pattern is given in Equation 4.10 and presented in Figure 4.4.

$$|E_\theta| = \eta_0 \frac{l\beta I_0}{4\pi r} \tag{4.16}$$

At a given point $P(r, \theta, \varphi)$ the dipole *H* plane radiation pattern is given in Equation 4.17.

$$|E_\theta| = \eta_0 \frac{l\beta I_0 |\sin\theta|}{4\pi r} = A$$

$$\text{Choose} \quad A = 1 \tag{4.17}$$

$$|E_\theta| = 1$$

The dipole *H* plane radiation pattern in the *xy* plane is a circle with $r = 1$.

The radiation pattern of a vertical dipole is omnidirectional. It radiates equal power in all azimuthal directions perpendicular to the axis of the antenna. Figure 4.4 shows the dipole *H* plane radiation pattern in a spherical coordinate system

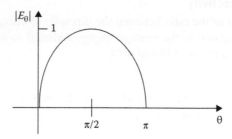

FIGURE 4.2 Dipole *E* plane radiation pattern.

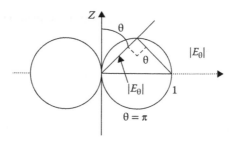

FIGURE 4.3 Dipole *E* plane radiation pattern in a spherical coordinate system.

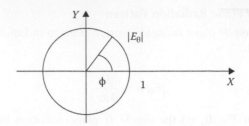

FIGURE 4.4   Dipole *H* plane radiation pattern for θ = π/2.

4.3.1.4   Antenna Radiation Pattern

Figure 4.5 shows a typical antenna radiation pattern. The antenna main beam is measured between the points that the maximum relative field intensity *E* decays to 0.707*E*. Half of the radiated power is concentrated in the antenna main beam. The antenna main beam is called the 3 dB beam width. Radiation to an undesired direction is concentrated in the antenna side lobes.

For a dipole, the power intensity varies as $\left(\sin^2\theta\right)$. At θ = 45° and θ = 135° the radiated power is equal to half the power radiated toward θ = 90°. The dipole beam width is θ = (135–45) = 90°.

4.3.1.5   Dipole Directivity

Directivity is defined as the ratio between the amounts of energy propagating in a certain direction compared to the average energy radiated to all directions over a sphere as written in Equations 4.18 and 4.19.

$$D \; = \; \frac{P(\theta,\phi)\text{maximal}}{P(\theta,\phi)\text{average}} = 4\pi\frac{P(\theta,\phi)\text{maximal}}{P \text{ rad}} \tag{4.18}$$

$$P(\theta,\phi)\text{average} = \frac{1}{4\pi}\iint P(\theta,\phi)\sin\theta\, d\theta\, d\phi = \frac{P \text{ rad}}{4\pi} \tag{4.19}$$

The radiated power from a dipole is calculated by computing the pointing vector *P* as given in Equation 4.20.

$$P \; = \; 0.5(E \times H^*) \; = \; \frac{15\pi I_0^2 l^2 \sin^2\theta}{r^2\lambda^2}$$

$$W_T \; = \; \int_s P\cdot ds \; = \; \frac{15\pi I_0^2 l^2}{\lambda^2}\int_0^\pi \sin^3\theta\, d\theta \int_0^{2\pi} d\varphi \; = \; \frac{40\pi^2 I_0^2 l^2}{\lambda^2} \tag{4.20}$$

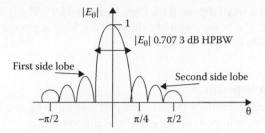

FIGURE 4.5 Antenna typical radiation pattern.

The overall radiated energy is W_T. W_T is computed by integration of the power flow over an imaginary sphere surrounding the dipole. The power flow of an isotropic radiator is equal to W_T divided by the surrounding area of the sphere, $4\pi r^2$, as given in Equation 4.21. The dipole directivity at $\theta = 90°$ is 1.5 or 1.76 dB as shown in Equation 4.22.

$$\oint_s ds = r^2 \int_0^\pi \sin\theta\,d\theta \int_0^{2\pi} d\phi = 4\pi r^2$$

$$P_{\text{iso}} = \frac{W_T}{4\pi r^2} = \frac{10\pi I_0^2 l^2}{r^2 \lambda^2} \tag{4.21}$$

$$D = \frac{P}{P_{\text{iso}}} = 1.5\sin^2\theta$$

$$G_{\text{dB}} = 10\log_{10} G = 10\log_{10} 1.5 = 1.76\,\text{dB} \tag{4.22}$$

For small antennas or for antennas without losses, $D = G$, losses are negligible. For a given θ and ϕ for small antennas the approximate directivity is given by Equation 4.23.

$$D = \frac{41,253}{\theta_{3\text{dB}}\phi_{3\text{dB}}}$$

$$\tag{4.23}$$

$$G = \xi D \qquad \xi = \text{Efficiency}$$

Antenna losses degrade the antenna efficiency. They consist of conductor loss, dielectric loss, radiation loss, and mismatch losses. For resonant small antennas, $\xi = 1$. For reflector and horn antennas the efficiency varies from $\xi = 0.5$ to $\xi = 0.7$.

The beam width of a small dipole, 0.1 λ long, is around 90°. The 0.1 λ dipole impedance is around 2 Ω. The beam width of a dipole 0.5 λ long is around 80°. The impedance of a 0.5 λ dipole is around 73 Ω.

4.3.1.6 Antenna Impedance

Antenna impedance determines the efficiency of transmitting and receiving energy in antennas. The dipole impedance is given in Equation 4.24.

$$R_{\mathrm{rad}} = \frac{2W_T}{I_0^2}$$

$$\text{For a dipole: } R_{\mathrm{rad}} = \frac{80\pi^2 l^2}{\lambda^2}$$

(4.24)

4.3.1.7 Impedance of a Folded Dipole

A folded dipole is a half-wave dipole with an additional wire connecting its two ends. If the additional wire has the same diameter and cross-section as the dipole, two nearly identical radiating currents are generated. The resulting far-field emission pattern is nearly identical to the one for the single-wire dipole described above, but at resonance its feed point impedance $R_{\mathrm{rad}-f}$ is four times the radiation resistance of a dipole. This is because for a fixed amount of power, the total radiating current I_0 is equal to twice the current in each wire and thus equal to twice the current at the feed point. Equating the average radiated power to the average power delivered at the feed point, we obtain $R_{\mathrm{rad}-f} = 4\,R_{\mathrm{rad}} = 300\ \Omega$. The folded dipole has a wider bandwidth than a single dipole.

4.4 MONOPOLE ANTENNA FOR WEARABLE COMMUNICATION SYSTEMS

A monopole antenna is usually a one-quarter wavelength long conductor mounted above a ground plane or the earth. Based on image theory, the monopole image is located behind the ground plane. The monopole antenna and the monopole image form a dipole antenna (Figure 4.6).

A monopole antenna is half a dipole and radiates electromagnetic fields above the ground plane. The impedance of a 0.5 λ monopole antenna is around 37 Ω. The beam width of a monopole 0.25 λ long is around 40°. The directivity of a monopole 0.25 λ long is around 3 dBi to 5 dBi. Usually in wireless communication systems very short monopole antennas are employed. The impedance of a 0.05 λ monopole antenna is around 1 Ω with capacitive reactance. The beam width of a monopole 0.05 λ long is around 45°. The directivity of a monopole 0.05 λ long is around 3 dBi.

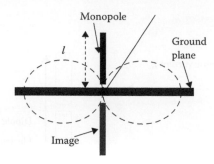

FIGURE 4.6   Monopole antenna.

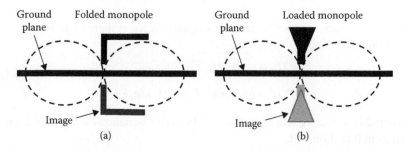

FIGURE 4.7   (a) Inverted monopole antenna. (b) Loaded monopole antenna.

An inverted monopole antenna is shown in Figure 4.7a. A loaded monopole antenna is shown in Figure 4.7b. Monopole antennas can be printed on a dielectric substrate as part of wearable communication devices.

4.5   LOOP ANTENNAS FOR WIRELESS COMMUNICATION SYSTEMS

Loop antennas are compact, low profile, and low cost antennas. They are employed in wearable wireless communication systems.

4.5.1   Duality Relationship between Dipole and Loop Antennas

The loop antenna is referred to as the dual of the dipole antenna, because if a small dipole had magnetic current flowing (as opposed to electric current as in a regular dipole), the fields would resemble a small loop. The short dipole has a capacitive impedance (the imaginary part of the impedance is negative). The impedance of a small loop is inductive (positive imaginary part).

Duality means combining two different things that are closely linked (Figure 4.8). In antennas, the duality theory means it is possible to write the fields of one antenna from the field expressions of the other antenna by interchanging linked parameters. Electric current can be interchanged by an equivalent magnetic current. The variation of electromagnetic waves as a function of time can be written as $e^{j\omega t}$. The derivative

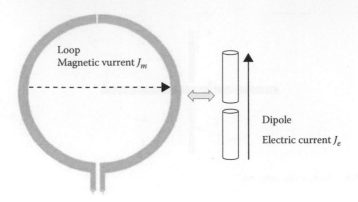

FIGURE 4.8 Duality relationship between dipole and loop antennas.

as a function of time is $j\omega e^{j\omega t}$. Maxwell's equations for system 1 can be written as in Equation 4.25:

$$\nabla X E_1 = -j\omega\mu_1 H_1$$

$$\nabla X H_1 = (\sigma + j\omega\varepsilon_1)E = J_e + j\omega\varepsilon_1 E_1$$

(4.25)

System 2 is a dual system to system 1. Maxwell's equations for system 2 can be written as in Equation 4.26:

$$\nabla X H_2 = j\omega\varepsilon_2 E_2$$

$$\nabla X E_2 = -J_m - j\omega\mu_2 H_2$$

(4.26)

System 1 Electric Current Source	System 2 Magnetic Current Source
J_e	J_m
E_1	H_2
μ_1	ε_2
H_1	$-E_2$
ε_1	μ_2

By using the duality principle the far electromagnetic fields of the loop antenna are given in Equation 4.27.

$$E_r = H_\varphi = E_\theta = 0$$

$$H_\theta = j\eta_0 \frac{l\beta I_m \sin\theta}{4\pi r} e^{j(\omega t - \beta r)}$$

$$E_\varphi = -j \frac{l\beta I_m \sin\theta}{4\pi r} e^{j(\omega t - \beta r)}$$

(4.27)

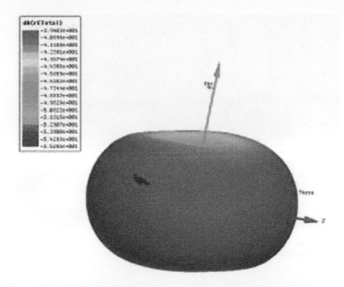

FIGURE 4.9 *H* plane radiation pattern of loop antenna in free space.

The directivity of a loop antenna with circumference 0.5 λ long is around 1 dBi. The directivity of a loop antenna with circumference 1 λ long is around 4 dBi. The *H* plane 3D radiation pattern of a loop antenna with circumference 0.45 λ in free space is shown in Figure 4.9.

4.5.2 APPLICATIONS OF LOOP ANTENNAS

Loop antennas have low radiation resistance and high reactance. It is difficult to match the antenna to a transmitter. Loop antennas are most often used as receiving antennas, where impedance mismatch loss can be accepted. Small loop antennas are used in medical devices as field strength probes, in pagers, and in wireless measurements.

A BALUN transformer is connected to the loop feed lines. A BALUN transformer is a transformer from a balance transmission line to and unbalanced transmission line. The transformer can be used to match the loop antenna to the communication system. Figure 4.10 shows loop antennas. The loop antenna can be inserted to a sleeve as shown in Figure 4.10. The sleeve electrical properties were chosen to match the loop antenna to a human body. The sleeve also provides protection from the environment to the loop antenna. Figure 4.11 shows a four loop antenna array inside a belt. The loop antenna can be tuned by adding a capacitor or a varactor as shown in Figure 4.11.

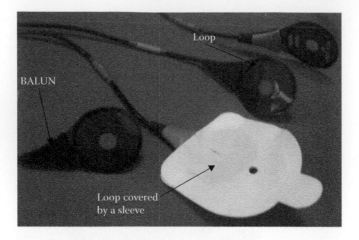

FIGURE 4.10   Loop antennas.

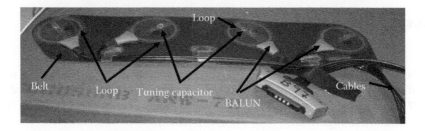

FIGURE 4.11   Loop antenna array inside a belt.

4.6 CONCLUSIONS

Antennas are a major component in wearable communication systems. In this chapter basic antenna theory was presented. Radiating elements for wearable communication systems was also presented. Dipole, monopole, and loop antennas can be used in wearable wireless communication systems. These are compact antennas with directivity around 1 dBi to 4 dBi. Dipole, monopole, and loop antennas can be printed on a dielectric substrate as part of wearable communication devices.

REFERENCES

1. C. A. Balanis, *Antenna Theory: Analysis and Design*, 2nd Edition, Hoboken, NJ: Wiley, 1996.
2. L. C. Godara, ed., *Handbook of Antennas in Wireless Communications*, Boca Raton, FL: CRC Press LLC, 2002.
3. J. D. Kraus and R . J. Marhefka, *Antennas for All Applications*, 3rd Edition, New Delhi, India: McGraw Hill, 2002.
4. J. R. James, P . S. Hall and C. Wood, *Microstrip Antenna Theory and Design*, London: Institution of Engineering and Technology, 1981.

5. A. Sabban and K. C. Gupta, Characterization of radiation loss from microstrip discontinuities using a multiport network modeling approach, *IEEE Transactions on Microwave Theory and Techniques*, vol. 39, no. 4, 705–712, April 1991.
6. A. Sabban, PhD Thesis, Multiport network model for evaluating radiation loss and coupling among discontinuities in microstrip circuits, University of Colorado at Boulder, CO, January 1991.
7. A. Sabban, Inventor, *Microstrip antenna arrays*, U.S. Patent US 1986/4,623,893, 1986.
8. A. Sabban. A new wideband stacked microstrip antenna, IEEE Antenna and Propagation Symposium, Houston, TX, June 1983.
9. A. Sabban, *Low Visibility Antennas for Communication Systems*, New York: Taylor & Francis Group, 2015.
10. A. Sabban, Wideband microstrip antenna arrays, IEEE Antenna and Propagation Symposium MELCOM, Tel-Aviv, Israel, June 1981.
11. A. Sabban, *RF Engineering, Microwave and Antennas*, Israel: Saar Publications, 2014.
12. K. Fujimoto, J. R. James, eds., *Mobile Antenna Systems Handbook*, Boston, MA: Artech House, 1994.
13. A. Sabban, New wideband notch antennas for communication systems, *Wireless Engineering and Technology*, 75–82, April 2016.
14. A. Sabban, Inventor, *Dual polarized dipole wearable antenna*, U.S. Patent US 8203497, June 19, 2012, USA.
15. A. Sabban. New wideband printed antennas for medical applications, *IEEE Transactions on Antennas and Propagation*, vol. 61, no. 1, 84–91, January 2013.
16. A. Sabban, Comprehensive study of printed antennas on human body for medical applications, *International Journal of Advance in Medical Science (AMS)*, vol. 1, 1–10, February 2013.

5 Wearable Printed Antennas for Wireless Communication Systems

Wireless communication and the medical industry have undergone continuous growth in the last few years. Low-profile compact antennas are crucial in the development of wearable human biomedical systems. Printed antennas are the perfect antenna solution for wireless and medical communication systems. Printed antennas possess attractive features such as low profile, light weight, small volume, and low production cost. These features are crucial for wireless compact wearable communication systems. In addition, the benefit of a compact low-cost feed network is attained by integrating the feed structure with the radiating elements on the same substrate. Printed antennas are used in communication systems that employ MIC and MMIC technologies.

5.1 WEARABLE PRINTED ANTENNAS

Printed antennas possess attractive features such as low profile, flexible, light weight, small volume, and low production cost. They may be used as wearable antennas. Printed antennas have been widely presented in books and papers in the last decade [1–19]. The most popular type of printed antennas are microstrip antennas. However, PIFA, slot, and dipole printed antennas are widely used in communication systems. Printed antennas may be employed in communication links, seekers, and medical systems.

Applications of wearable antennas

- Medical
- Wireless communication
- WLAN
- HIPER LAN
- GPS
- Military applications

5.1.1 WEARABLE MICROSTRIP ANTENNAS

Microstrip antennas are printed on a dielectric substrate with low dielectric losses. Figure 5.1 shows a cross section of a microstrip antenna. Microstrip antennas are thin patches etched on a dielectric substrate ε_r. The substrate thickness, H, is less than 0.1 λ. Microstrip antennas are widely presented in [1–8]. The printed antenna may be attached to the human body or inserted inside a wearable belt.

95

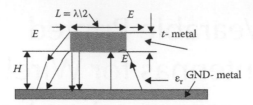

FIGURE 5.1   Microstrip antenna cross section.

Advantages of microstrip antennas

- Low cost to fabricate.
- Conformal structures are possible.
- Easy to form a large uniform array with half-wavelength spacing.
- Light weight and low volume.

These features are crucial for wearable communication systems.

Disadvantages of microstrip antennas

- Limited bandwidth (usually 1% to 5%, but much more is possible with increased complexity)
- Low power handling

The electric field along the radiating edges is shown in Figure 5.2. The magnetic field is perpendicular to the E-field according to Maxwell's equations. At the edge of the strip ($X/L = 0$ and $X/L = 1$) the H-field drops to zero, because there is no conductor to carry the RF current; it is maximum in the center. The E-field intensity is at maximum magnitude (and opposite polarity) at the edges ($X/L = 0$ and $X/L = 1$) and zero at the center. The ratio of E to H field is proportional to the impedance that we see when we feed the patch. Microstrip antennas may be fed by a microstrip line or by a coaxial line or probe feed. By adjusting the location of the feed point between the center and the edge, we can get any impedance, including 50 Ω. The shape of a microstrip antenna can be square, rectangular, trianglular, circlular, or any arbitrary shape as shown in Figure 5.3.

The dielectric constant that controls the resonance of the antenna is the effective dielectric constant of the microstrip line. The antenna dimension W is given by Equation 5.1.

$$W = \frac{c}{2f\sqrt{\epsilon_{\text{eff}}}} \tag{5.1}$$

The antenna bandwidth is given in Equation 5.2.

$$BW = \frac{H}{\sqrt{\epsilon_{\text{eff}}}} \tag{5.2}$$

The gain of a microstrip antenna is between 0 dBi to 7 dBi. The microstrip antenna gain is a function of the antenna dimensions and configuration. We may increase

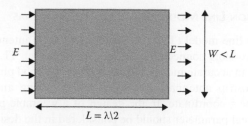

FIGURE 5.2 Rectangular microstrip antenna.

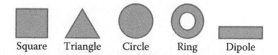

Square   Triangle   Circle   Ring   Dipole

FIGURE 5.3 Microstrip antenna shapes.

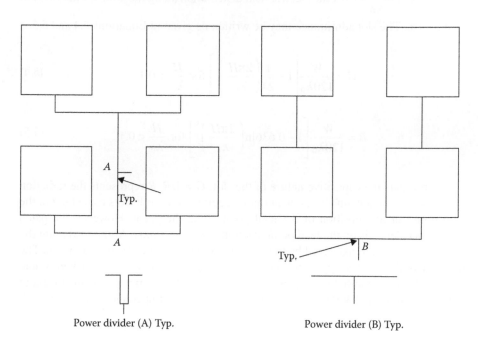

Power divider (A) Typ.   Power divider (B) Typ.

FIGURE 5.4 Configuration of microstrip antenna array. (a) Parallel feed network. (b) Parallel series feed network.

printed antenna gain by using a microstrip antenna array configuration. In a microstrip antenna array the benefit of a compact low cost feed network is attained by integrating the RF feed network with the radiating elements on the same substrate. Microstrip antenna feed networks are presented in Figure 5.4. Figure 5.4a presents a parallel feed network. Figure 5.4b presents a parallel series feed network.

5.1.2 Transmission Line Model of Microstrip Antennas

In the transmission line model (TLM) of patch microstrip antennas the antenna is represented as a two slots connected by a transmission line. TLM is presented in Figure 5.5. It is not an accurate model. However it gives a good physical understanding of patch microstrip antennas. The electric field along and underneath the patch depend on the z coordinate. In the design of a wearable patch antennas the human body electrical parameter should be considered in the design.

$$E_x \sim \cos\left(\frac{\pi z}{L_{\text{eff}}}\right) \tag{5.3}$$

At $z = 0$ and $z = L_{\text{eff}}$ the electric field is maximum. At $z = \dfrac{L_{\text{eff}}}{2}$ the electric field equals zero. For $\dfrac{H}{\lambda_0} < 0.1$ the electric field distribution along the x-axis is assumed to be uniform. The slot admittance may be written as given in Equations 5.4 and 5.5.

$$G = \frac{W}{120\lambda_0}\left[1 - \frac{1}{24}\left(\frac{2\pi H}{\lambda_0}\right)^2\right] \text{ for } \frac{H}{\lambda_0} < 0.1 \tag{5.4}$$

$$B = \frac{W}{120\lambda_0}\left[1 - 0.636\ln\left(\frac{2\pi H}{\lambda_0}\right)^2\right] \text{ for } \frac{H}{\lambda_0} < 0.1 \tag{5.5}$$

B represents the capacitive nature of the slot. $G = 1/R$. R represents the radiation losses. When the antenna is resonant the susceptances of both slots cancel out at the feed point for any position of the feed point along the patch. However, the patch admittance depends on the feed point position along the z-axis. At the feed point the slot admittance is transformed by the equivalent length of the transmission line. The width W of the microstrip antenna controls the input impedance. Larger widths can increase the bandwidth. For a square patch antenna fed by a microstrip line, the input impedance is around 300 Ω. By increasing the width, the impedance can be reduced.

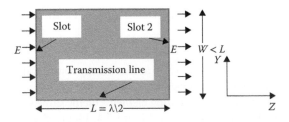

FIGURE 5.5   Transmission line model of patch microstrip antennas.

$$Y(l_1) = Z_0 \frac{1 + j\dfrac{Z_L}{Z_0}\tan\beta l_1}{\dfrac{Z_L}{Z_0} + j\tan\beta l_1} = Y_1 \tag{5.6}$$

$$Y_{in} = Y_1 + Y_2$$

5.1.3 Higher-Order Transmission Modes in Microstrip Antennas

In order to prevent higher-order transmission modes we should limit the thickness of the microstrip substrate to 10% of a wavelength. The cutoff frequency of the higher-order mode is given in Equation 5.7.

$$f_c = \frac{c}{4H\sqrt{\varepsilon - 1}} \tag{5.7}$$

5.1.4 Effective Dielectric Constant

Part of the field in the microstrip antenna structure exists in air and the other part of the field exists in the dielectric substrate. The effective dielectric constant is somewhat less than the substrate's dielectric constant.

The effective dielectric constant of the microstrip line may be calculated by Equations 5.8 and 5.9 as a function of W/H:

For $\left(\dfrac{W}{H}\right) < 1$

$$\varepsilon_e = \frac{\varepsilon_r + 1}{2} + \frac{\varepsilon_r - 1}{2}\left[\left(1 + 12\left(\frac{H}{W}\right)\right)^{-0.5} + 0.04\left(1 - \left(\frac{W}{H}\right)\right)^2\right] \tag{5.8}$$

For $\left(\dfrac{W}{H}\right) \geq 1$

$$\varepsilon_e = \frac{\varepsilon_r + 1}{2} + \frac{\varepsilon_r - 1}{2}\left[\left(1 + 12\left(\frac{H}{W}\right)\right)^{-0.5}\right] \tag{5.9}$$

This calculation ignores strip thickness and frequency dispersion, but their effects are negligible.

5.1.5 Losses in Microstrip Antennas

Losses in microstrip lines are due to conductor loss, radiation loss, and dielectric loss.
Conductor loss
Conductor loss may be calculated by using Equation 5.10.

$$\alpha_c = 8.686 \log(R_S/(2WZ_0)) \qquad \text{dB/Length}$$

$$R_S = \sqrt{\pi f \mu \rho} \qquad \text{Skin resistance}$$

(5.10)

Conductor losses may also be calculated by defining an equivalent loss tangent δc, given by $\delta c = \delta s/h$, where $\delta s = \sqrt{2/\omega \mu \sigma}$. σ is the strip conductivity, h is the substrate height, and μ is the free space permeability.

Dielectric loss

Dielectric loss may be calculated by using Equation 5.11.

$$\alpha_d = 27.3 \, \frac{\varepsilon_r}{\sqrt{\varepsilon_{eff}}} \frac{\varepsilon_{eff} - 1}{\varepsilon_r - 1} \frac{tg\delta}{\lambda_0} \qquad \text{dB/cm}$$

(5.11)

$tg\delta$ = dielectric loss coefficient

5.1.6 PATCH RADIATION PATTERN

The patch width, W, controls the antenna radiation pattern. The coordinate system is shown in Figure 5.6. The normalized radiation pattern is approximately given by:

$$E_\theta = \frac{\sin\left(\frac{k_0 W}{2} \sin\theta \sin\varphi\right)}{\frac{k_0 W}{2} \sin\theta \sin\varphi} \cos\left(\frac{k_0 L}{2} \sin\theta \cos\varphi\right) \cos\varphi$$

(5.12)

$$k_0 = 2\pi/\lambda$$

$$E_\varphi = \frac{\sin\left(\frac{k_0 W}{2} \sin\theta \sin\varphi\right)}{\frac{k_0 W}{2} \sin\theta \sin\varphi} \cos\left(\frac{k_0 L}{2} \sin\theta \cos\varphi\right) \cos\theta \sin\varphi$$

(5.13)

$$k_0 = 2\pi/\lambda$$

The magnitude of the fields is given by:

$$f(\theta, \varphi) = \sqrt{E_\theta^2 + E_\varphi^2}$$

(5.14)

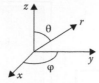

FIGURE 5.6 Coordinate system.

5.2 TWO-LAYER WEARABLE STACKED MICROSTRIP ANTENNAS

Two-layer microstrip antennas were first presented in [1–3, 5–8]. The major disadvantage of single layer microstrip antennas is narrow bandwidth. By designing a double-layer microstrip antenna we can achieve a wider bandwidth. Two-layer microstrip antennas may be the best antenna choice for wideband wearable systems.

In the first layer, the antenna feed network and a resonator are printed. In the second layer, the radiating element is printed. The electromagnetic field is coupled from the resonator to the radiating element. The resonator and the radiating element shape may be square, rectangular, triangular, circular, or any arbitrary shape. The distance between the layers is optimized to get maximum bandwidth with the best antenna efficiency. The spacing between the layers may be air or foam with low dielectric losses.

A circular polarization double layer antenna was designed at 2.2 GHz. The resonator and the feed network were printed on a substrate with relative dielectric constant of 2.5 with thickness of 1.6 mm. The resonator is a square microstrip resonator with dimensions $W = L = 45$ mm. The radiating element was printed on a substrate with relative dielectric constant of 2.2 with thickness of 1.6 mm. The radiating element is a square patch with dimensions $W = L = 48$ mm. The patch was designed as a circular polarized antenna by connecting a 3 dB 90° branch coupler to antenna feed-lines, as shown in Figure 5.7. The antenna bandwidth is 10% for VSWR better than 2:1. The measured antenna beam width is around 72°. The measured antenna gain is 7.5 dBi. This antenna may be applied in wideband wireless wearable systems.

Measured results of stacked microstrip wearable antennas are listed in Table 5.1. The antennas listed in Table 5.1 may be used in wearable communication systems.

The results in Table 5.1 indicate that the bandwidth of a two-layer microstrip antennas may be around 9% to 15% for VSWR better than 2:1. In Figure 5.13, a stacked microstrip antenna is shown. The antenna feed network is printed on FR4 dielectric substrate with a dielectric constant of 4 that is 1.6 mm thick. The radiator is printed on RT-DUROID 5880 dielectric substrate with dielectric constant of 2.2 that is 1.6 mm thick. The antenna electrical parameters were calculated and optimized by using ADS software. The dimensions of the microstrip stacked patch antenna shown in Figure 5.8 are $33 \times 20 \times 3.2$ mm. The computed S11 parameters are presented in Figure 5.9. The radiation pattern of the microstrip stacked patch is shown in Figure 5.10. The antenna bandwidth is around 5% for VSWR better than 2.5:1. The antenna bandwidth is improved to 10% for VSWR better than 2.0:1 by adding 8 mm air spacing between the layers. The antenna beam width is around 72°. The antenna gain is around 7 dBi.

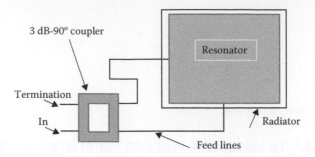

FIGURE 5.7   Circular polarized microstrip stacked patch antenna.

TABLE 5.1
Measured Results of Stacked Microstrip Antennas

Antenna	F (GHz)	Bandwidth %	Beam width °	Gain dBi	Side lobe dB	Polarization
Square	2.2	10	72	7.5	−22	Circular
Circular	2.2	15	72	7.9	−22	Linear
Annular disc	2.2	11.5	78	6.6	−14	Linear
Rectangular	2.0	9	72	7.4	−25	Linear
Circular	2.4	9	72	7	−22	Linear
Circular	2.4	10	72	7.5	−22	Circular

FIGURE 5.8   A microstrip stacked patch antenna.

5.3   STACKED MONO-PULSE KU BAND PATCH ANTENNA

A mono-pulse double-layer antenna was designed at 15 GHz. The mono-pulse double-layer antenna consists of four circular patch antennas as shown in Figure 5.11. The resonator and the feed network were printed on a substrate with relative dielectric constant of 2.5 and thickness of 0.8 mm. The resonator is a circular microstrip resonator with diameter $a = 4.2$ mm. The radiating element was printed on a substrate with relative dielectric constant of 2.2 and thickness of 0.8 mm. The radiating element

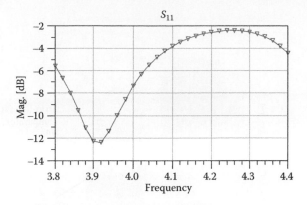

FIGURE 5.9 Computed S_{11} of the microstrip stacked patch.

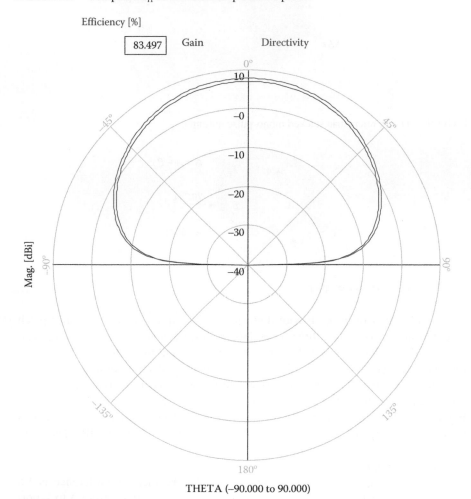

FIGURE 5.10 Radiation pattern of the microstrip stacked patch.

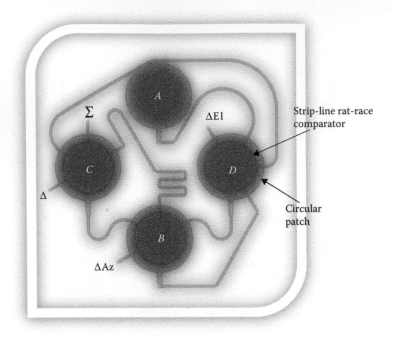

FIGURE 5.11   A microstrip stacked mono-pulse antenna.

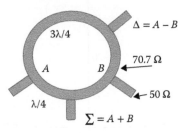

FIGURE 5.12   Rat-race coupler.

is a circular microstrip patch with diameter $a = 4.5$ mm. The four circular patch antennas are connected to three 3 dB 180° rat-race couplers via the antenna feed lines, as shown in Figure 5.11. The comparator consists of three strip-line 3 dB 180° rat-race couplers printed on a substrate with relative dielectric constant of 2.2 and thickness of 0.8 mm. The comparator has four output ports: a sum port Σ, difference port Δ, elevation difference port ΔEl, and azimuth difference port ΔAz, as shown in Figure 5.16. The antenna bandwidth is 10% for VSWR better than 2:1. The antenna beam width is around 36°. The measured antenna gain is around 10 dBi. The comparator losses are around 0.7 dB.

Rat-race coupler

A rat-race coupler is shown in Figure 5.12. The rat-race circumference is 1.5 wavelengths. The distance from A to Δ port is 3 $\lambda/4$. The distance from A to Σ port is $\lambda/4$. For an equal-split rat-race coupler, the impedance of the entire ring is fixed at

$1.41 \times Z_0$, or 70.7 Ω for $Z_0 = 50$ Ω. For an input signal V, the outputs at ports 2 and 4 are equal in magnitude, but 180° out of phase.

5.4 WEARABLE LOOP ANTENNAS

Loop antennas are used as receiving antennas in wearable communication and medical systems. They may be printed on a dielectric substrate or manufactured as a wired antenna. In this section, several loop antennas are presented.

5.4.1 SMALL LOOP ANTENNA

The small loop antenna is shown in Figure 5.13. The shape of the loop antenna may be circular or rectangular. These antennas have low radiation resistance and high reactance. It is difficult to match the antenna to a transmitter. Loop antennas are most often used as receiving antennas, where an impedance mismatch loss can be accepted. Small loop antennas are used as field strength probes, in pagers, and in wireless measurements. The loop lies in the x-y plane. The radius a of the small loop antenna is smaller than a wavelength ($a \ll \lambda$). The loop antenna electric field is given by Equation 5.11. The loop antenna magnetic field is given in Equations 5.15 and 5.16.

$$E_\phi = \eta \frac{(ak)^2 I_0 \sin\theta}{4r} e^{j(\omega t - \beta r)} \tag{5.15}$$

$$H_\theta = -\frac{(ak)^2 I_0 \sin\theta}{4r} e^{j(\omega t - \beta r)} \tag{5.16}$$

The variation of the radiation pattern with direction is $\sin\theta$, the same as for a dipole antenna. The fields of a small loop have the E and H fields switched relative to that of a short dipole. The E-field is horizontally polarized in the x-y plane.

The small loop is often referred to as the dual of the dipole antenna, because if a small dipole had magnetic current flowing (as opposed to electric current as in a regular dipole), the fields would resemble that of a small loop. The short dipole has a capacitive impedance (imaginary part of the impedance is negative). The impedance of a small loop is inductive (positive imaginary part). The radiation resistance (and ohmic loss resistance) can be increased by adding more turns to the loop. If

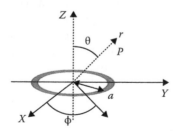

FIGURE 5.13 Small loop antenna.

there are N turns of a small loop antenna, each with a surface area S, the radiation resistance for small loops can be approximated as given in Equation 5.17.

$$R_{rad} = \frac{31,329 N^2 S^2}{\lambda^4} \qquad (5.17)$$

For a small loop, the reactive component of the impedance can be determined by finding the inductance of the loop. For a circular loop with radius a, and wire radius r, the reactive component of the impedance is given by Equation 5.18.

$$X = 2\pi a f\mu(\ln\left(\frac{8a}{r}\right) - 1.75) \qquad (5.18)$$

Loop antennas behave better in the vicinity of the human body than dipole antennas. The reason is that the electric near fields in a dipole antenna are very strong. For $r \ll 1$, the dominant component of the field varies as $\frac{1}{r^3}$. This fields are the dipole near fields. In this case the waves are standing waves and the energy oscillates in the antenna near zone and is not radiated to the open space. The real part of the Poynting vector is equal to zero. Near the body the electric fields decay rapidly. However, the magnetic fields are not affected near the body. The magnetic fields are strong in the near field of the loop antenna. These magnetic fields give rise to the loop antenna radiation. The loop antenna radiation near the human body is stronger than the dipole radiation near the human body. Several loop antennas are used as "wearable antennas."

5.4.2 Wearable Printed Loop Antenna

The diameter of a printed loop antenna is around half a wavelength. A loop antenna is dual to a half wavelength dipole. Several loop antennas were designed for medical systems at a frequency range between 400 MHz and 500 MHz. In Figure 5.14a a printed loop antenna is presented. A photo of a printed loop antenna with a BALUN transformer is presented in Figure 5.14b. A BALUN transformer is a transformer from a balance transmission line to an unbalanced transmission line. The loop may be attached to a human body or inserted inside a wearable belt. The antenna was printed on FR4 with 0.5 mm thickness. The loop diameter is 45 mm. The loop antenna VSWR is around 4:1. The printed loop antenna radiation pattern at 435 MHz is shown in Figure 5.15. The loop antenna gain is around 1.8 dBi. The antenna with a tuning capacitor is shown in Figure 5.16. The loop antenna VSWR without the tuning capacitor was 4:1. This loop antenna may be tuned by adding a capacitor or varactor as shown in Figure 5.17. Matching stubs are employed to tune the antenna to the resonant frequency. Tuning the antenna allows us to work in a wider bandwidth as shown in Figure 5.18. Loop antennas are used as receiving antennas in medical systems. The loop antenna radiation pattern on the human body is shown in Figure 5.19.

The computed 3D radiation pattern and the coordinates used in this chapter are shown in Figure 5.19.

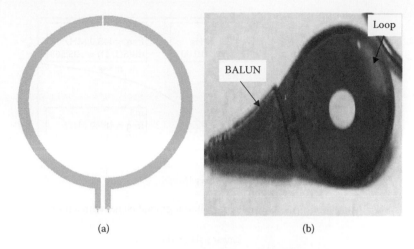

(a)   (b)

FIGURE 5.14   (a) Printed loop antenna. (b) Photo of a printed loop antenna.

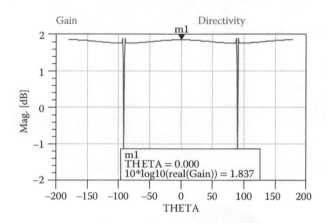

FIGURE 5.15   Printed loop antenna radiation pattern at 435 MHz.

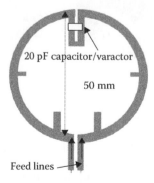

FIGURE 5.16   Tunable loop antenna without ground plane.

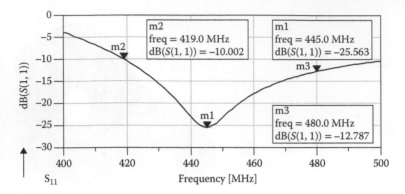

FIGURE 5.17 Computed S_{11} of loop antenna, without ground plane, with a tuning capacitor.

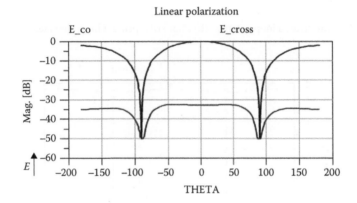

FIGURE 5.18 Radiation pattern of a loop antenna on human body.

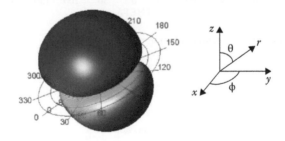

FIGURE 5.19 Loop antenna 3D radiation pattern.

5.4.3 WEARABLE RFID LOOP ANTENNAS

RFID loop antennas are widely used. Several RFID loop antennas are presented in [10]. RFID loop antennas have low efficiency and narrow bandwidth. As an example the measured impedance of a square four-turn loop at 13.5 MHz is 0.47 + j107.5 Ω. A matching network is used to match the antenna to 50 Ω. The matching network consists of a 56 pF shunt capacitor, 1 kΩ shunt resistor, and another 56 pF capacitor. This matching network has a narrow bandwidth. The antenna is printed on a FR4 substrate. The antenna dimensions are $32 \times 52.4 \times 0.25$ mm. The antenna layout is shown in Figure 5.20. A photo of the RFID antenna is shown in Figure 5.21. S_{11} results of the printed loop antenna are shown in Figure 5.22. The antenna S_{11} parameter is better than −9.5 dB without an external matching network. The computed radiation pattern is shown in Figure 5.23. The RFID antenna beam width is around 160°.

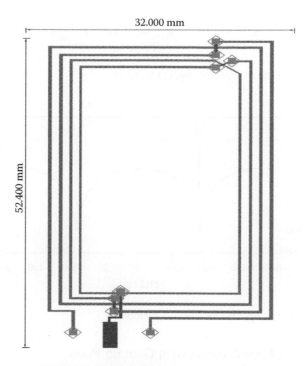

FIGURE 5.20 A square four-turn loop antenna.

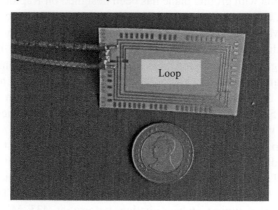

FIGURE 5.21 Four-turn 13.5 MHz loop rectangular antenna.

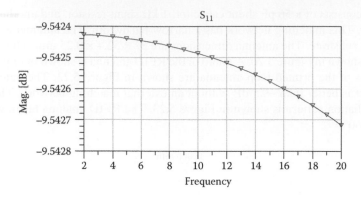

FIGURE 5.22 RFID loop antenna computed S_{11} results.

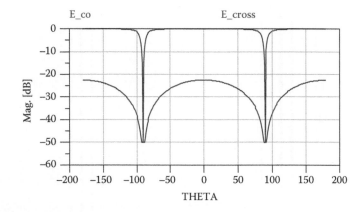

FIGURE 5.23 RFID loop antenna radiation pattern.

5.4.4 Wearable Loop Antenna with Ground Plane

A new loop antenna with ground plane has been designed on Kapton substrates with relative dielectric constant of 3.5 and thickness of 0.25 mm. The antenna is presented in Figure 5.24. Matching stubs are employed to tune the antenna to the resonant frequency. The diameter of the loop antenna with ground plane is 45 mm. The antenna was designed by employing ADS software. The antenna center frequency is 427 MHz. The antenna bandwidth for VSWR better than 2:1 is around 12%, as shown in Figure 5.25. The printed loop antenna radiation pattern at 435 MHz is shown in Figure 5.26. The loop antenna gain is around 1.8 dBi. The beam width of the loop antenna with ground plane is around 100°.

A printed loop antenna with ground plane with shorter tuning stubs is shown in Figure 5.27. The diameter of the loop antenna with ground plane with shorter tuning stubs is 45 mm. The antenna center frequency is 438 MHz. The antenna bandwidth for VSWR better than 2:1 is around 12% as shown in Figure 5.28. The printed loop antenna with shorter tuning stubs radiation pattern at 435 MHz is shown in

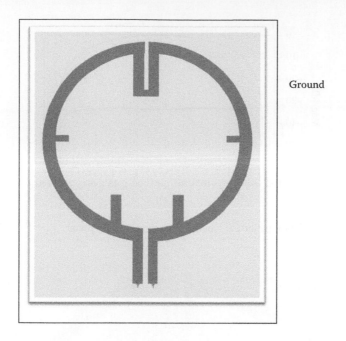

FIGURE 5.24 Printed loop antenna with ground plane.

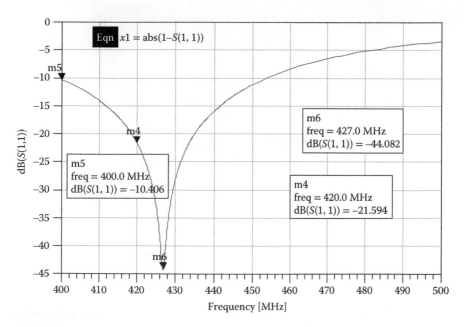

FIGURE 5.25 Computed S_{11} of loop antenna with ground plane.

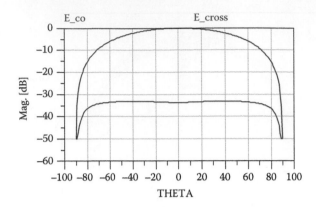

FIGURE 5.26   Radiation pattern of loop antenna with ground plane.

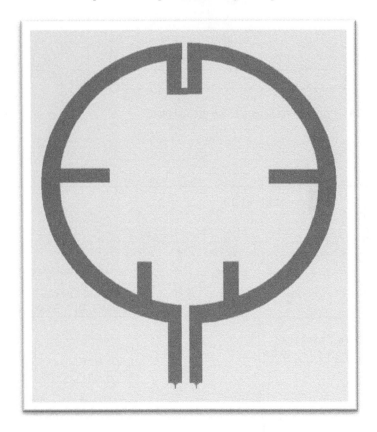

FIGURE 5.27   Printed loop antenna with ground plane and short tuning stubs.

Figure 5.29. The loop antenna gain is around 1.8 dBi. The loop antenna with ground plane beam width is around 100°. The printed loop antenna with shorter tuning stubs 3D radiation pattern at 430 MHz is shown in Figure 5.30.

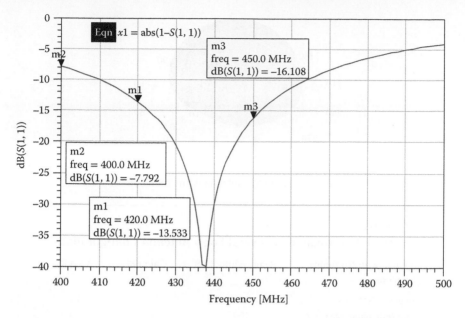

FIGURE 5.28　Computed S11 of loop antenna with ground plane and short tuning stubs.

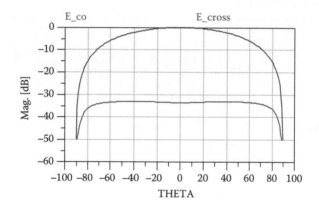

FIGURE 5.29　Radiation pattern of loop antenna with ground plane and short tuning stubs.

Table 5.2 compares the electrical performance of a loop antenna with ground plane with a loop antenna without ground plane.

5.5　WIRED LOOP ANTENNA

A wire seven-turn loop antenna is shown in Figure 5.31. The antenna length $l = 4.5$ mm. The loop diameter is 3.5 mm. Equation 5.19 is an approximation to calculate the inductance value for an air coil loop antenna with N turns, diameter r, and length l.

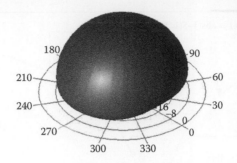

FIGURE 5.30 3D radiation pattern of loop antenna with ground plane.

TABLE 5.2

Electrical Performance of Several Loop Antenna Configurations

Antenna with No Tuning Capacitor	Beam Width 3 dB	Gain dBi	VSWR
Loop no GND	100°	0	4:1
Loop with tuning capacitor (no GND)	100°	0	2:1
Wearable loop with GND	100°	0 to 2	2:1
Loop with GND in free space	100° to 110°	−3	5:1

$$L(nH) = \frac{3.94 r_{\text{mm}} N^2}{0.9\dfrac{l}{r}+1} = \frac{0.1 r_{\text{mil}} N^2}{0.9\dfrac{l}{r}+1} \tag{5.19}$$

An approximation to calculate the inductance value for an air coil loop antenna with N turns, diameter r, and length l is given in Equation 5.20.

$$L(nH) \approx \frac{r_{\text{mm}}^2 N^2}{2l+r} \tag{5.20}$$

For length $l = 4.5$ mm, wire diameter 0.6 mm, loop diameter 3.5 mm, and $N = 7$ the inductance is around $L = 52$ nH. The quality factor of this seven-turn wire loop is around 100.

For length $l = 1.7$ mm, wire diameter 0.6 mm, loop diameter 6.5 mm, and $N = 2$, the inductance is around $L = 45$ nH.

For length $l = 2$ mm, wire diameter 0.6 mm, loop diameter 7.62 mm, and $N = 2$ the inductance is around $L = 42.1$ nH.

For length $l = 0.5$ mm, wire diameter 0.6 mm, loop diameter 7 mm, and $N = 2$ the inductance is around $L = 87$ nH.

For length $l = 2.5$ mm, wire diameter 0.6, loop diameter 5 mm, and $N = 2$ the inductance is around $L = 20.7$ nH.

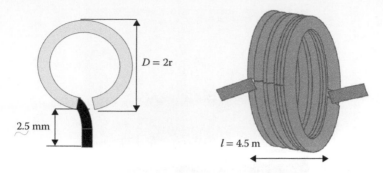

FIGURE 5.31   Wire seven-turn loop antenna.

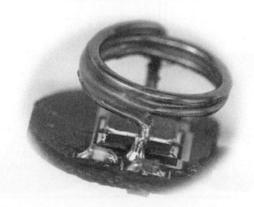

FIGURE 5.32   Wire loop antenna on PCB board.

The wire loop antenna has very low radiation efficiency. The amount of power radiated is a small fraction of the input power. The antenna efficiency is around 0.01%, −41 dB. The ratio between the antenna's dimension and wavelength is around 1:100. Small antennas are characterized by radiation resistance Rr. The radiated power is given by I^2Rr, where I is the current through the coil. Remember that the current through the coil is Q times the current through the antenna. For example, for a current of 2 mA and Q of 20, if Rr = 10^{-3} Ohm, the radiated power is around −32 dBm.

Figure 5.32 presents a wire loop antenna with 2.5 turns on a PCB board. Figure 5.33 presents a wire loop antenna with 7 turns on a PCB board.

5.6   RADIATION PATTERN OF A LOOP ANTENNA NEAR A METAL SHEET

The *E* and *H* plane 3D radiation pattern of a wire loop antenna in free space is shown in Figure 5.34.

The *E* and *H* plane 3D radiation pattern of a wire loop antenna near a metal sheet as shown in Figure 5.35 was computed by employing HFSS software.

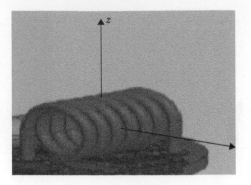

FIGURE 5.33   Seven-turn loop antenna on PCB board.

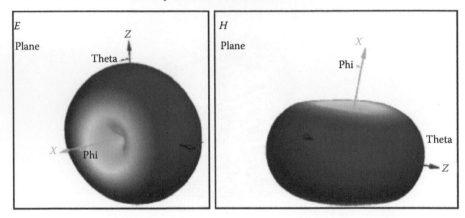

FIGURE 5.34   *E* and *H* plane radiation pattern of loop antenna in free space.

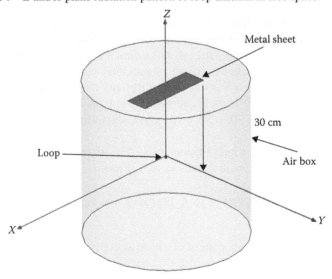

FIGURE 5.35   Loop antenna located near a metal sheet.

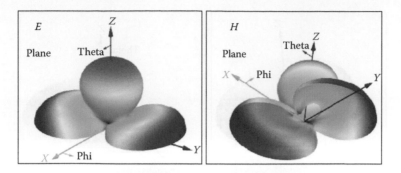

FIGURE 5.36 *E* and *H* plane radiation pattern of a loop antenna for distance of 30 cm from a metal sheet.

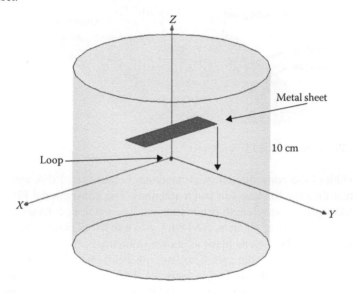

FIGURE 5.37   Loop antenna located 10 cm from a metal sheet.

Figure 5.36 presents the *E* and *H* plane radiation pattern of a loop antenna for a distance of 30 cm from a metal sheet. We can see that a metal sheet in the vicinity of the antenna split the main beam and creates holes of around 20 dB in the radiation pattern.

Figure 5.37 presents a loop antenna located 10 cm from a metal sheet, and the *E* and *H* plane radiation pattern for this antenna is presented in Figure 5.38. We can see that a metal sheet in the vicinity of the antenna splits the main beam and creates holes up to 15 dB in the radiation pattern.

5.7 WEARABLE PLANAR INVERTED-F ANTENNA (PIFA)

The planar inverted-F antenna possess attractive features such as low profile, small size, and low fabrication costs [16–18]. The PIFA antenna bandwidth is higher than

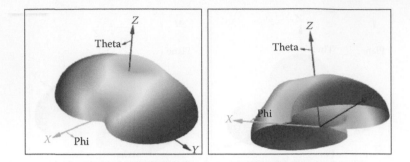

FIGURE 5.38   *E* and *H* plane radiation pattern of a loop antenna for a distance of 10 cm from a metal sheet.

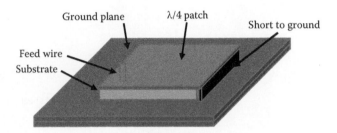

FIGURE 5.39   Conventional PIFA antenna.

the bandwidth of the conventional patch antenna, because the PIFA antenna thickness is larger than the thickness of patch antennas. The conventional PIFA antenna is a grounded quarter-wavelength patch antenna. The antenna consists of a ground plane, a top plate radiating element, feed wire, and a shorting plate or holes from the radiating element to the ground plane as shown in Figure 5.39.

The patch is shorted at the end. The fringing fields, which are responsible for radiation, are shorted on the far end, so only the fields nearest the transmission line radiate. Consequently, the gain is reduced, but the patch antenna maintains the same basic properties as a half-wavelength patch. However the antenna length is reduced by 50%. The feed location may be placed between the open and shorted end. The feed location controls the antenna input impedance.

5.7.1   GROUNDED QUARTER-WAVELENGTH PATCH ANTENNA

A grounded quarter-wavelength patch antenna was designed on FR4 substrate with relative dielectric constant of 4.5 and 1.6 mm thickness at 3.85 GHz. The antenna is shown in Figure 5.40. The antenna was designed using ADS software. The antenna dimensions are 34 × 17 × 1.6 mm. The S11 results of the antenna are shown in Figure 5.41. The antenna bandwidth is around 6% for VSWR better than 3:1 without a matching network. The radiation pattern is shown in Figure 5.42. The antenna beam width is around 76°. The grounded quarter-wavelength patch antenna gain is around 6.7 dBi. The antenna efficiency is around 92%. The compact PIFA antenna may be attached to the human body or inserted inside a wearable belt.

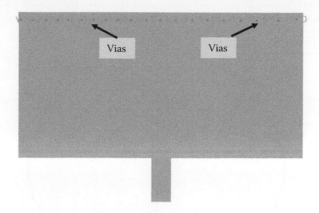

FIGURE 5.40 Grounded quarter-wavelength patch antenna.

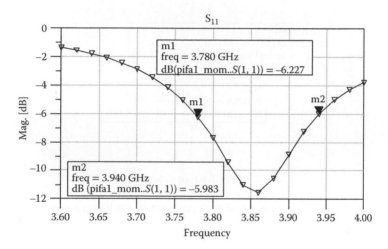

FIGURE 5.41 Grounded quarter-wavelength patch antenna S_{11} results.

5.7.2 A WEARABLE DOUBLE-LAYER PIFA ANTENNA

A new double-layer PIFA antenna was designed. The first layer is a grounded quarter-wavelength patch antenna printed on FR4 substrate with relative dielectric constant of 4.5 and 1.6 mm thickness. The second layer is a rectangular patch antenna printed on Dorouid substrate with relative dielectric constant of 2.2 and 1.6 mm thickness. The antenna is shown in Figure 5.43. The antenna was designed using ADS software. The dimensions are $34 \times 17 \times 3.2$ mm. The S_{11} results of the antenna are shown in Figure 5.44. It is a dual-band antenna. The first resonant frequency is 3.48 GHz. The second resonant frequency is 4.02 GHz. The radiation pattern is shown in Figure 5.45. The antenna beam width is around 74°. The antenna gain is around 7.4 dBi, while the efficiency is around 83.4%.

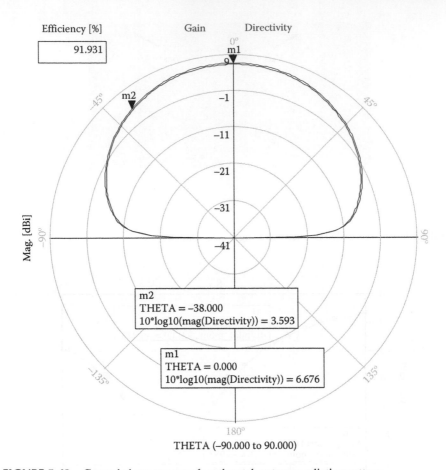

FIGURE 5.42 Grounded quarter-wavelength patch antenna radiation pattern.

FIGURE 5.43 Double-layer PIFA antenna.

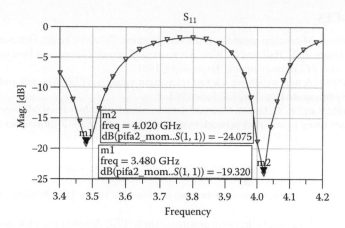

FIGURE 5.44 Double-layer PIFA antenna S_{11} results.

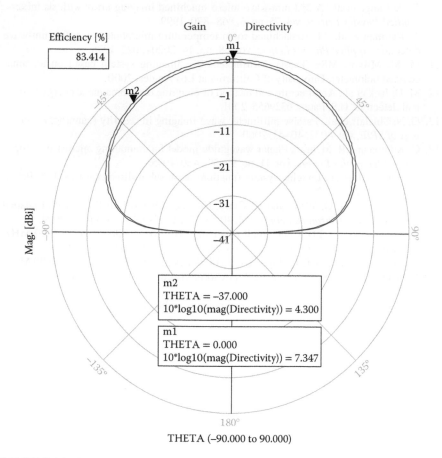

FIGURE 5.45 Double-layer PIFA antenna radiation pattern.

REFERENCES

1. A. Sabban, Microstrip antennas, IEEE Symposium, Tel-Aviv, Israel, October 1979.
2. J. R. James, P. S. Hall and C. Woo, *Microstrip Antenna Theory and Design*, London: Institution of Engineering and Technology, 1981.
3. A. Sabban, A new wideband stacked microstrip antenna, IEEE Antenna and Propagation Symposium, Houston, TX, June 1983.
4. A. Sabban and K. C. Gupta, Characterization of radiation loss from microstrip discontinuities using a multiport network modeling approach, *IEEE Transactions on Microwave Theory and Techniques*, vol. 39, no. 4, 705–712, April 1991.
5. A. Sabban, PhD Thesis, Multiport network model for evaluating radiation loss and coupling among discontinuities in microstrip circuits, University of Colorado at Boulder, CO, January 1991.
6. A. Sabban, Inventor, *Microstrip antenna arrays*, U.S. Patent US 1986/4,623,893, 1986, USA.
7. A. Sabban, Wideband microstrip antenna arrays, IEEE Antenna and Propagation Symposium MELCOM, Tel-Aviv, Israel, June 1981.
8. A. Sabban, *Low Visibility Antennas for Communication Systems*, New York: Taylor & Francis Group, 2015.
9. G. de Lange et al., A 3*3 mm-wave micro machined imaging array with sis mixers, *Applied Physics Letters*, vol. 75, no. 6, 868–870, 1999.
10. A. Rahman et al., Micromachined room temperature microbolometers for mm-wave detection, *Applied Physics Letters*, vol. 68, no. 14, 2020–2022, 1996.
11. M. M. Milkov, MSc. Thesis, Millimeter-wave imaging system based on antenna-coupled bolometer, University of California at Los Angles, 2000.
12. M. D. Jack et al., Architecture and method of coupling electromagnetic energy to thermal detectors, U.S. Patent 6329655, 2001.
13. G. N. Sinclair et al., Passive millimeter wave imaging in security scanning, *Proceedings of SPIE*, vol. 4032, 40–45, 2000.
14. G. Kompa and R. Mehran, Planar waveguide model for computing microstrip components, *Electronics Letters*, vol. 11, no. 9, 459–460, 1975.
15. A. Luukanen et al., Imaging system functioning on submillimeter waves, U.S. Patent 6242740, 2001.
16. F. Wang, Z. Du, Q. Wang and K. Gong, Enhanced-bandwidth PIFA with T-shaped ground plane, *Electronics Letters*, vol. 40, no. 23, 1504–1505, November 2004.
17. B. Kim, J. Hoon and H. Choi, Small wideband PIFA for mobile phones at 1800 MHz, Vehicular Technology Conference, Milan, Italy, vol. 1, May 2004, pp. 27–29.
18. B. Kim, J. Park and H. Cho, Tapered type PIFA design for mobile phones at 1800 MHz, Vehicular Technology Conference, Stockholm, Sweden, vol. 2, April 2005, pp. 1012–1014.
19. A. Sabban, Inventor, Dual polarized dipole wearable antenna, U.S Patent 8203497, June 19, 2012, USA.

6 Wideband Wearable Antennas for Communication and Medical Applications

The communication and biomedical industry have been in continuous growth in the last few years. Wearable compact antennas are a major part of every wearable communication and biomedical system. Compact efficient wideband antennas affect significantly the electrical performance of wearable communication and biomedical systems. This chapter presents design considerations, computational results and measured results on the human body of several compact wideband microstrip antennas with high efficiency. For example, the compact dually polarized antenna dimensions are 5 × 5 × 0.05 cm. The antenna beam width is around 100°. The antenna's gain is around 0 dBi to 4 dBi. The proposed antennas can be used in wearable communication and medical radio frequency (RF) systems. The S_{11} results for different belt thicknesses, shirt thicknesses, and air spacing between the antennas and the human body are presented in this chapter.

6.1 INTRODUCTION

Microstrip antennas are widely employed in communication systems and seekers. They posseess attractive features that are crucial to communication and medical systems. Microstrip antennas features are low profile, flexible, light weight, and have low production cost. In addition, the benefit of a compact low-cost feed network is attained by integrating the RF frontend with the radiating elements on the same substrate. Microstrip antennas have been widely presented in books and papers in the last decade [1–7]. However, the effect of the human body on the electrical performance of wearable antennas at 434 MHz is not presented [8–13]. The RF transmission properties of human tissues have been investigated in several articles [8–9]. Several wearable antennas have been presented in the last decade [10–16]. A review of wearable and body-mounted antennas designed and developed for various applications at different frequency bands over the last decade can be found in [10]. In [11], meander wearable antennas in close proximity of a human body are presented in the frequency range between 800 MHz and 2700 MHz. In [12], the performance of a textile antenna in the vicinity of the human body is presented at 2.4 GHz. In [13], the effect of the human body on wearable 100 MHz portable radio antennas is studied. In [13], the authors concluded that wearable antennas need to be shorter by 15% to

25% from the antenna length in free space. Measurement of the antenna gain in [13] shows that a wide dipole (116 × 10 cm) has −13 dBi gain. The antennas presented in [10–13] were developed mostly for cellular applications. The requirements and frequency range for medical applications are different from those for cellular applications.

This chapter presents a new class of wideband compact wearable antennas for communication and medical RF systems. It also discusses numerical results in free space and in the presence of the human body.

6.2 WIDEBAND WEARABLE PRINTED DIPOLE ANTENNAS

This section presents two wearable antennas, first a dual polarized printed microstrip dipole and second a dual polarized folded printed microstrip dipole. The compact microstrip loaded dipole antenna has been designed to provide horizontal polarization. The antenna dimensions have been optimized to operate on the human body employing Agilent Advanced Design System (ADS) software [17]. The antenna consists of two layers. The first layer consists of RO3035 0.8 mm dielectric substrate. The second layer consists of RT-Duroid 5880 0.8 mm dielectric substrate. The substrate thickness determines the antenna bandwidth. However, thinner antennas are flexible. Thicker antennas have been designed with wider bandwidth. The printed slot antenna provide vertical polarization. In several medical systems, the required polarization can be vertical or horizontal. The proposed antenna is dually polarized. The printed dipole and the slot antenna provide dual orthogonal polarizations. The dimensions and current distribution of the dual polarized wearable antenna are presented in Figure 6.1. The antenna dimensions are 26 × 6 × 0.16 cm. The antenna can be used as a wearable antenna on a human body. It can be attached to the patient's shirt, stomach, or in the back zone. The antenna has been analyzed using Agilent ADS software. There is good agreement between measured and computed results. The antenna bandwidth is around 10% for VSWR better than 2:1. The antenna beam width is around 100°, and the gain is around 2 dBi. The computed S_{11} and S_{22} parameters are presented in Figure 6.2. Figure 6.3 presents the measured S_{11} parameters for the antenna. The computed radiation patterns are shown in Figure 6.4. The co-polar radiation pattern belongs to the yz plane. The cross-polar radiation pattern belongs to the xz plane. The antenna's cross-polarized field strength may be adjusted by varying the slot feed location. The dimensions and current distribution of

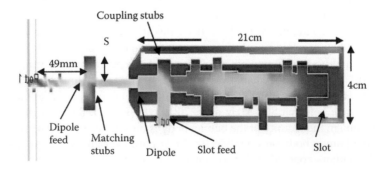

FIGURE 6.1 Current distribution of the wearable antenna.

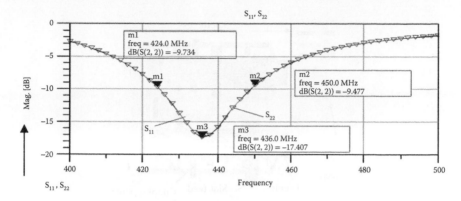

FIGURE 6.2 Computed S_{11} and S_{22} results on human body.

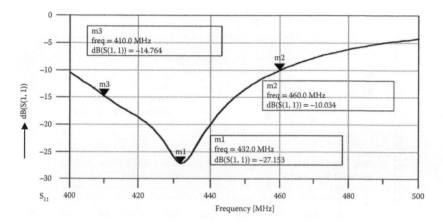

FIGURE 6.3 Measured S_{11} on human body.

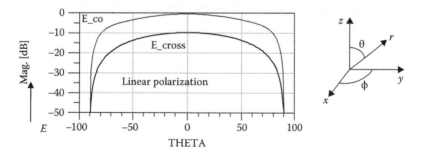

FIGURE 6.4 Antenna radiation patterns.

the folded dually polarized antenna are presented in Figure 6.5. The antenna dimensions are 6 × 5 × 0.16 cm. Figure 6.6 presents computed S_{11} and S_{22} parameters for the antenna. The computed radiation patterns of the folded dipole are shown in Figure 6.7. The antenna's radiation characteristics on the human body have been measured by using

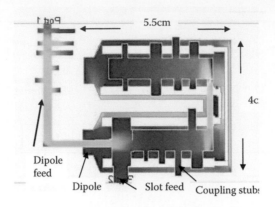

FIGURE 6.5   Current distribution of the folded dipole antenna, 6 × 5 × 0.16 cm.

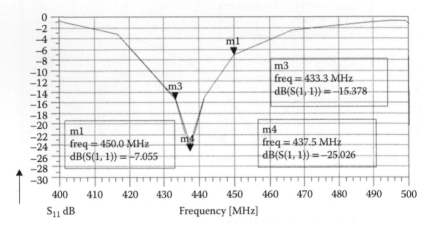

FIGURE 6.6   Folded antenna computed S_{11} and S_{22} results on the human body.

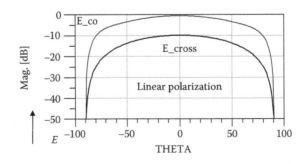

FIGURE 6.7   Folded antenna radiation patterns.

a phantom. The phantom's electrical characteristics represent the human body's electrical characteristics.

The phantom has a cylindrical shape with a 40 cm diameter and a length of 1.5 m. The phantom contains a mix of 55% water, 44% sugar, and 1% salt. The antenna under test was placed on the phantom during the measurements of the antenna's radiation characteristics. The S_{11} and S_{12} parameters were measured directly on human body by using a network analyzer. The measured results were compared to a known reference antenna.

6.3 WEARABLE LOOP ANTENNA WITH GROUND PLANE

Wearable loop antennas with ground plane are presented in this section. A wearable loop antenna with ground plane has been designed on Kapton substrates with thicknesses of 0.25 mm and 0.4 mm. The antenna without ground plane is shown in Figure 6.8a. A photo of wearable antennas is presented in Figure 6.8b. The loop antenna VSWR without the tuning capacitor was 4:1. This loop antenna can be tuned by adding a capacitor or varactor as shown in Figure 6.9. Tuning the antenna allows us to work in a wider bandwidth. Figure 6.10 presents the loop antenna with ground plane computed S_{11} on human body. There is a good agreement between measured and computed results for several loop antennas electrical parameters on human body.

The results presented in Table 6.1 indicates that the loop antenna with ground plane is matched to the human body environment, without the tuning capacitor, better than the loop antenna without ground plane. Comparison of electrical perfor-

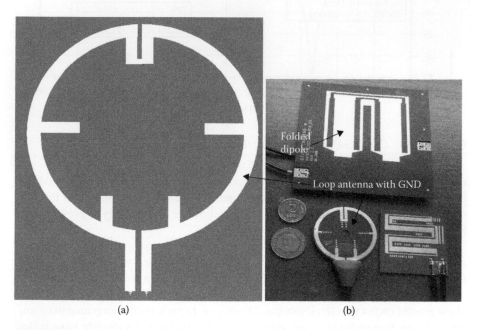

(a)   (b)

FIGURE 6.8   (a) Printed loop antenna with ground. (b) Photo of wearable antennas.

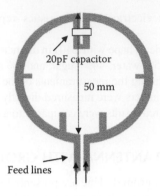

FIGURE 6.9   Tunable loop antenna without ground plane.

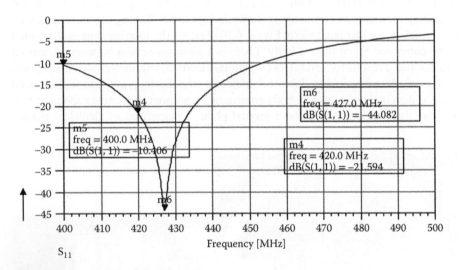

FIGURE 6.10   Computed S_{11} of a loop antenna with ground.

mance of several wearable printed antennas is given in Table 6.1. Computed S_{11} parameters of the Loop Antenna with ground, in free space, are shown in Figures 6.11. Loop Antenna with ground Radiation pattern on human body is presented in Figures 6.12.

The computed 3D radiation pattern and the coordinate system used in this chapter are shown in Figures 6.13. Computed S_{11} of the Loop Antenna with a tuning capacitor is given in Figures 6.14. Figures 6.15 presents the radiation pattern of loop antenna without ground on human body. Figures 6.16 presents a loop antenna with ground plane printed on 0.4 mm thick substrate. Figures 6.17 presents the loop antenna computed S_{11} on human body. Loop antennas printed on thicker substrate have wider bandwidth as presented in Figures 6.17. Figures 6.18 presents the loop antenna printed on 0.4mm thick substrate, radiation pattern.

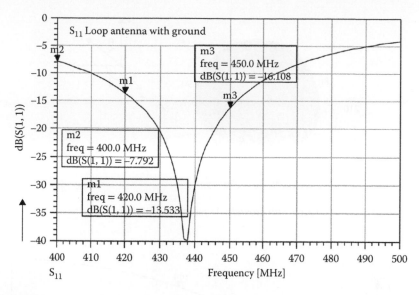

FIGURE 6.11 Computed S_{11} parameters of the loop antenna with ground in free space.

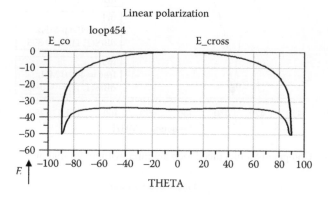

FIGURE 6.12 Radiation pattern on human body of loop antenna presented in Figure 6.8.

TABLE 6.1
Comparison of Electrical Performance of Several Printed Antennas

Parameter	Beam Width (3 Db)	Gain (dBi)	VSWR	Dimensions (cm)
Printed loop antenna	100°	0	4:1	$6 \times 5 \times 0.05$
Printed microstrip dipole	100°	2	2:1	$26 \times 6 \times 0.16$
Wearable loop with ground	100°	0–2	2:1	$6 \times 5 \times 0.05$
Folded printed microstrip dipole	100°	2–3	2:1	$6 \times 5 \times 0.16$

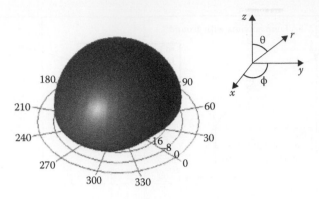

FIGURE 6.13   Loop antenna with ground, 3D radiation pattern.

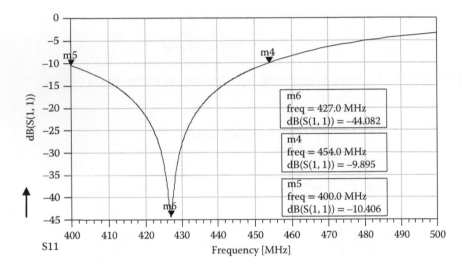

FIGURE 6.14   Computed S_{11} of a tuned loop antenna, without ground plane.

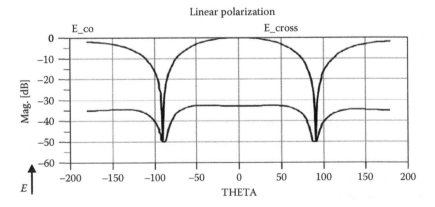

FIGURE 6.15   Radiation pattern of loop antenna without ground on human body.

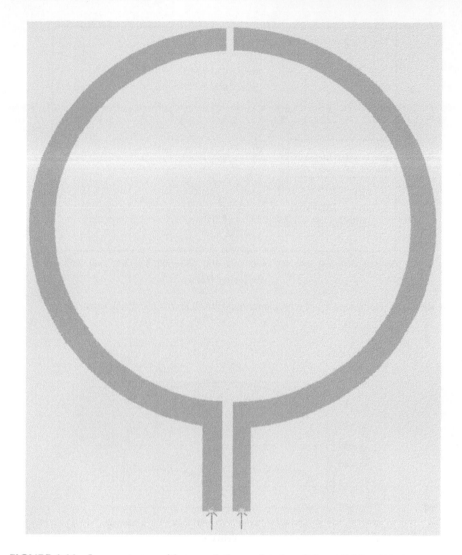

FIGURE 6.16 Loop antenna with ground plane printed on 0.4 mm thick substrate.

6.4 WEARABLE ANTENNAS IN VICINITY OF HUMAN BODY

The antenna's input impedance variation as a function of distance from the body was computed using ADS software. The analyzed structure is presented in Figure 6.19a. The antenna was placed inside a belt with a thickness between 1 and 4 mm as shown in Figure 6.19b. The patient's body thickness varied from 15 mm to 300 mm. The dielectric constant of the body varied from 40 to 50. The antenna was placed inside a belt with a thickness between 2 and 4 mm and with a dielectric constant from 2 to 4. The air layer between the belt and the patient's shirt varied from 0 mm to 8 mm. The shirt thickness varied from 0.5 mm to 1 mm. The dielectric constant of

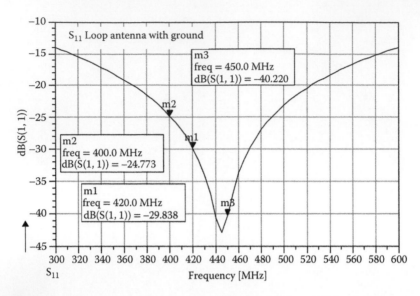

FIGURE 6.17 Computed S_{11} of a loop antenna printed on 0.4 mm thick substrate.

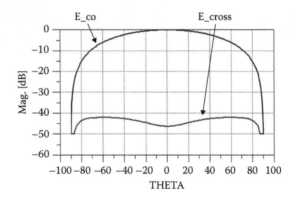

FIGURE 6.18 Loop antenna radiation pattern, printed on 0.4 mm thick Kapton substrate.

the shirt varied from 2 to 4. The properties of human body tissues are listed in Table 6.2, see [8]. These properties were employed in the antenna design. Figure 6.20 presents the S_{11} results (of the antenna shown in Figure 6.1) for different belt thicknesses, shirt thicknesses, and air spacing between the antennas and the human body.

One can conclude from the results shown in Figure 6.20 that the antenna has VSWR of better than 2.5:1 for air spacing up to 8 mm between the antennas and the patient's body. For frequencies ranging from 415 MHz to 445 MHz the antenna has VSWR better than 2:1 when there is no air spacing between the antenna and the patient's body. Results shown in Figure 6.21 indicate that the folded antenna

TABLE 6.2

Properties of Human Body Tissues

Tissue	Property	434 MHz	800 MHz	1000 MHz
Prostate	σ	0. 75	0.90	1.02
	ε	50.53	47.4	46.65
Stomach	σ	0.67	0.79	0.97
	ε	42.9	40.40	39.06
Colon, heart	σ	0.98	1.15	1.28
	ε	63.6	60.74	59.96
Kidney	σ	0.88	0.88	0.88
	ε	117.43	117.43	117.43
Nerve	σ	0.49	0.58	0.63
	ε	35.71	33. 68	33. 15
Fat	σ	0.045	0.056	0.06
	ε	5.02	4.58	4.52
Lung	σ	0.27	0.27	0.27
	E	38.4	38.4	38.4

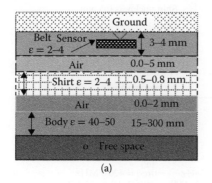
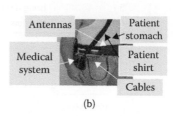

FIGURE 6.19 (a) Analyzed structure model. (b) Medical system on patient.

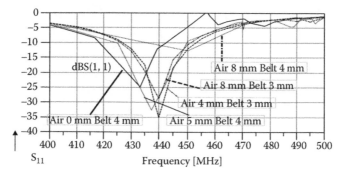

FIGURE 6.20 S_{11} results for different antenna positions relative to the human body.

(the antenna shown in Figure 6.5) has VSWR of better than 2.0:1 for air spacing up to 5 mm between the antennas and the patient's body. Figure 6.21 presents the S_{11} results of the folded antenna for different positions relative to the human body. The explanation of Figure 6.21 is given in Table 6.3. If the air spacing between the sensors and the human body increases from 0 mm to 5 mm the antenna resonant frequency shifts by 5%. The loop antenna with ground plane has VSWR better than 2.0:1 for air spacing up to 5 mm between the antennas and the patient's body. If the air spacing between the sensors and the human body increases from 0 mm to 5 mm the computed antenna resonant frequency shifts by 2%.

However, if the air spacing between the sensors and the human body increases up to 5 mm the measured loop antenna resonant frequency shifts by 5%. The explanation of Figure 6.22 is given in Table 6.4.

TABLE 6.3
Explanation of Figure 6.21

Picture #	Line Type	Sensor Position
1	Dot	Shirt thickness 0.5 mm
2	Line	Shirt thickness 1 mm
3	Dash dot	Air spacing 2 mm
4	Dash	Air spacing 4 mm
5	Long dash	Air spacing 1 mm
6	Big dots	Air spacing 5 mm

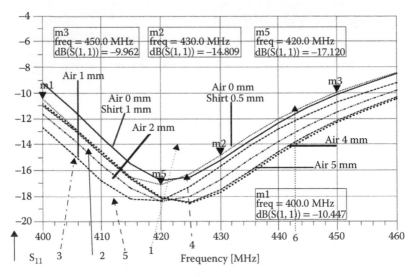

FIGURE 6.21   Folded antenna S_{11} results for different antenna position relative to the human body.

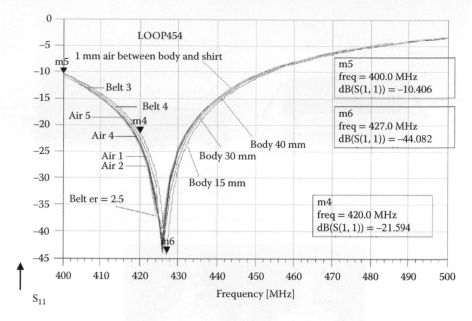

FIGURE 6.22 Loop antenna S_{11} results for different antenna positions relative to the body.

TABLE 6.4
Explanation of Figure 6.22

Plot Color	Sensor Position
Red	Body 15 mm, air spacing 0 mm
Blue	Air spacing 5 mm, body 15 mm
Pink	Body 40 mm, air spacing 0 mm
Green	Body 30 mm, air spacing 0 mm
Sky	Body 15 mm, air spacing 2 mm
Purple	Body 15 mm, air spacing 4 mm

6.5 WEARABLE ANTENNA ARRAYS

An application of the proposed antenna is shown in Figure 6.23a. Three to four folded dipole or loop antennas can be assembled in a belt and attached to the patient's stomach. The cable from each antenna is connected to a recorder. The received signal is routed to a switching matrix. The signal with the highest level is selected during the medical test. The antennas receive a signal that is transmitted from various positions in the human body. Folded antennas may be also attached on the patient's back in order to improve the level of the received signal from different locations in the human body. Wearable antennas inside a belt are shown in Figure 6.23b. Figures 6.24 and 6.25 show various antenna locations on the back and front of the human body for different medical applications. In several applications the distance separating the transmitting and receiving antennas is less than $2D^2/\lambda$. D is the largest dimension of the radiator. In these applications, the

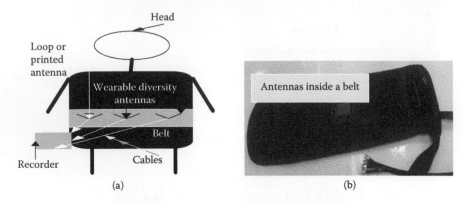

FIGURE 6.23 (a) Printed wearable antenna. (b) Wearable antennas inside a belt.

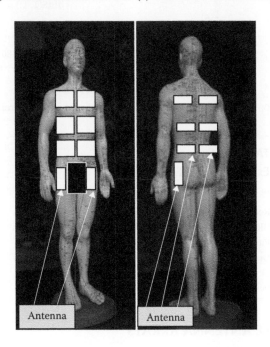

FIGURE 6.24 Printed patch antenna locations for various medical applications.

amplitude of the electromagnetic field close to the antenna may be quite powerful, but because of rapid falloff with distance, the antenna does not radiate energy to infinite distances; instead the radiated power remains trapped in the region near to the antenna. Thus, the near fields only transfer energy to close distances from the receivers. The receiving and transmitting antennas are magnetically coupled. Change in current flow through one wire induces a voltage across the ends of the other wire through electromagnetic induction. The amount of inductive coupling between two conductors is measured by their mutual inductance. In these applications, we have to refer to the near field and not to the far field radiation.

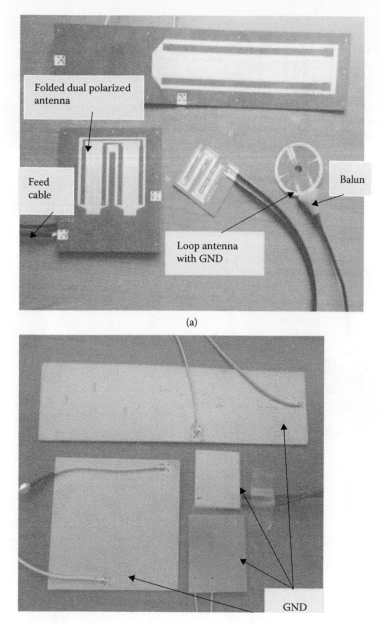

FIGURE 6.25 (a) Microstrip antennas for medical applications. (b) Backside of the antennas.

Figures 6.25 and 6.26 show several microstrip antennas for medical applications at 434 MHz. The backside of the antennas is presented in Figure 6.25b. The diameter of the loop antenna presented in Figure 6.26 is 50 mm. The dimensions of the folded dipole antenna are 7 × 6 × 0.16 cm. The dimensions of the compact folded dipole presented in Figure 6.26 are 5 × 5 × 0.05 cm.

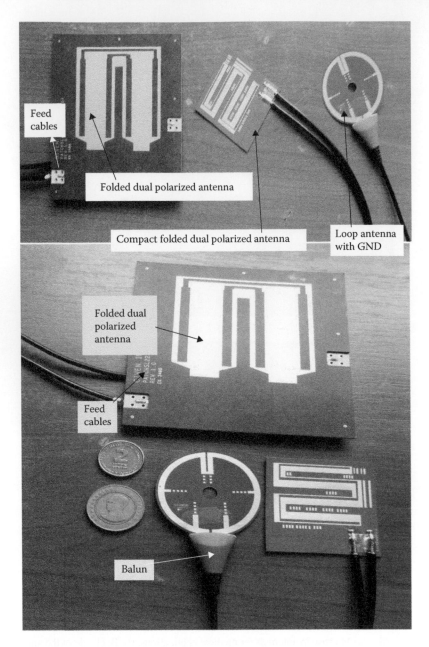

FIGURE 6.26   Microstrip antennas for medical applications.

6.6   COMPACT DUAL POLARIZED PRINTED ANTENNA

A compact microstrip loaded dipole antennas has been designed. The antenna consists of two layers. The first layer consists of FR4 0.25 mm dielectric substrate. The
second layer consists of Kapton 0.25 mm dielectric substrate. The substrate thickness

determines the antenna's bandwidth. However, with a thinner substrate we may achieve better flexibility. The proposed antenna is dual polarized. The printed dipole and the slot antenna provide dual orthogonal polarizations. The dual polarized antenna is shown in Figure 6.27. The antenna dimensions are $5 \times 5 \times 0.05$ cm.

The antenna can be attached to the patient's shirt, stomach, or back zone. It has been analyzed using Agilent ADS software. There is a good agreement between measured and computed results. The antenna bandwidth is around 10% for VSWR better than 2:1. The antenna beam width is around 100°. The antenna gain is around 0 dBi. The computed S_{11} parameters are presented in Figure 6.28. Figure 6.29 presents the antenna measured S_{11} parameters. The antenna cross-polarized field strength

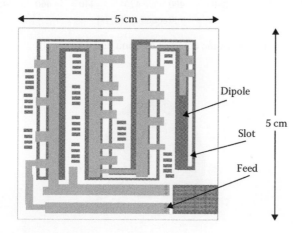

FIGURE 6.27   Printed compact dual polarized antenna.

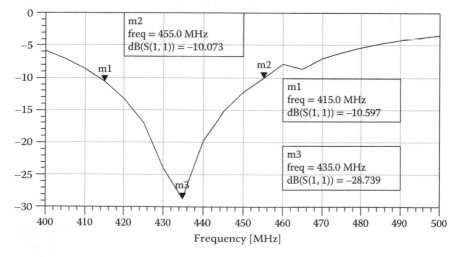

FIGURE 6.28   Computed S_{11} results of compact antenna.

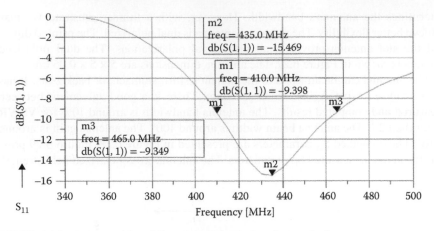

FIGURE 6.29   Measured S_{11} of the compact antenna on human body.

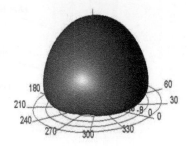

FIGURE 6.30   Compact antenna 3D radiation pattern.

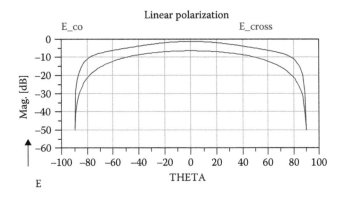

FIGURE 6.31   Compact dual polarized antenna radiation pattern.

may be adjusted by varying the slot feed location. The computed 3D radiation pattern of the antenna is shown in Figure 6.30. The computed radiation pattern is shown in Figure 6.31.

6.7 HELIX ANTENNA PERFORMANCE ON HUMAN BODY

In order to compare the variation of the antenna input impedance as a function of distance from the body to other antennas a helix antenna has been designed. A helix antenna with 9 turns is shown in Figure 6.32. The backside of the circuit is copper under the microstrip matching stubs. However, in the helix antenna area there is no ground plane. The antenna has been designed to operate on the human body. A matching microstrip line network has been designed on RO4003 substrate with 0.8 mm thickness. The helix antenna has VSWR better than 3:1 in the frequency range from 440 MHz to 460 MHz. The antenna dimensions are $4 \times 4 \times 0.6$ cm. Figure 6.33 presents the measured S_{11} parameters on human body. The computed E and H radiation plane of the helix antenna is shown in Figure 6.34. The helix antenna input impedance variation as a function of distance from the body is very sensitive. If the air spacing between the helix antenna and the human body increases from 0 mm to 2 mm the antenna resonant frequency shifts by 5%.

However, if the air spacing between the dual polarized antenna and the human body increases from 0 mm to 5 mm the antenna resonant frequency shifts only by 5%.

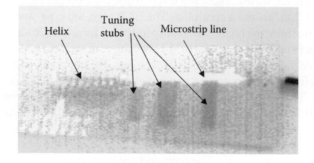

FIGURE 6.32   Helix antenna for medical applications.

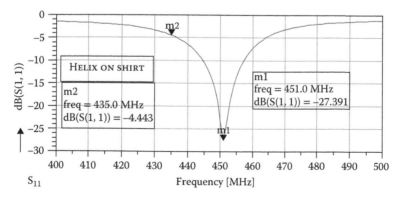

FIGURE 6.33   Measured S_{11} of the helix antenna on human body.

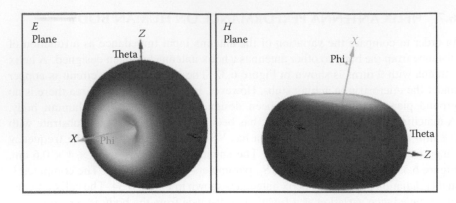

FIGURE 6.34   *E* and *H* plane radiation pattern of the helix antenna.

6.8   COMPACT WEARABLE RFID ANTENNAS

Radio **F**requency **Id**entification (RFID) is an electronic method of exchanging data over radio frequency waves. There are three major components in an RFID system: a transponder (Tag), an and a controller. The RFID tag, antenna, and controller can be assembled on the same board. Microstrip antennas have been widely presented in books and papers in the last decade [1–7]. However, compact wearable printed antennas are not widely used in 13.5 MHz RIFD systems. HF tags work best at close range but are more effective at penetrating non-metal objects, especially objects with high water content. This chapter presents wideband compact wearable printed antennas for RFID applications. The RF transmission properties of human tissues have been investigated in papers [8–9]. The effect of the human body on the antenna's performance is investigated in this chapter. The proposed antennas can be used as wearable antennas on persons or animals. The proposed antennas can also be attached to cars, trucks, containers, and various other objects.

6.8.1   Dual Polarized 13.5 MHz Compact Printed Antenna

One of the most critical elements of any RFID system is the electrical performance of its antenna. The antenna is the main component for transferring energy from the transmitter to the passive RFID tags to receive the transponder's reply signal and to avoid in-band interference from electrical noise and other nearby RFID components. Low profile compact printed antennas are crucial in the development of RIFD systems.

A compact microstrip loaded dipole antenna has been designed at 13.5 MHz to provide horizontal polarization. The antenna consists of two layers, first a layer of FR4 0.8 mm dielectric substrate and second a layer of Kapton 0.8 mm dielectric substrate. The substrate thickness determines the antenna bandwidth. A printed slot antenna provides vertical polarization. The proposed antenna is dual polarized. The printed dipole and the slot antenna provide dual orthogonal polarizations. The dual polarized RFID antenna is shown in Figure 6.35. The antenna's dimensions are 6.4 × 6.4 × 0.16 cm.

The antenna can be attached to the customer's shirt in the customer's stomach or back zone. The antenna has been analyzed using Agilent ADS software.

The antenna's S_{11} parameter is better than −21 dB at 13.5 MHz. The antenna gain is around −10 dBi. The beam width is around 160°. The computed S_{11} parameters are presented in Figure 6.36. There is good agreement between the measured and computed results. Figure 6.37 presents the measured S_{11} parameters for the antenna. The

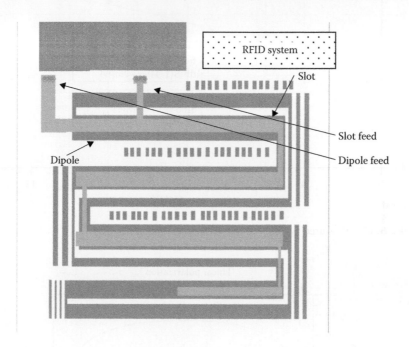

FIGURE 6.35 Printed compact dual polarized antenna, 64 × 64 × 1.6 mm.

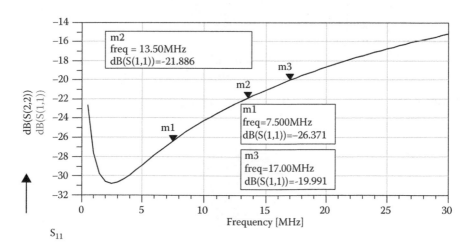

FIGURE 6.36 Computed S_{11} results.

antenna's cross-polarized field strength can be adjusted by varying the slot feed location. The computed radiation pattern is shown in Figure 6.38. The computed 3D radiation pattern of the antenna is shown in Figure 6.39.

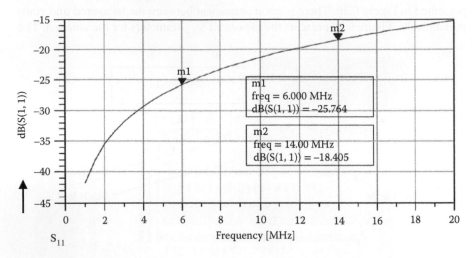

FIGURE 6.37   Measured S_{11} of the 13.5MHz antenna on human body.

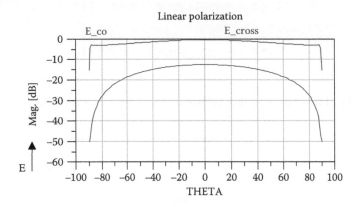

FIGURE 6.38   Radiation pattern of the 13.5MHz antenna.

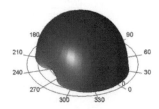

FIGURE 6.39   3D antenna radiation pattern.

6.8.2 VARYING THE ANTENNA FEED NETWORK

Several designs with different feed networks have been developed. A compact antenna with a different feed network is shown in Figure 6.40. The antenna dimensions are 8.4 × 6.4 × 0.16 cm. Figure 6.41 presents the computed S_{11} parameters for the antenna on a human body. There is good agreement between the measured and computed results. The computed radiation pattern is shown in Figure 6.42. Table 6.5 compares the electrical performance of a loop antenna with the compact dual polarized antenna.

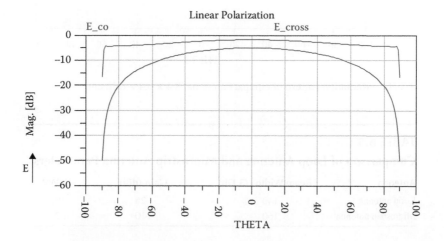

FIGURE 6.40   RFID printed antenna, 8.4 × 6.4 × 0.16 cm.

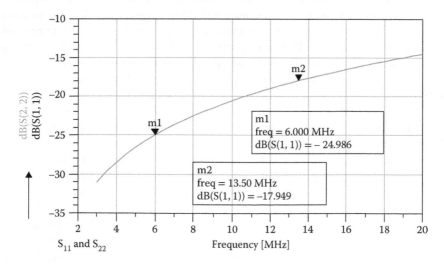

FIGURE 6.41   RFID antenna computed S_{11} and S_{22} results.

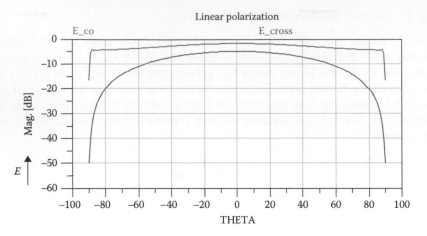

FIGURE 6.42   Radiation pattern of compact antenna, 8.4 × 6.4 × 0.16 cm.

TABLE 6.5
Comparison of Loop Antenna and Microstrip Antenna Parameters

Antenna	Beam Width° (3 Db)	Gain (dBi)	VSWR
Loop antenna	140	−25	2:1
Microstrip antenna	160	−10	1.2:1

6.8.3   RFID WEARABLE LOOP ANTENNAS

Several RFID loop antennas are presented in [15]. The disadvantages of loop antennas with number of turns are low efficiency and narrow bandwidth. The real part of the loop antenna impedance approaches 0.5 Ω. The image part of the loop antenna impedance can be represented as high inductance. A matching network can be used to match the antenna to 50 Ω. The matching network consists of an RLC matching that has narrow bandwidth. The loop antenna efficiency is lower than 1%.

A square four-turn loop antenna has been designed at 13.5 MHz by using Agilent ADS software. The antenna is printed on a FR4 substrate. The antenna dimensions are 32 × 52.4 × 0.25 mm, and the layout is shown in Figure 6.43a. A photo of the antenna is shown in Figure 6.43b. The S_{11} results of the printed loop antenna are shown in Figure 6.44. The antenna's S_{11} parameter is better than −9.5 dB without an external matching network. The computed radiation pattern is shown in Figure 6.45. The computed radiation pattern takes into account an infinite ground plane.

The microstrip antenna input impedance variation as a function of distance from the body has been computed employing ADS software. The analyzed structure is presented in Figure 6.19 and the properties of human body tissues are listed in Table 6.2, see [8]. These properties were used in the antenna design. The S_{11} parameters for different human body thicknesses have been computed. Note that the differences in the results for body thickness of 15 mm to 100 mm are

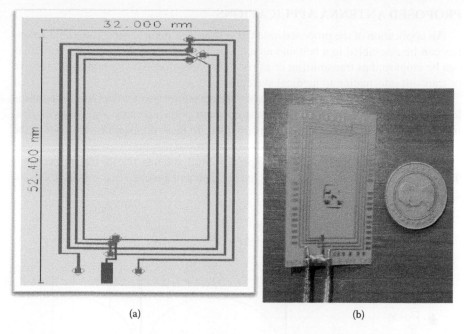

(a)   (b)

FIGURE 6.43   A square four-turn loop antenna. (a) Layout. (b) Photo.

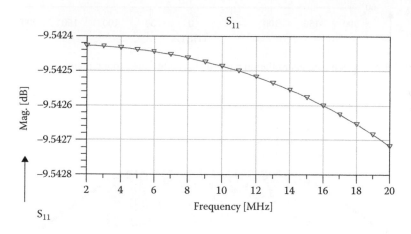

FIGURE 6.44   Loop antenna computed S_{11} results.

negligible. The S_{11} parameters for different positions relative to the human body have been computed. If the air spacing between the antenna and the human body is increased from 0 mm to 10 mm, the antenna S_{11} parameters can change by less than 1%. The VSWR is better than 1.5:1.

PROPOSED ANTENNA APPLICATIONS

An application of the proposed antenna is shown in Figure 6.46. The RFID antennas can be assembled in a belt and attached to the customer stomach. The antennas can be employed as transmitting or as receiving antennas. The antennas can receive or transmit information to medical systems.

In RFID systems, the distance between the transmitting and receiving antennas is less than $2D^2/\lambda$, where D is the largest dimension of the antenna. The receiving and transmitting antennas are magnetically coupled. In these applications we refer to the near field and not to the far field radiation pattern.

Figures 6.47 and 6.48 present compact printed antenna for RFID applications. The presented antennas can be assembled in a belt and attached to the patient's stomach or back.

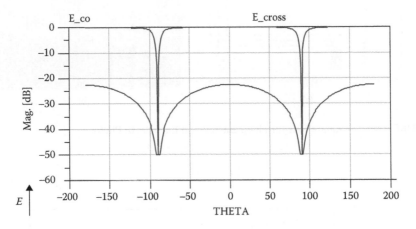

FIGURE 6.45   Loop antenna radiation patterns for an infinite ground plane.

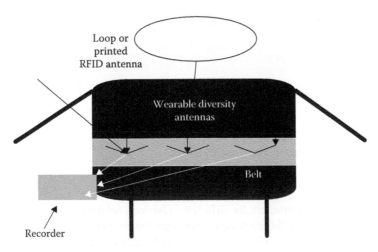

FIGURE 6.46   Wearable RFID antenna.

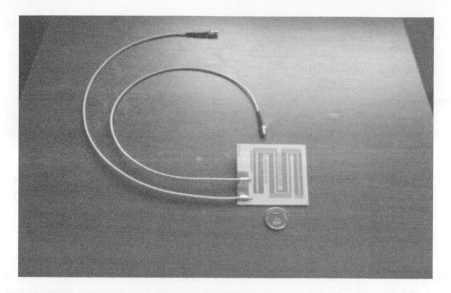

FIGURE 6.47   A microstrip antenna for RFID applications.

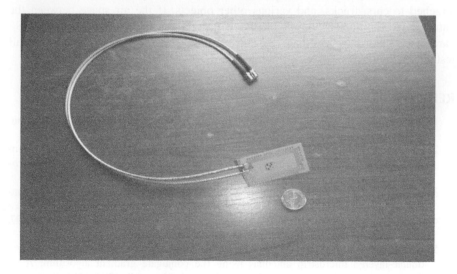

FIGURE 6.48   Loop antenna for RFID applications.

6.9   CONCLUSIONS

This chapter presents wideband microstrip antennas with high efficiency for medical applications. The antenna dimensions vary from $26 \times 6 \times 0.16$ cm to $5 \times 5 \times 0.05$ cm according to the medical system specifications. The antenna's bandwidth is around 10% for VSWR better than 2:1. The antenna's beam width is around 100°, and the gain varies from 0 to 4 dBi. The S_{11} results for different belt thicknesses, shirt thicknesses, and air spacing between the antennas and human body are presented in this chapter. If the air spacing between the dual polarized antenna and the human body is increased from 0 mm to 5 mm, the antenna resonant frequency is shifted by 5%. However, if the air spacing between the helix antenna and the human body is increased only from 0 mm to 2 mm, the antenna resonant frequency is shifted by 5%. The effect of the antenna location on the human body should be considered in the antenna design process. The proposed antenna can be used in medical RF systems.

Wideband tunable microstrip antennas with high efficiency for medical applications has been presented in this chapter. The antenna dimensions may vary from $26 \times 6 \times 0.16$ cm to $5 \times 5 \times 0.05$ cm according to the medical system specifications. The antenna's bandwidth is around 10% for VSWR better than 2:1, and the beam width width is around 100°. The antenna's gain varies from 0 to 2 dBi. If the air spacing between the dual polarized antenna and the human body increases from 0 mm to 5 mm, the antenna resonant frequency shifts by 5%. A varactor is employed to compensate for variations in the antenna resonant frequency at different locations on the human body.

This chapter also presents wideband compact printed antennas and microstrip and loop antennas for RFID applications. The beam width for the antennas is around 160°, and the gain. The antenna gain is around −10 dBi. The proposed antennas can be used as wearable antennas on persons or animals. The proposed antennas can be attached to cars, trucks, and various other objects. If the air space between the antenna and the human body is increased from 0 mm to 10 mm, the antenna S_{11} parameters change by less than 1%. The antenna VSWR is better than 1.5:1 for all tested environments.

REFERENCES

1. J. R. James, P. S. Hall and C. Wood, *Microstrip Antenna Theory and Design*, London: Institution of Engineering and Technology, 1981.
2. A. Sabban and K. C. Gupta, Characterization of radiation loss from microstrip discontinuities using a multiport network modeling approach, *IEEE Transactions on Microwave Theory and Techniques*, vol. 39, no. 4, 705–712, April 1991.
3. A. Sabban, A new wideband stacked microstrip antenna, IEEE Antenna and Propagation Symposium, Houston, TX, June 1983.
4. A. Sabban, Inventor, Dual polarized dipole wearable antenna, U.S. Patent 8203497, June 19, 2012, USA.
5. R. Kastner, E. Heyman, A. Sabban, Spectral domain iterative analysis of single and double-layered microstrip antennas using the conjugate gradient algorithm, *IEEE Transactions on Antennas and Propagation*, vol. 36, no. 9, 1204–1212, September 1988.
6. A. Sabban, Wideband microstrip antenna arrays, IEEE Antenna and Propagation Symposium MELCOM, Tel-Aviv, Israel, June 1981.
7. A. Sabban, *Microstrip Antenna Arrays, Microstrip Antennas*, N. Nasimuddin (Ed.), ISBN: 978-953-307-247-0, Croatia: InTech, pp. 361–384, 2011, Available from: http://www.intechopen.com/articles/show/title/microstrip-antenna-arrays.
8. L. C. Chirwa, P. A. Hammond, S. Roy, and D. R. S. Cumming, Electromagnetic radiation from ingested sources in the human intestine between 150 MHz and 1.2 GHz, *IEEE Transaction on Biomedical Engineering*, vol. 50, no. 4, 484–492, April 2003.

9. D. Werber, A. Schwentner, E. M. Biebl, Investigation of RF transmission properties of human tissues, *Advances in Radio Science*, vol. 4, 357–360, 2006.
10. B. Gupta, S. Sankaralingam, S. Dhar, Development of wearable and implantable antennas in the last decade, Mediterranean Microwave Symposium (MMS), 2010, Guzelyurt, Turkey, pp. 251–267.
11. T. Thalmann, Z. Popovic, B. M. Notaros, J. R. Mosig, Investigation and design of a multi-band wearable antenna, 3rd European Conference on Antennas and Propagation, EuCAP, 2009, Berlin, Germany, pp. 462–465.
12. P. Salonen, Y. Rahmat-Samii, M. Kivikoski, Wearable antennas in the vicinity of human body, IEEE Antennas and Propagation Society International Symposium, vol. 1, 2004, pp. 467–470.
13. T. Kellomaki, J. Heikkinen, M. Kivikoski, Wearable antennas for FM reception, First European Conference on Antennas and Propagation, EuCAP, 2006, Hague, Netherlands, pp. 1–6.
14. A. Sabban, Wideband printed antennas for medical applications, Asian Pacific Microwave Conference, APMC 2009, Singapore, 12/2009.
15. Y. Lee, *Antenna Circuit Design for RFID Applications*, Microchip Technology, Microchip AN 710c.
16. A. Sabban, *Low Visibility Antennas for Communication Systems*, New York: Taylor & Francis Group, 2015.
17. ADS software, Agilent, Available at: http://www.keysight.com/en/pc-1297113/advanced-design-system-ads?cc=IL&lc=eng

7 Base Station Aperture Antennas for Communication Systems

Reflector antennas, horn antennas, and antenna arrays are usually used as transmitting antennas in wireless communication base station systems. Reflector and horn antennas are defined as *aperture antennas*. The longest dimension of an aperture antenna is longer than several wavelengths.

7.1 PARABOLIC REFLECTOR ANTENNA CONFIGURATION

The *parabolic reflector* antenna [1] consists of a radiating feed that is used to illuminate a reflector that is curved in the form of an accurate parabola with diameter D, as presented in Figure 7.1. This shape enables a very narrow beam to be obtained. To provide the optimal illumination of the reflecting surface, the level of the parabola illumination should be 10 dB greater in the center than that at the parabola edges.

The reflector geometry is presented in Figure 7.2. The following relations given in Equations 7.1 through 7.4 can be derived from the reflector geometry.

Parabolic reflector antenna gain

$$G \cong 10\log_{10}\left(\alpha\frac{(\pi D)^2}{\lambda^2}\right) \tag{7.1}$$

$$PQ = r'\cos\theta' \tag{7.2}$$

$$2f = r'(1+\cos\theta') \tag{7.3}$$

$$2f = r' + r'\cos\theta' = \sqrt{(x')^2 + (y')^2 + (z')^2} + z' \tag{7.4}$$

The relation between the reflector diameter D and θ is given in Equations 7.5 through 7.8.

$$\theta_0 = \tan^{-1}\frac{\dfrac{D}{2}}{z_0} \tag{7.5}$$

153

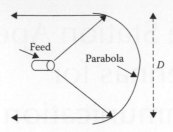

FIGURE 7.1   Parabolic antenna.

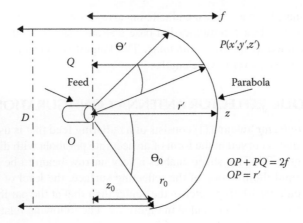

FIGURE 7.2   Reflector geometry.

$$z_0 = f - \frac{\left(\dfrac{D}{2}\right)^2}{4f} \tag{7.6}$$

$$\theta_0 = \tan^{-1}\left|\frac{\dfrac{D}{2}}{z_0}\right| = \tan^{-1}\left|\frac{\dfrac{D}{2}}{f - \dfrac{\left(\dfrac{D}{2}\right)^2}{4f}}\right| = \tan^{-1}\left|\frac{\dfrac{f}{2D}}{\left(\dfrac{f}{D}\right)^2 - \dfrac{1}{16}}\right| \tag{7.7}$$

$$f = \frac{D}{4}\cot\left(\frac{\theta_0}{2}\right) \tag{7.8}$$

7.2   REFLECTOR DIRECTIVITY

Reflector directivity is a function of the reflector geometry and feed radiation characteristics as given in Equations 7.9 and 7.10.

$$D_0 = \frac{4\pi U_{max}}{P_{rad}} = \frac{16\pi^2}{\lambda^2} f^2 \left| \int_0^{\theta_0} \sqrt{G_F(\theta')} \tan\left(\frac{\theta'}{2}\right) d\theta' \right|^2 \tag{7.9}$$

$$D_0 = \frac{(\pi D)^2}{\lambda^2} \left[\cot^2\left(\frac{\theta_0}{2}\right) \left| \int_0^{\theta_0} \sqrt{G_F(\theta')} \tan\left(\frac{\theta'}{2}\right) d\theta' \right|^2 \right] \tag{7.10}$$

The reflector aperture efficiency is given in Equation 7.11. The feed radiation pattern can be presented as in Equation 7.12.

$$\epsilon_{ap} = \left[\cot^2\left(\frac{\theta_0}{2}\right) \left| \int_0^{\theta_0} \sqrt{G_F(\theta')} \tan\left(\frac{\theta'}{2}\right) d\theta' \right|^2 \right] \tag{7.11}$$

$$G_F(\theta') = G_0^n \cos^n(\theta') \quad \text{for } 0 \le \theta' \le \frac{\pi}{2} \tag{7.12}$$

$$G_F(\theta') = 0 \quad \text{for } \frac{\pi}{2} < \theta' \le \pi$$

$$\int_0^{\frac{\pi}{2}} G_0^n \cos^n(\theta') \sin(\theta') d\theta' = 2$$

where $G_0^n = 2(n+1)$

Uniform illumination of the reflector aperture can be achieved if $G_F(\theta')$ is given by Equation 7.13.

$$G_F(\theta') = \sec^4\left(\frac{\theta'}{2}\right) \quad \text{for } 0 \le \theta' \le \frac{\pi}{2} \tag{7.13}$$

$$G_F(\theta') = 0 \quad \text{for } \frac{\pi}{2} < \theta' \le \pi$$

The reflector aperture efficiency is computed by multiplying all the antenna efficiencies due to spillover, blockage, taper, phase error, cross polarization losses, and random error over the reflector surface. $\epsilon_{ap} = \epsilon_s \epsilon_t \epsilon_b \epsilon_x \epsilon_p \epsilon_r$.

ϵ_s −spillover efficiency, written in Equation 7.14
ϵ_t −taper efficiency, written in Equation 7.15
ϵ_b −blockage efficiency
ϵ_p −phase efficiency
ϵ_x −cross polarization efficiency
ϵ_r −random error over the reflector surface efficiency

$$\epsilon_s = \frac{\int_0^{\theta_0} G_F\left(\theta'\right)\sin\theta' d\theta'}{\int_\pi^{\theta_0} G_F\left(\theta'\right)\sin\theta' d\theta'} \tag{7.14}$$

$$\epsilon_t = 2\cot^2\left(\frac{\theta_0}{2}\right)\frac{\left|\int_0^{\theta_0}\sqrt{G_F\left(\theta'\right)}\tan\left(\frac{\theta'}{2}\right)d\theta'\right|^2}{\int_0^{\theta_0} G_F\left(\theta'\right)\sin\theta' d\theta'} \tag{7.15}$$

In the literature [1] we can find graphs that present reflector antenna efficiencies as a function of reflector antenna geometry and feed radiation pattern. However, Equations 7.10 through 7.16 give us a good approximation of reflector directivity.

$$D_0 = \frac{(\pi D)^2 \epsilon_{ap}}{\lambda^2} \tag{7.16}$$

7.3   CASSEGRAIN REFLECTOR

The parabolic reflector or dish antenna consists of a radiating element which can be either a simple dipole or a waveguide horn antenna. It is placed at the center of the metallic parabolic reflecting surface as shown in Figure 7.3. The energy from the radiating element is arranged so that it illuminates the sub-reflecting surface. The energy from the sub-reflector is arranged so that it illuminates the main reflecting surface. Once the energy is reflected it leaves the antenna system in a narrow beam.

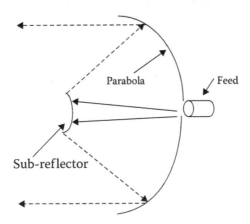

FIGURE 7.3   Cassegrain feed system.

7.4 HORN ANTENNAS

Horn antennas are used as a feed element for radio astronomy, satellite tracking, and communication reflector antennas, as phased array radiating elements, and in antenna calibration and measurements. Figure 7.4a presents an E-plane sectoral horn. Figure 7.4b presents an H-plane sectoral horn. Figure 7.4c presents a pyramidal horn. Figure 7.4d presents a conical horn.

7.4.1 E-PLANE SECTORAL HORN

Figure 7.5 presents a E-plane sectoral horn. Horn antennas are fed by a waveguide. The excited mode is TE_{10}. Fields expressions over the horn aperture are similar to the fields of a TE_{10} mode in a rectangular waveguide with the aperture dimensions of a, b_1. The fields in the antenna aperture are given in Equations 7.17 through 7.19.

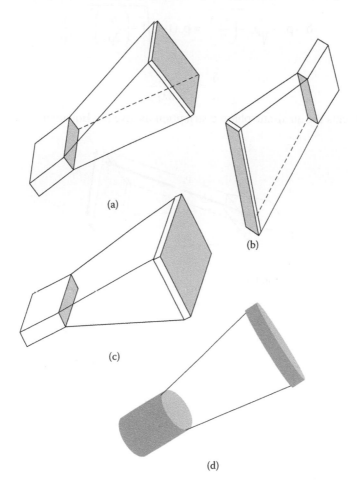

(a)

(b)

(c)

(d)

FIGURE 7.4 (a) E-plane sectoral horn. (b) H-plane sectoral horn. (c) Pyramidal horn. (d) Conical horn.

$$E_y'(x',y') \approx E_1 \cos\left(\frac{\pi}{a}x'\right)e^{-j\left[ky'^2/(2\rho_1)\right]} \tag{7.17}$$

$$H_x'(x',y') \approx \frac{E_1}{\eta} \cos\left(\frac{\pi}{a}x'\right)e^{-j\left[ky'^2/(2\rho_1)\right]} \tag{7.18}$$

$$H_z'(x',y') \approx jE_1\left(\frac{\pi}{ka\eta}\right)\sin\left(\frac{\pi}{a}x'\right)e^{-j\left[ky'^2/(2\rho_1)\right]} \tag{7.19}$$

The horn length is ρ_1, as shown in Figure 7.6. The extra distance along the aperture sides compared with the distance to the center is δ and is given by Equations 7.20 through 7.23.

$$\delta = \rho_e - \sqrt{\rho_e - \left(\frac{b_1}{2}\right)^2} = \rho_e\left(1 - \sqrt{1 - \left(\frac{b_1}{2\rho_e}\right)^2}\right) = \frac{b_1^2}{8\rho_e} \tag{7.20}$$

$$\frac{\delta}{\lambda} = S = \frac{b_1^2}{8\lambda\rho_e} \tag{7.21}$$

S represents the quadratic phase distribution as given in Equation 7.21.

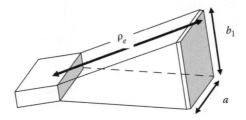

FIGURE 7.5 *E*-plane sectoral horn.

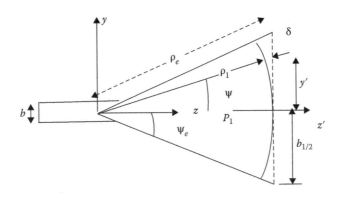

FIGURE 7.6 *E*-plane sectoral horn geometry.

$$(\delta(y') + \rho_1)^2 = \rho_1^2 + (y')^2 \qquad (7.22)$$

$$\delta(y') = -\rho_1 + \sqrt{\rho_1^2 + (y')^2} = -\rho_1 + \rho_1\sqrt{1 + \left(\frac{y'}{\rho_1}\right)^2} \qquad (7.23)$$

The maximum phase deviation at the aperture $\varnothing_{max}$ is given by Equation 7.24.

$$\varnothing_{max} = k\delta(y'):\left(y' = \frac{b_1}{2}\right) = \frac{kb_1^2}{8\rho_1} \qquad (7.24)$$

The total flare angle of the horn, $2\psi_e$, is given in Equation 7.25.

$$2\psi_e = 2\tan^{-1}\left(\frac{b_1}{2\rho_1}\right) \qquad (7.25)$$

Directivity of the E-plane horn

The maximum radiation is given by Equations 7.26 through 7.28.

$$U_{max} = \frac{r^2}{2\eta}|E|_{max}^2 \qquad (7.26)$$

$$U_{max} = \frac{2ka^2\rho_1}{\pi^3\eta}|E|^2|F(t)|^2 \qquad (7.27)$$

$$|F(t)|^2 = \left[C^2\left(\frac{b_1}{\sqrt{2\lambda\rho_1}}\right) + S^2\left(\frac{b_1}{\sqrt{2\lambda\rho_1}}\right)\right] \qquad (7.28)$$

C and S are Fresnel integers and are given in Table 7.1.
The total radiated power by the horn is given in Equation 7.29.

$$P_{rad} = \frac{ab_1}{4\eta}|E|^2 \qquad (7.29)$$

The directivity of E-plane horn D_E is given in Equation 7.30.

$$D_E = \frac{4\pi U_{max}}{P_{rad}} = \frac{64a\rho_1}{\pi\lambda b_1}\left[C^2\left(\frac{b_1}{\sqrt{2\lambda\rho_1}}\right) + S^2\left(\frac{b_1}{\sqrt{2\lambda\rho_1}}\right)\right] \qquad (7.30)$$

Figure 7.7 presents the H-plane horn radiation pattern as a function of S where $S = \frac{b_1^2}{8\lambda\rho_e}$.

TABLE 7.1
Fresnel Integers

X	$C_1(x)$	$S_1(x)$	$C(x)$	$S(x)$
0.0	0.62666	0.62666	0.0	0.0
0.1	0.52666	0.62632	0.10000	0.00052
0.2	0.42669	0.62399	0.19992	0.00419
0.3	0.32690	0.61766	0.29940	0.01412
0.4	0.22768	0.60536	0.39748	0.03336
0.5	0.12977	0.58518	0.49234	0.06473
0.6	0.03439	0.55532	0.58110	0.11054
0.7	− 0.05672	0.51427	0.65965	0.17214
0.8	− 0.14119	0.46092	0.72284	0.24934
0.9	− 0.21606	0.39481	0.76482	0.33978
1.0	− 0.27787	0.31639	0.77989	0.43826
1.1	− 0.32285	0.22728	0.76381	0.53650
1.2	− 0.34729	0.13054	0.71544	0.62340
1.3	− 0.34803	0.03081	0.63855	0.68633
1.4	− 0.32312	− 0.06573	0.54310	0.71353
1.5	− 0.27253	− 0.15158	0.44526	0.69751
1.6	− 0.19886	− 0.21861	0.36546	0.63889
1.7	− 0.10790	− 0.25905	0.32383	0.54920
1.8	− 0.00871	− 0.26682	0.33363	0.45094
1.9	0.08680	− 0.23918	0.39447	0.37335
2.0	0.16520	− 0.17812	0.48825	0.34342
2.1	0.21359	− 0.09141	0.58156	0.37427
2.2	0.22242	0.00743	0.63629	0.45570
2.3	0.18833	0.10054	0.62656	0.55315
2.4	0.11650	0.16879	0.55496	0.61969
2.5	0.02135	0.19614	0.45742	0.61918
2.6	− 0.07518	0.17454	0.38894	0.54999
2.7	− 0.14816	0.10789	0.39249	0.45292
2.8	− 0.17646	0.01329	0.46749	0.39153
2.9	− 0.15021	− 0.08181	0.56237	0.41014
3.0	− 0.07621	− 0.14690	0.60572	0.49631
3.1	0.02152	− 0.15883	0.56160	0.58181
3.2	0.10791	− 0.11181	0.46632	0.59335
3.3	0.14907	− 0.02260	0.40570	0.51929
3.4	0.12691	0.07301	0.43849	0.42965
3.5	0.04965	0.13335	0.53257	0.41525
3.6	− 0.04819	0.12973	0.58795	0.49231
3.7	− 0.11929	0.06258	0.54195	0.57498
3.8	− 0.12649	− 0.03483	0.44810	0.56562
3.9	− 0.06469	− 0.11030	0.42233	0.47521
4.0	0.03219	− 0.12048	0.49842	0.42052
4.1	0.10690	− 0.05815	0.57369	0.47580
4.2	0.11228	0.03885	0.54172	0.56320

(Continued)

TABLE 7.1 (*Continued*)
Fresnel Integers

X	$C_1(x)$	$S_1(x)$	$C(x)$	$S(x)$
4.3	0.04374	0.10751	0.44944	0.55400
4.4	− 0.05287	0.10038	0.43833	0.46227
4.5	− 0.10884	0.02149	0.52602	0.43427
4.6	− 0.08188	− 0.07126	0.56724	0.51619
4.7	0.00810	− 0.10594	0.49143	0.56715
4.8	0.08905	− 0.05381	0.43380	0.49675
4.9	0.09277	0.04224	0.50016	0.43507
5.0	0.01519	0.09874	0.56363	0.49919
5.1	− 0.07411	0.06405	0.49979	0.56239
5.2	− 0.09125	− 0.03004	0.43889	0.49688
5.3	− 0.01892	− 0.09235	0.50778	0.44047
5.4	0.07063	− 0.05976	0.55723	0.51403
5.5	0.08408	0.03440	0.47843	0.55369
5.6	0.00641	0.08900	0.45171	0.47004
5.7	− 0.07642	0.04296	0.53846	0.45953
5.8	− 0.06919	− 0.05135	0.52984	0.54604
5.9	0.01998	− 0.08231	0.44859	0.51633
6.0	0.08245	− 0.01181	0.49953	0.44696
6.1	0.03946	0.07180	0.54950	0.51647
6.2	− 0.05363	0.06018	0.46761	0.53982
6.3	− 0.07284	− 0.03144	0.47600	0.45555
6.4	0.00835	− 0.07765	0.54960	0.49649
6.5	0.07574	− 0.01326	0.48161	0.54538
6.6	0.03183	0.06872	0.46899	0.46307
6.7	− 0.05828	0.04658	0.54674	0.49150
6.8	− 0.05734	− 0.04600	0.48307	0.54364
6.9	0.03317	− 0.06440	0.47322	0.46244
7.0	0.06832	0.02077	0.54547	0.49970
7.1	− 0.00944	0.06977	0.47332	0.53602
7.2	− 0.06943	0.00041	0.48874	0.45725
7.3	− 0.00864	0.06793	0.53927	0.51894
7.4	0.06582	− 0.01521	0.46010	0.51607
7.5	0.02018	0.06353	0.51601	0.46070
7.6	− 0.06137	0.02367	0.51564	0.53885
7.7	− 0.02580	− 0.05958	0.46278	0.48202
7.8	0.05828	− 0.02668	0.53947	0.48964
7.9	0.02638	0.05752	0.47598	0.53235
8.0	− 0.05730	0.02494	0.49980	0.46021
8.1	− 0.02238	− 0.05752	0.52275	0.53204
8.2	0.05803	− 0.01870	0.46384	0.48589
8.3	0.01387	0.05861	0.53775	0.49323
8.4	− 0.05899	0.00789	0.47092	0.52429
8.5	− 0.00080	− 0.05881	0.51417	0.46534

(*Continued*)

TABLE 7.1 (*Continued*)
Fresnel Integers

X	$C_1(x)$	$S_1(x)$	$C(x)$	$S(x)$
8.6	0.05767	0.00729	0.50249	0.53693
8.7	− 0.01616	0.05515	0.48274	0.46774
8.8	− 0.05079	− 0.02545	0.52797	0.52294
8.9	0.03461	− 0.04425	0.46612	0.48856
9.0	0.03526	0.04293	0.53537	0.49985
9.1	− 0.04951	0.02381	0.46661	0.51042
9.2	− 0.01021	− 0.05338	0.52914	0.48135
9.3	0.05354	0.00485	0.47628	0.52467
9.4	− 0.02020	0.04920	0.51803	0.47134
9.5	− 0.03995	− 0.03426	0.48729	0.53100
9.6	0.04513	− 0.02599	0.50813	0.46786
9.7	0.00837	0.05086	0.49549	0.53250
9.8	− 0.04983	− 0.01094	0.50192	0.46758
9.9	0.02916	− 0.04124	0.49961	0.53215
10.0	0.02554	0.04298	0.49989	0.46817
10.1	− 0.04927	0.00478	0.49961	0.53151
10.2	0.01738	− 0.04583	0.50186	0.46885
10.3	0.03233	0.03621	0.49575	0.53061
10.4	− 0.04681	0.01094	0.50751	0.47033
10.5	0.01360	− 0.04563	0.48849	0.52804

7.4.2 *H*-Plane Sectoral Horn

An *H*-plane sectoral horn is shown in Figure 7.8. The *H*-plane sectoral horn geometry is shown in Figure 7.9.

Field expressions over the horn aperture are similar to the fields of a TE_{10} mode in a rectangular waveguide with the aperture dimensions of *a*, *b*. The fields in the antenna aperture are written in Equations 7.31 and 7.32.

$$E'_y(x',y') \approx E_2 \cos\left(\frac{\pi}{a}x'\right)e^{-j\left[kx'^2/(2\rho_2)\right]}$$ (7.31)

$$H'_x(x',y') \approx \frac{E_2}{\eta}\cos\left(\frac{\pi}{a}x'\right)e^{-j\left[kx'^2/(2\rho_2)\right]}$$ (7.32)

The horn length is ρ_l. The extra distance along the aperture sides compared with the distance to the center is δ and is given by Equations 7.33 through 7.36.

$$\delta = \rho_h - \sqrt{\rho_h - \left(\frac{a_1}{2}\right)^2} = \rho^h\left(1 - \sqrt{1 - \left(\frac{a_1}{2\rho_h}\right)^2}\right) = \frac{a_1^2}{8\rho_h}$$ (7.33)

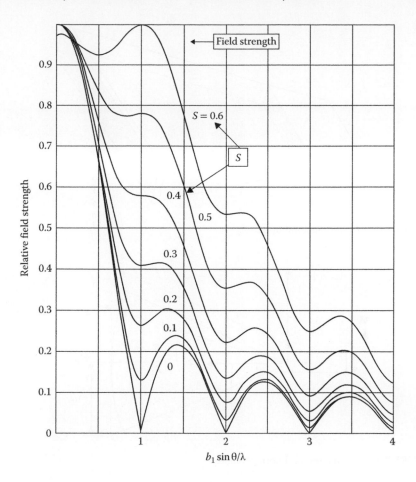

FIGURE 7.7 H-plane horn radiation pattern as function of S, $S = \dfrac{b_1^2}{8\lambda\rho_e}$.

$$\frac{\delta}{\lambda} = S = \frac{a_1^2}{8\lambda\rho_h} \tag{7.34}$$

S represents the quadratic phase distribution as written in Equation 7.34.

$$(\delta(x') + \rho_2)^2 = \rho_2^2 + (x')^2 \tag{7.35}$$

$$\delta(x') = -\rho_2 + \sqrt{\rho_2^2 + (x')^2} = -\rho_2 + \rho_1\sqrt{1 + \left(\frac{x'}{\rho_2}\right)^2} \tag{7.36}$$

The maximum phase deviation at the aperture $\varnothing_{max}$ is given by Equation 7.37.

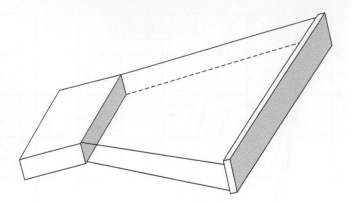

FIGURE 7.8   *H*-plane sectoral horn.

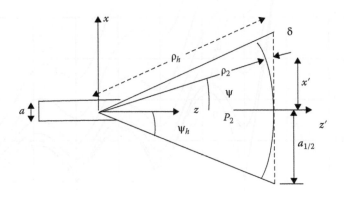

FIGURE 7.9   *H*-plane sectoral horn geometry.

$$\varnothing_{max} = k\delta(x'){:}\left(x' = \frac{a_1}{2}\right) = \frac{ka_1^2}{8\rho_2} \qquad (7.37)$$

The total flare angle of the horn, $2\psi_e$, is given in Equation 7.38.

$$2\psi_h = 2\tan^{-1}\left(\frac{a_1}{2\rho_2}\right) \qquad (7.38)$$

Directivity of the *H*-plane horn

The maximum radiation is given by Equations 7.39 and 7.41.

$$U_{max} = \frac{r^2}{2\eta}|E|_{max}^2 \qquad (7.39)$$

$$U_{max} = \frac{b^2\rho_2}{4\lambda\eta}|E|^2|F(t)|^2 \qquad (7.40)$$

$$|F(t)|^2 = [(C(u) - C(v))^2 + (S(u) - S(v))^2]$$ (7.41)

where $u = \dfrac{1}{\sqrt{2}} \left(\dfrac{\sqrt{\rho_2\lambda}}{a_1} - \dfrac{a_1}{\sqrt{\rho_2\lambda}} \right)$ and $v = \dfrac{1}{\sqrt{2}} \left(\dfrac{\sqrt{\rho_2\lambda}}{a_1} + \dfrac{a_1}{\sqrt{\rho_2\lambda}} \right)$

C and S are Fresnel integers.

The total radiated power by the horn is given in Equation 7.42.

$$P_{rad} = \frac{ab_1}{4\eta}|E|^2$$ (7.42)

The directivity of H-plane horn D_H is given in Equation 7.43.

$$D_H = \frac{4\pi U_{max}}{P_{rad}} = \frac{4b\pi\rho_2}{\lambda a_1}\left[(C(u) - C(v))^2 + (S(u) - S(v))^2\right]$$ (7.43)

The H-plane horn radiation pattern as a function of S, $S = \dfrac{a_1^2}{8\lambda\rho_h}$, is shown in Figure 7.10.

7.4.3 PYRAMIDAL HORN ANTENNA

The pyramidal horn antenna is a combination of the E and H horns as shown in Figure 7.11. The pyramidal horn antenna is realizable only if $\rho_h = \rho_e$.

The directivity of a pyramidal horn antenna D_P is given in Equation 7.44.

$$D_P = \frac{4\pi U_{max}}{P_{rad}} = \frac{\pi\lambda^2}{32ab}D_E D_H$$ (7.44)

Kraus [3] gives the following approximation, Equations 7.45 through 7.48, for pyramidal horn beam width.

$$\theta_{3dB}^e = \frac{56}{A_{e\lambda}}$$ (7.45)

$$\theta_{3dB}^h = \frac{67}{A_{h\lambda}}$$ (7.46)

$$\theta_{10dB}^e = \frac{100.8}{A_{e\lambda}}$$ (7.47)

$$\theta_{10dB}^h = \frac{120.6}{A_{h\lambda}}$$ (7.48)

The aperture dimension in wavelength in the E plane is $A_{e\lambda}$. The aperture dimension in wavelength in the H plane is $A_{h\lambda}$. The pyramidal horn gain is given by Equation 7.49.

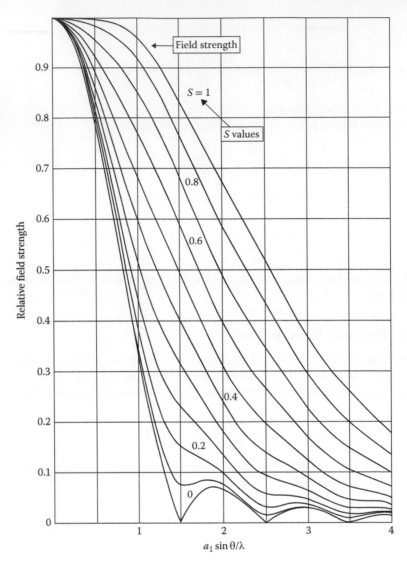

FIGURE 7.10 H-plane horn radiation pattern as function of S, $S = \dfrac{a_1^2}{8\lambda\rho_h}$.

$$G = 10\log_{10} 4.5 A_{h\lambda} A_{e\lambda} \quad \text{dBi} \tag{7.49}$$

The relative power at any angle, $P_{dB}^h (\theta)$, is given approximately by Equation 7.50.

$$P_{dB}^h(\theta) = 10 \left(\frac{\theta}{\theta_{10dB}^h} \right)^2 \tag{7.50}$$

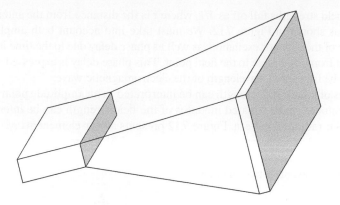

FIGURE 7.11   Pyramidal horn antenna.

7.5   ANTENNA ARRAYS FOR WIRELESS COMMUNICATION SYSTEMS

7.5.1   INTRODUCTION

An array of antenna elements is a set of antennas used for transmitting or receiving electromagnetic waves. An array of antennas is a collection of N similar radiators with the same three-dimensional radiation pattern. All the radiating elements are fed with the same frequency and with a specified amplitude and phase relationship for the drive voltage of each element. The array functions as a single antenna, generally with higher antenna gain than would be obtained from the individual elements. In antenna arrays electromagnetic wave interference is used to enhance an electromagnetic signal in one desired direction at the expense of other directions. It can also be used to null the radiation pattern in one particular direction. Antenna array theory is presented in [1–11]. Several printed arrays and the gain limitations of printed array are presented in [4–10]. Analysis and computations of losses in microstrip lines is given in [4–10]. MM wave arrays are presented in [7–10].

7.5.2   ARRAY RADIATION PATTERN

The polar radiation pattern of a single element is called the *element pattern* (EP). The array pattern is the polar radiation pattern that would result if the elements were replaced by isotropic radiators with the same amplitude and phase of excitation as the actual elements and spaced at points on a grid corresponding to the far-field phase centers of the radiators. If we assume that all the polar radiation patterns of the elements taken individually are identical (within a certain tolerance) and that the patterns are all aligned in the same direction in azimuth and elevation, then the total array antenna pattern is obtained by multiplying the array factor, AF, by the element pattern. The total array antenna pattern, ET, is ET = AF·EP.

The radiated field strength at a certain point in space in the far field is calculated by adding the contributions of each element to the total radiated fields. The summation of the contribution of each element to the total radiated fields is called the *array factor*

(AF). The field strengths fall off as $1/r$ where r is the distance from the antenna to the field point as shown in Figure 7.12. We must take into account both amplitude and phase angle of the radiator excitation, as well as phase delay due to the time it takes the signal to get from the source to the field point. This phase delay is expressed as $2\pi r/\lambda$ where λ is the free space wavelength of the electromagnetic wave.

Contours of equal field strength can be interpreted as an amplitude polar radiation pattern. Contours of the squared modulus of the field strength can be interpreted as a power polar radiation pattern. Figure 7.12 presents a four-element array. The array factor of an N-element array is given in Equation 7.51. β presents the phase difference between the elements in the array.

Figure 7.13 presents a two-element.

$$AF = 1 + e^{j\varphi} + e^{j2\varphi} + \ldots + e^{j\varphi(N-1)} = \sum_{n=1}^{N} e^{j\varphi(n-1)} \qquad (7.51)$$

where $\varphi = kd\cos\theta + \beta$ and $k = \dfrac{2\pi}{\lambda}$.

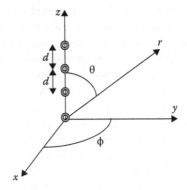

FIGURE 7.12 Coordinate system for external field calculations.

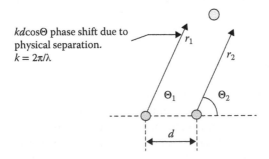

FIGURE 7.13 Two-element array.

The series summation is given in Equation 7.52.

$$AF = \frac{\sin\left(\dfrac{N\varphi}{2}\right)}{\sin\left(\dfrac{\varphi}{2}\right)} \tag{7.52}$$

The array factor is zero when $\sin\left(\dfrac{N\varphi}{2}\right) = 0$. The array nulls occur as given in Equation 7.53.

$$\theta_n = \cos^{-1}\left[\frac{\lambda}{2\pi d}\left(-\beta \pm \frac{2n}{N}\pi\right)\right] \quad n \neq N = 1,2,3\ldots \tag{7.53}$$

For $\varphi = \pm 2m\pi$, the array maximum level is given in Equation 7.54.

$$\theta_m = \cos^{-1}\left[\frac{\lambda}{2\pi d}(-\beta \pm 2m\pi) \; m = 0, 1, 2, 3\ldots\right] \tag{7.54}$$

The array 3 dB beam width is given in Equation 7.55.

$$\theta_{3\,dB} = \cos^{-1}\left[\frac{\lambda}{2\pi d}\left(-\beta \pm \frac{2.782}{N}\right)\right] \tag{7.55}$$

The peak value of the side lobe is given in Equation 7.56.

$$\theta_{SL} = \cos^{-1}\left[\frac{\lambda}{2\pi d}\left(-\beta \pm \frac{3\pi}{N}\right)\right] \tag{7.56}$$

The side-lobe level for $\beta = 0$ is -13.46 dB, as calculated in Equation 7.57.

$$AF_{SL} = 20\log_{10}\left(\frac{2}{3\pi}\right) = -13.46 \text{ dB} \tag{7.57}$$

7.5.3 BROADSIDE ARRAY

In a broadside array, the main beam is perpendicular to the array. The array radiates maximum energy perpendicular to the array if all elements in the array are fed with the same amplitude and phase level, $\beta = 0$.

The array factor is zero when $\sin\left(\dfrac{N\varphi}{2}\right)$. The array nulls occur as given in Equation 7.58.

$$\theta_n = \cos^{-1}\left(\pm\frac{n\lambda}{Nd}\right) \quad n \neq N = 1,2,3\ldots \tag{7.58}$$

For $\varphi = \pm 2m\pi$, the array maximum level is given in Equation 7.59.

$$\theta_m = \cos^{-1}\left(\frac{m\lambda}{d}\right) \quad m = 0,1,2,3\ldots \tag{7.59}$$

The array 3 dB beam width is given in Equation 7.60 when $\pi d/\lambda \ll 1$.

$$\theta_{3dB} = \cos^{-1}\left(\frac{1.391\lambda}{\pi Nd}\right) \quad \pi d/\lambda \ll 1 \tag{7.60}$$

The peak value of the side lobe is given in Equation 7.61.

$$\theta_{SL} = \cos^{-1}\left[\frac{\lambda}{2d}\left(\pm\frac{(2s+1)}{N}\right)\right] \quad s = 0, 1, 2, 3\ldots \tag{7.61}$$

7.5.4 END-FIRE ARRAY

In an end-fire array, the main beam is in the direction of the array axis. The array radiates maximum energy in the direction of the array axis, that is, $\theta = 0$ if $\beta = -kd$. The array radiates maximum energy in the direction $\theta = 180$ if $\beta = kd$.

The array nulls occur as given in Equation 7.62.

$$\theta_n = \cos^{-1}\left(1 - \frac{n\lambda}{Nd}\right) \quad n \neq N = 1,2,3\ldots \tag{7.62}$$

For $\varphi = \pm 2m\pi$, the array maximum level is given in Equation 7.63.

$$\theta_m = \cos^{-1}\left(1 - \frac{m\lambda}{d}\right) \quad m = 0,1,2,3\ldots \tag{7.63}$$

The array 3 dB beam width is given in Equation 7.64 when $\frac{\pi d}{\lambda \ll 1}$.

$$\theta_{3\,dB} = \cos^{-1}\left(1 - \frac{1.391\lambda}{\pi Nd}\right) \quad \frac{\pi d}{\lambda \ll 1} \tag{7.64}$$

The peak value of the side lobe is given in Equation 7.65.

$$\theta_{SL} = \cos^{-1}\left[\frac{\lambda}{2d}\left(1 - \frac{(2s+1)}{N}\right)\right] \quad s = 0, 1, 2, 3\ldots \tag{7.65}$$

7.5.5 PRINTED ARRAYS

In Figure 7.14a, a microstrip antenna array with a parallel feed network is shown. In Figure 7.14b a microstrip antenna array with a parallel-series feed network is presented.

Array directivity, D, can be written as $D = D_0 = \frac{U_{max}}{U_0} \sim AF\,max^2 = N$.

The half power beam width (HPBW) can be written as $2*(90 - \arccos(1.39\lambda/\pi Nd))$.

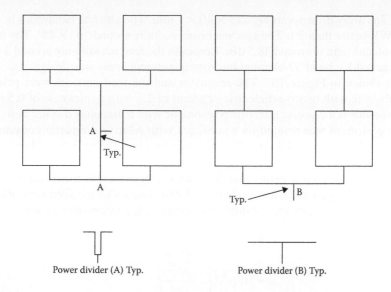

FIGURE 7.14 Configuration of microstrip antenna array. (a) Parallel feed network. (b) Parallel-series feed network.

TABLE 7.2
Array Directivity as Function of Number of Elements

No. of Elements	D_0, dB	HPBW, θ_{3dB}
4	6	26°
8	9	10°
12	10.8	9°
16	12	7°
32	15	3.5°
64	18.1	1.75°

In Table 7.2, array directivity and beam width as a function of the number of elements are listed. The radiation pattern of a 16-element broadside array is shown in Figure 7.15. The array directivity is 12 dB.

7.5.6 STACKED MICROSTRIP ANTENNA ARRAYS

A stacked Ku band 16-element microstrip antenna array was designed at 14.5 GHz as shown in Figure 7.16. The resonator and the feed network were printed on a substrate with relative dielectric constant of 2.5 with a thickness of 0.5 mm. The resonator is a circular microstrip resonator with a diameter $a = 4.2$ mm. The radiating element was printed on a substrate with a relative dielectric constant of 2.2 and with a thickness of 0.5 mm. The distance between the radiating elements is around

0.75 λ .The array dimensions are 125 × 40 × 1 mm. The antenna bandwidth is 10% for VSWR better than 2:1. The antenna beam width is around 10° × 25°. The measured antenna gain is around 18.5 dBi. Losses in the feed network are around 1 dB.

A stacked Ku band 32-element microstrip antenna array was designed at 14.5 GHz as shown in Figure 7.17. The resonator and the feed network were printed on a substrate with relative dielectric constant of 2.5 with a thickness of 0.5 mm. The resonator is a circular microstrip resonator with a diameter $a = 4.2$ mm. The radiating element was printed on a substrate with relative dielectric constant of 2.2 with a thickness of 0.5 mm. The distance between the radiating elements is around 0.75λ. The array dimensions are 125 × 125 × 1 mm. The antenna bandwidth is 10% for VSWR better than 2:1, and the beam width is around 10 × 20. The measured antenna gain is around 20.5 dBi. Losses in the feed network are around 1.5 dB. The measured results of several stacked microstrip antenna arrays

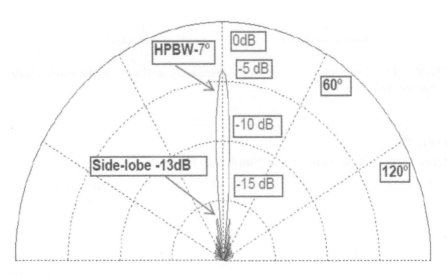

FIGURE 7.15   Radiation pattern of a 16 broadside element array.

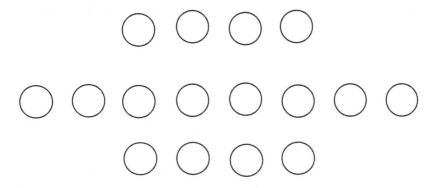

FIGURE 7.16   Stacked Ku band 16 elements microstrip antenna arrays.

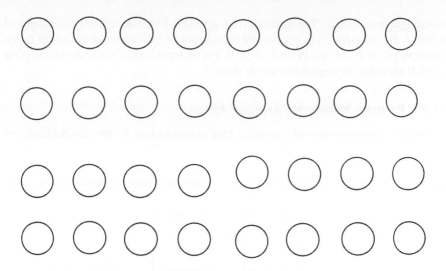

FIGURE 7.17 Stacked Ku band 32 elements microstrip antenna array.

TABLE 7.3

Measured Results of Stacked Microstrip Antenna Array

Array	F (GHz)	Bandwidth (%)	Beam Width	Gain (dBi)	Dimensions (mm)
16	14.5	10	10×25	18.5	$125 \times 40 \times 1$
32	14.5	10	10×20	20.5	$125 \times 125 \times 1$
16	10	13.5	23×23	17.0	$60 \times 60 \times 1.6$
64	34	10	10×10	23.5	$55 \times 55 \times 0.5$

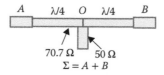

FIGURE 7.18 Power combiner/splitter.

are listed in Table 7.3. The measured gain of the 64-element array at 34 GHz is around 23.5 dBi.

A basic configuration of a power combiner/splitter is shown in Figure 7.18. This configuration of a power combiner/splitter is used in the feed network of several printed arrays. The power combiner/splitter consists of two sections of a quarter wavelength transformer. The distance from A to O is $\lambda\backslash 4$. The impedance at point O is 100 Ω. For an equal-split splitter the impedance of the quarter-wavelength transformer is $1.41 \times Z_0$, or 70.7 Ω for $Z_0 = 50$ Ω. For an input signal V, the outputs at ports A and B are equal in magnitude and in phase.

7.5.7   KA BAND MICROSTRIP ANTENNA ARRAYS

Microstrip antenna arrays with integral feed networks can be broadly divided into arrays fed by parallel feeds and series-fed arrays. Usually series-fed arrays are more efficient than parallel-fed arrays. However, parallel-fed arrays have a well-controlled aperture distribution. Two Ka band microstrip antenna arrays consisting of 64 radia-

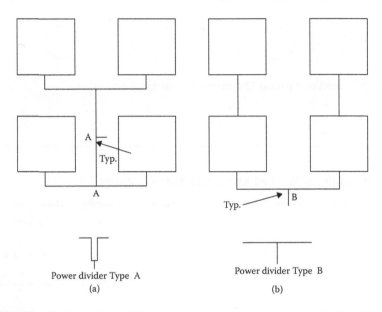

FIGURE 7.19   Configuration of 64-element microstrip antenna arrays. (a) Parallel feed network. (b) Parallel-series feed network.

TABLE 7.4
Performance of 64-Element Microstrip Antenna Arrays

PARAMETER	Corporate Feed	Parallel Feed	Corporate Feed Mix
Number of elements	64	64	64
Beam width	8.5	8.5	8.5
Computed gain (dBi)	26.3	26.3	26.3
Microstrip line loss (dB)	1.1	1.2	0.5
Radiation losses (dB)	0.7	1.3	0.7
Mismatch loss (dB)	0.5	0.5	0.5
Expected gain	24.0 dBi	23.3 dBi	24.6 dBi
Efficiency (%)	58.9	50.7	67.6

ing elements have been designed on a 10 mil Duroid substrate with $\varepsilon r = 2.2$. The first array uses a parallel feed network and the second uses a parallel-series feed network as shown in Figure 7.19a and b. Comparison of the performance of the arrays is given in Table 7.4. The results given in Table 7.4 verify that the parallel-series fed array is more efficient than the parallel-fed array due to minimization of the number of discontinuities in the parallel-series feed network.

The parallel-series fed array has been modified using a 5-cm coaxial line to replace the same length of microstrip line. The results are given in Table 7.4. i indicate that the efficiency of the parallel-series fed array that incorporates coaxial line in the feed network is around 67.6% due to minimization of the microstrip line length. Two microstrip antenna arrays that consist of 256 radiating elements have een

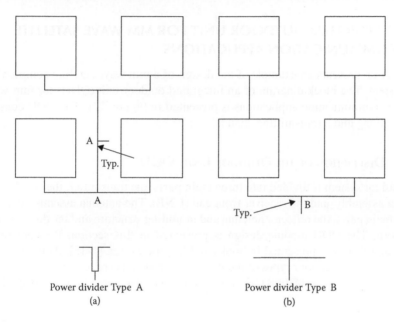

FIGURE 7.20 Configuration of 256-element microstrip antenna arrays. (a) Parallel feed network. (b) Parallel-series feed network.

TABLE 7.5

Performance of 256-Element Microstrip Antenna Arrays

Parameter	Type A	Type B	Type C
Number of elements	256	256	256
Beam width	4.2	4.2	4.2
Computed gain (dBi)	32	32	32
Microstrip line loss (dB)	3.1	3.1	1.5
Radiation losses (dB)	1	1.9	1
Mismatch loss (dB)	0.5	0.5	0.5
Expected gain (dBi)	27.43	26.5	29.03
Efficiency (%)	34.9	28.2	50.47

designed. In the first array, as shown in Figure 7.20a, using power divider Type A minimizes the number of microstrip discontinuities. The second array, Type B, as shown in Figure 7.20b, incorporates more bend discontinuities in the feed network. Comparison of the performance of the arrays is given in Table 7.5. The Type A array with 256 radiating elements has been modified using a ten-centimeter coaxial line to replace the same length of microstrip line. The performance comparison of the arrays given in Table 7.5 shows that the gain of the modified array has increased by 1.6 dB. The results given in Table 7.5 verify that the Type A array is more efficient than the Type B array due to minimization of the number of bend discontinuities in the Type A array feed network. The measured gain results are very close to the computed gain results and verify the loss computation.

7.6 INTEGRATED OUTDOOR UNIT FOR MM WAVE SATELLITE COMMUNICATION APPLICATIONS

This section presents an example of the design of a mm wave satellite communication system. The block diagram of an integrated outdoor unit (ODU) for mm wave satellite communication applications is presented in Figure 7.21. The ODU consists of a receiving and a transmitting channel.

7.6.1 DESCRIPTION OF THE OUTDOOR UNIT, ODU

The outdoor system is divided into three main parts: the transmitter, the "ODU," the antenna assembly, and the receiver front end (LNB). The antenna assembly consists of two main parts: the reflector antenna and mounting structure and the dual channel feed horn. The ODU module design is presented in this section. RF component design and theory is presented in books and in articles, see [1–15]. At the low frequency I/O terminal, four types of input and output signals are fed: transmitting, Tx, input IF signal (in 2500–3000 GHz frequency band), DC input power supply (28 V

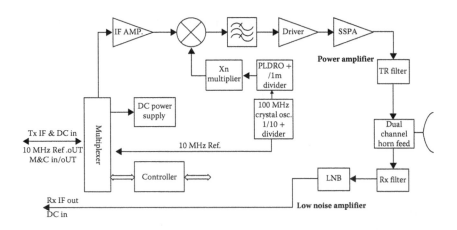

FIGURE 7.21 ODU basic block diagram

±10%), output reference (10 MHz), and monitor and control (22 KHz) IN/OUT signal.

The DC input is fed through the multiplexer to the power supply, from which regulated voltages are supplied to the different parts of the ODU. The output 10 MHz reference signal is obtained from a 100 MHz internal crystal oscillator by a 1:10 frequency divider and is routed to the I/O connector through the multiplexer. The monitor and control (22 KHz) signal is separated from the other signals by the multiplexer between the I/O connector and the controller. The control command ON/OFF is processed by the controller and applied to the SSPA supply ON/OFF switch. The monitoring signals, originating from different parts of the ODU, are processed by the controller and installed in the 22 KHz serial link. The PLDRO Lock/Unlock monitoring signal is used (via the controller) for switching the SSPA supply ON/ OFF accordingly (automatic shutdown). Additional alarm monitoring signals are provided by switching the 10 MHz signal from ON to OFF state (by the controller) if any of the alarm signals (PLDRO unlocked, SSPA supply in the OFF state, or power-supply alarm) appears at the controller inputs. The input IF signal (in frequency band 2500–3000 GHz) is separated from the other inputs by the multiplexer and is fed to the IF amplifier. The IF signal is amplified to an appropriate level (the IF amplifiers amplify the input IF signal from the minimum input level to the nominal level at the mixer input) and is fed to the mixer input.

The frequency band of the input signal is converted to the transmitted frequency band by the mixer and the LO signal. The band-pass filter, following the mixer output, attenuates the LO signal leaking (at 27 GHz), image signal, and other spurious products. The filtered Tx signal is amplified by the driver and the power amplifier (PA) to the appropriate output power level. The Tx band pass following the power amplifier attenuates all the spurious signal levels below the relevant specified levels and also the output noise, in the receiving (Rx) frequency band, below the thermal noise at the LNB (Rx link) input. The LO source consists of a PLDRO, multiplier, and a band-pass filter. The PLDRO is locked to a 100 MHz (internal) crystal oscillator. The output signal (at 9 or 13.5 GHz) is multiplied by the frequency multiplier to the specified frequency (27 GHz) and filtered to eliminate the spurious signals. All the above-mentioned components are installed in a mechanical enclosure that protects them from the outside environment and dissipates the heat, by convection, to the air outside the enclosure. Two connectors are mounted on the enclosure (box): input I/O (Type F connector) and output (ISO PBR 320 for WR-28 waveguide). The ODU box is mounted directly to the dual channel feed horn through the waveguide flange. The ODU, dual channel feed horn, and the LNB are assembled on a special mounting cradle, which is mounted on the antenna boom and allows the rotation of the ODU, the LNB, and the antenna feed around the feed axis for polarization adjustment. The ODU specifications are listed in Table 7.1.

7.6.2 The Low Noise unit, LNB

The LNB is of universal standard one with a circular C-120 Flange at the input. The LNB is mounted directly to the Dual Channel Feed Horn through the C-120 flange.

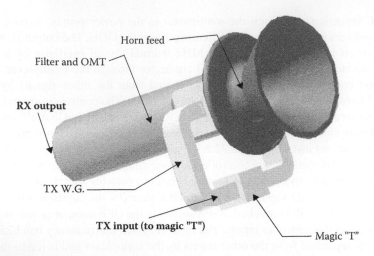

FIGURE 7.22 Outdoor unit drawing.

This LNB is produced by several manufacturers and is available on the commercial market. The full description and specification of the LNB is listed in Table 7.6 with an exception that the maximum Noise figure should be 0.9 dB for both receiving bands. The LNB output may be connected through the ODU to enable the use of only one coaxial cable between the indoor unit, IDU, and the outdoor assembly. For that purpose, a special power supply must be added into the ODU enclosure, an appropriate protocol must be specified and the Multiplexer must be redesigned to allow the filtering of the different signals at the ODU's I/O terminal (Figure 7.22). The antenna assembly losses up to the antenna feed output are 0.8 dB as presented and listed here.

Calculations of the antenna assembly losses

- Dual Band Feed Horn's Insertion loss:	0.5 dB max.
- Transmitter Filter and WG28 W.G Loss	0.2 dB max.
- Mismatch Loss (WSWR<1.35):	0.1 dB max.
	Total Loss: 0.8 dB max.

Calculations of the Minimum SSPA Output power is listed here.

Calculations of the Minimum SSPA Output power

Reflector antenna	Antenna I	Antenna II	Antenna III
Antenna Gain at Ka band:	45.0dBi	47.0dBi	49.5dBi
Tx to Feed Output Loss:	0.8 dB	0.8 dB	0.8 dB
Net. Gain:	44.2dBi	46.2dBi	48.7dBi
Specified EIRP:	40.0dBW	45.0dBW	50.0dBW
Minimum SSPA Output:	-4.2dBw	-1.2dBW	+1.3dBW

TABLE 7.6
ODU Specifications

Description	Specification
Transmit Frequency range	29.5 ÷ 30.0 GHz
Receive Frequency range, in two bands:	10.7 ÷ 12.75 GHz
Low:	10.7 ÷ 11.7 GHz
High:	11.7 ÷12.75 GHz
Transmit: on one linear (Horizontal, H, or Vertical, V,) polarization plane. Receive dual linear orthogonal polarized signal by switching between H and V polarization	
Selecting the polarization orientation. Continuous adjustment of the polarization orientation: Identical antenna tilt angle.	H or V $\pm45^0$ Ka and Ku signals
min. EIRP & 1db gain compression:	
@max. antenna diameter 0.75 m:	40dBW
@max. antenna diameter 0.95 m:	45dBW
@max. antenna diameter 1.30 m:	50dBW
Off-axis EIRP density, max. :	10 W/m²
EIRP stability over temperature:	± 2 dB
G/T Figure of Merit:	> 14 dB/K
Description	Specification
Spurious Emission below the total EIRP:	
In /out 29.5 ÷ 30.0 GHz band.	60 dB max.
Noise Emission max. in 29.5÷30.0 GHz band:	
SSPA - ON:	-75dBW/Hz of EIRP
SSPA - OFF:	-105dBW/Hz of EIRP
Phase Noise, max.: Freq. Offset	
(For the transmitter) 10 Hz	-32dBC/Hz
100 Hz	-62dBC/Hz
1 kHz	-72dBC/Hz
10 kHz	-82dBC/Hz
> 100 kHz	-92dBC/Hz
Spurious phase noise at AC line frequency. Level of the sum of all phase noise components in frequency range from AC line freq. to 1MHz.	-32dBC max. -38dBC max.
Amplitude Variation (Transmitter only), in any 200 kHz band:	0.2 dB max.
2 MHz band:	0.4 dB max.
40 MHz band:	1.0 dB max.
500 MHz band:	2.5 dB max.
Group Delay Variations (transmitter only) in any 2 MHz band:	2 ns max. ptp
40 MHz band:	4 ns max. ptp
Radiation Pattern (Transmitter only),	
$1.8^0 < \Phi < 7^0$	29 ÷ 25logΦ dBi max.
$7^0 < \Phi < 9.2^0$	8dBi max.
$9.2^0 < \Phi < 48^0$	32 ÷ 25log ΦdBi max.
$48^0 < \Phi < 180^0$	0dBi max.
Tx cross polar gain: $1.8^0 < \Phi < 7^0$	19 ÷ 25logΦ dBi max.
$7^0 < \Phi < 9.2^0$	-2dBi max.

(Continued)

TABLE 7.6
ODU Specifications

Description	Specification
Tx Cross-pole Isolation within 1/10 dB beam contour:	-25/-22 dB max.
Antenna Pointing, manual adjustment: Elevation:	$10^0 \div 50^0$
Azimuth:	$0^0 \div 360^0$
Pointing Accuracy (mechanical coarse & fine adjustment)	10% of the 3dB beam-width
TX Power consumption: SIT I :	20 W
SIT II:	30 W
SIT III:	50 W
Safety SSPA Switch-OFF:	Automatic shut down
Avoiding interference to other users.	
Monitoring functions:	Lock Alarm
	SSPA ON/OFF Status
Control:	Power Supply Alarm
SSPA ON/OFF Indication on ODU	Presence det. Alarm
	SSPA ON/OFF. Green/Red
	LED.
Operation Environment: Temperature:	$-30^0 \div +50^0$
Solar Radiation:	500 W/m^2 max.
Humidity:	0÷100% (condensing)
Rain/ Wind	40 mm/h max/45 km/h max.
Survival Conditions: Temperature:	$-40^0 \div +60^0$
Solar Radiation:	1000 W/m^2
Humidity:	0÷100% (condensing)
Precipitation: Rain:	100 mm/h max.
Freezing rain:	12 mm/h max.
Snowfall:	50 mm/h max.
Static load:	25mm of ice on all surfaces
Wind:	120 km/h max.
Storage & Transportation:	$-40^0 \div +70^0$
Temperature:	As required for commercial
Shock and Vibration:	freights
IDU & ODU, DC-power supply:	28 V ± 10%
Tx IF IN (2.5÷3GHz):	-40dBm
M&C: 10 MHz Ref. Output Power:	22 kHz PWK
Freq. Stability: Connector: Tx Output Flange.	-40dBm±20 ppm
(Tx to antenna Feed):	Type F - ISO PBR 320
Storage & Transportation:	$-40^0 \div +70^0$
Temperature:	As required for commercial
Shock and Vibration:	freights
IDU & ODU, DC-power supply:	28 V ± 10%
Tx IF IN (2.5÷3 GHz):	-40 dBm
M&C: 10 MHz Ref. Output Power:	22 kHz PWK
Freq. Stability: Connector: Tx Output Flange.	-40 dBm±20 ppm
(Tx to antenna Feed):	Type F – ISO PBR 320

7.6.3 SOLID STATE POWER AMPLIFIER, SSPA, OUTPUT POWER REQUIREMENTS

	SIT I	SIT II	SIT III
Antenna Gain at Ka band:	45.0dBi	47.0dBi	49.5dBi
Tx to Feed Output Loss:	0.8 dB	0.8 dB	0.8 dB
Net. Gain:	44.2dBi	46.2dBi	48.7dBi
Specified EIRP:	40.0dBW	45.0dBW	50.0dBW
Minimum SSPA Output:	-4.2 dBw	-1.2dBW	+1.3dBW

7.6.4 ISOLATION BETWEEN RECEIVING, RX, AND TRANSMITTING, TX, CHANNELS

Since the Tx and the Rx signal can appear at the feed with the same polarization, the isolation between the transmitter (Tx) port and the receiver (Rx) port is mainly achieved by the Rx input filter. The main objectives of the Rx input filter are to prevent the gain degradation of the LNB, to eliminate spurious response (mixing with the harmonics of the LOs in the LNB), and to reject signals at the image frequencies.

The isolation can be estimated for the following data:

Maximum Tx signal level at the Tx Port: +33 dBm
Output 1 dB compression point of the LNB: +5 dBm
LNB gain (max): 60 dB

According to these assumptions the input 1 dB comp. point of the LNB is around 55 dBm and the isolation must be at least 88 dB. The LNA inside the LNB is tuned to the 10.7–12.75 GHz range. Following the LNA, a band-pass filter is used to reject the image signal.

7.7 SOLID STATE POWER AMPLIFIER, SSPA

7.7.1 SPECIFICATIONS

- Input power: −15 dBm
- The output power level result from the system parameters as listed in Table 7.7.

TABLE 7.7

Output Power Requirements for Three Situations (SIT)

	EIRP Spec. (dBW)	Required PA Output [a](1) dBm (dBW)	PA to Feed Output Loss	Antenna Gain (dBi)	Antenna Diameter (m)
SIT1	40	25.8 (−4.2 dBW)	0.8	45	0.6
SIT2	45	28.8 (−1.2 dBW)	0.8	47	0.75
SIT3	50	31.3 (+1.3 dBW)	0.8	49.5	1.35

[a](1) Output power required at P1 dB

Reflector antenna design

For 50 dBW EIRP the required antenna gain should be 49.5 dBi. By using Equations 7.1 through 7.16 we get that the antenna diameter should be 1.35 m. The antenna efficiency is around 50% and the reflector antenna beam width is around 0.4°. The focal point distance for $f/D = 0.3$ is around 0.4 m. The reflector antenna electrical parameters are listed in Table 7.8.

7.7.2   SSPA GENERAL DESCRIPTION

The module is an integral MIC assembly which includes the upconverter, SSPA, output power detector, and transition to the antenna as shown in Figure 7.23. The key element for the realization of the ODU SSPA is the output stage basic MMIC power amplifier.

TABLE 7.8
Reflector Antenna Electrical Parameters

	EIRP Spec. (dBW)	Antenna Gain (dBi)	Antenna Diameter (m)	Beam Width °
SIT1	40	45	0.8	0.65
SIT2	45	47	1	0.52
SIT3	50	49.5	1.35	0.4

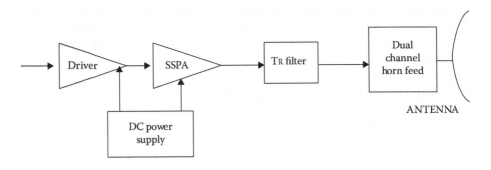

FIGURE 7.23   Block diagram of the SSPA unit.

TABLE 7.9
Situation 1

	P in	Low P.A	Medium P.A	High P.A
Power	−15 dBm	−5 dBm	13.5 dBm	26 dBm
Gain	−	10 dB	18.5 dB	12.5 dB
P1 dB	−	8 dBm	19 dBm	27 dBm

Power supply: ±5 v, 7 W

TABLE 7.10
Situation 2

	P in	Low P.A	Medium P.A	High P.A
Power	−15 dBm	−3 dBm	16 dBm	28.5 dBm
Gain		12 dB	19 dB	12.5 dB
P1 dB		8 dBm	19 dBm	29 dBm

Power supply: ±5 v, 10 W

TABLE 7.11
Situation 3

	P in	Low P.A	Medium P.A	High P.A
Power	−15 dBm	−1 dBm	18 dBm	31 dBm
Gain	−	14 dB	19 dB	13 dB
P1 dB	−	8 dBm	19 dBm	31.5 dBm

Power supply: ±5 v, 15 W

TABLE 7.12
Supplies

	Drain Voltage (V)	Gate Voltage (V)	DC Power (W)	Drain Current (Amp.)
SIT1	5	−5	7	1.4
SIT2	5	−5	10	2
SIT3	5	−5	15	3

7.7.3 SSPA Electrical Design

1. Input power: −15 dBm
2. The output power requirements result from the following system parameters:

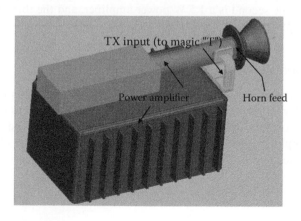

FIGURE 7.24 ODU package.

Power amplifier power and gain budget

1. Input power: −15 dBm
2. The output power requirements result from system parameters given in Tables 7.9 to Table 7.11.

The power supply requirements are listed in Table 7.12.

7.7.4   THE ODU MECHANICAL PACKAGE

The ODU package combines all antenna feed components and driving electronics. The RF chain consists of a horn feed, transducer, filter, and the LNB as shown in Figure 7.24. The ODU package is designed to ensure full compliance with the mechanical requirements listed in Table 7.6. The package houses the SSPA, up-converter, PLDRO, controller, and a power supply. The ODU is mounted on the boom of the antenna using mechanics that allow adjustment of the polarization angle, while maintaining accurate position of the horn on the antenna's focal point. The ODU's package is designed for cost effectiveness and large volume production, while it protects its inner components from precipitation, dissipates the heat generated within, and is coated and painted to absorb minimum solar radiation.

7.8   SOLID STATE HIGH POWER AMPLIFIERS, SSPA, FOR MM WAVE COMMUNICATION SYSTEM

This section describes the design and performance of new compact and low-cost Ka band power amplifiers. The main features of the power amplifiers are 27 dBm to 35 dBm minimum output power for −16 dBm input power over the frequency range of 27.5–31 GHz. To reduce losses MIC, MMIC, and waveguide technologies are employed in the development and fabrication of this set of power amplifiers. Employing waveguide technology has minimized losses in the power combiner.

Three power amplifiers are described in this section. The first amplifier is a 0.5 W power amplifier, the second is a 1.5 W power amplifier, and the third amplifier is a 3.2 W power amplifier.

7.8.1   INTRODUCTION

An increasing demand for wide bandwidth in communication links makes the Ka band attractive for future commercial systems. This section describes the design and performance of compact and low-cost Ka band power amplifiers. The main features of the power amplifiers are 27–35 dBm minimum output power for −16 dBm input power over the frequency range of 27.5–31 GHz.

7.8.2 POWER AMPLIFIER SPECIFICATIONS

The transmitting channel specifications were listed in Table 7.6. The power amplifier specifications are listed in Table 7.13.

7.8.3 DESCRIPTION OF THE 0.5 W AND 1.5 W POWER AMPLIFIERS

The block diagram of the 0.5 W and 1.5 W power amplifier is shown in Figure 7.25. The 0.5 W power amplifier consists of a low-power MMIC amplifier, band-pass filter, medium-power MMIC amplifier, and 0.5 W power amplifier. The 1.5 W power amplifier consists of the same modules as the 0.5 W power amplifier. The 0.5 W

TABLE 7.13
Power Amplifier Specifications

Parameter	Specification
Frequency range	27.5–31 GHz
Input power	−16 − −20 dBm
Output power, minimum	27, 32, 35 dBm minimum
Input VSWR	2:1
Output VSWR	2:1
Spurious level	−60 dBc
Supply voltage	±5 V
Connectors	K−connectors
Operating temperature	−30° C−60° C
Storage temperature	−50° C−80° C
Humidity	100%

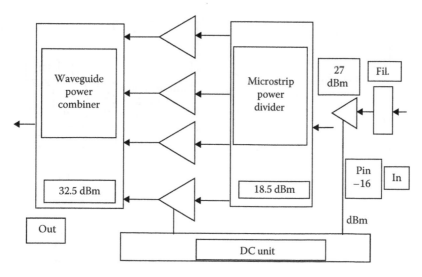

FIGURE 7.25   1.5 W power amplifier block diagram.

MMIC amplifier is connected to a four-way microstrip power divider, a high-power module with four MMIC power amplifiers, a four-way waveguide power combiner, and a DC supply unit. Three stages of MMIC power amplifiers amplify the input signal from −16 dBm to 18 dBm. The fourth stage, a 0.5 W MMIC power amplifier, is connected to a four-way hybrid ring microstrip power divider printed on 10 mil duroid. The output ports of the power divider are connected to four 0.5 W MMIC power amplifier. The 0.5 W power amplifiers are combined via a four-way waveguide power combiner to yield a 32.5 dBm minimum output power level. The DC bias voltages of each MMIC amplifier has been experimentally optimized to achieve the required gain and output power level.

TABLE 7.14
Transmitter Gain and Power Budget

Component	Gain/Loss (dB)	Pout (dBm) 0.5 W	Pout (dBm) 1.5 W
Input power	----	−16	−16
Amplifier	15	−1	−1
Filter	−1	−2	−2
Amplifier	20	18	18
Amplifier	9	27	27
4-way power divider	−7.5	−	19.5
Amplifier	8	−	27.5
4-way power combiner	5.5	−	33
Total	49	−	33

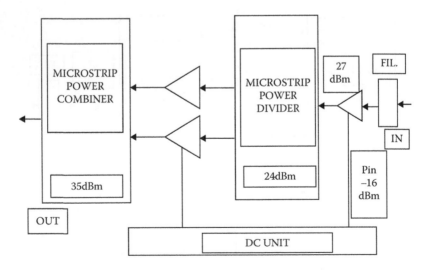

FIGURE 7.26   3.2 W power amplifier block diagram.

7.8.4 GAIN AND POWER BUDGET FOR THE 0.5 W AND 1.5 W AMPLIFIRES

The power amplifier's gain and power budget is listed in Table 7.14. The expected large signal gain of the 1.5 W amplifier is 49 dB. The expected output power is 33 dBm.

7.8.5 DESCRIPTION OF THE 3.2 W POWER AMPLIFIER

The block diagram of the 3.2 W power amplifier is shown in Figure 7.26. The 3.2 W power amplifier consists of the same modules as the 0.5 W power amplifier. The 0.5 W MMIC amplifier is connected to a two-way microstrip power divider, a high power module with two 2 W MMIC power amplifiers, and a two-way microstrip power combiner. Three stages of MMIC power amplifiers amplify the input signal from –16 dBm to 18 dBm. The fourth stage, a 0.5 W MMIC power amplifier, is connected to a two-way microstrip power divider printed on 5 mil alumina substrate. The output ports of the power divider are connected to two 2 W MMIC power amplifiers. The 2 W output power is combined via a two-way low loss power combiner to yield a 35 dBm minimum output power level. The DC bias voltages of each MMIC amplifier have been experimentally optimized to achieve the required gain and output power level.

7.8.6 MEASURED TEST RESULTS

Two different 1.5 W power amplifier modules were fabricated and tested. The first power amplifier is a modular unit and consists of seven modules. The unit consists of a band-pass filter, low power amplifier, medium power amplifier, four-way microstrip power divider module, four 0.5 W power amplifiers, a four-way microstrip power

---

TABLE 7.15
Measured Test Results of the Modular and Integrated Power Amplifier

Parameter	Measured Results Modular 1.5 W Amp.	Measured Results Integrated 1.5 W Amp.
Frequency range (GHz)	27–31	27–31
Input power (dBm)	–16	–16
Output power (dBm)	31.5	31.5
Spurious level (dBc)	> –50	> –50
VSWR (input/output)	2:1	2:1

TABLE 7.16
Measured Test Results of the Four-Way Waveguide Power Combiner

Parameter	Measured Results
Frequency range	27–31 GHz
Insertion loss	0.5 dB
Amplitude balance	0.2 dB max.
Phase balance	±5 max.
VSWR (input/output)	1.5:1

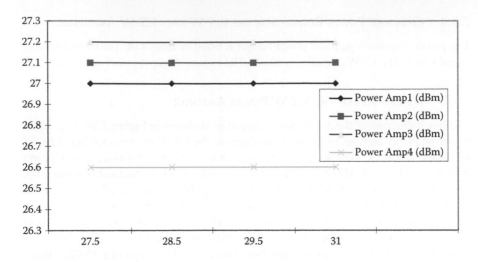

FIGURE 7.27 Output power balance of the 0.5 W power amplifier.

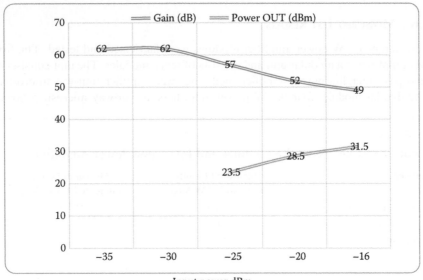

FIGURE 7.28 Output power and gain of the 1.5 W power amplifier.

combiner, and a DC supply unit. The second power amplifier is an integrated power amplifier as described in Section 7.7.5. Test results of the modular and integrated power amplifier are given in Table 7.15. The measured test results of the four-way waveguide power combiner are listed in Table 7.16.

Figure 7.27 presents the output power balance of the 0.5 W power amplifier. Figure 7.28 presents the output power and gain of the 1.5 W power amplifier. A photo

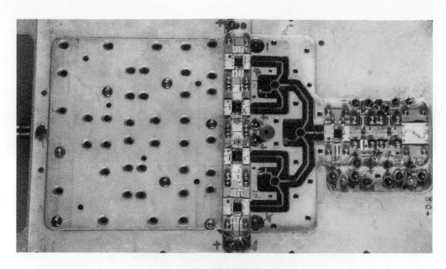

FIGURE 7.29 Photo of the 1.5 W power amplifier.

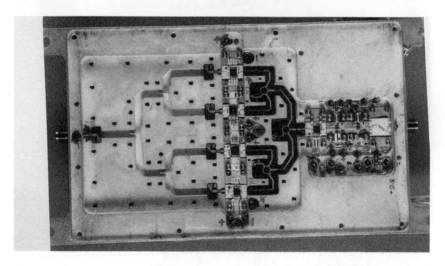

FIGURE 7.30 Photo of the 1.5 W power amplifier with a four-way waveguide power combiner.

of the 1.5 W power amplifier is shown in Figure 7.29. The four-way waveguide power combiner is covered by a metallic cover.

Figure 7.29 presents the low-power and medium-power MMIC amplifiers. A microstrip four-way power divider is used to supply the power to each of the four 0.5 W MMIC amplifiers. The output power of the 0.5 W MMIC amplifiers is combined by a four-way waveguide power combiner. A photo of the 1.5 W power amplifier with a four-way waveguide power combiner is shown in Figure 7.30.

A photo of the 1.5 W power amplifier without the four-way waveguide power combiner is shown in Figure 7.31. The first carrier in this photo is a side-coupled

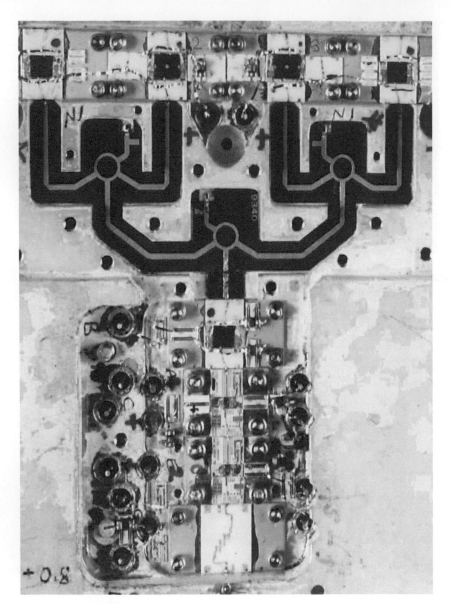

FIGURE 7.31 Photo of the 1.5 W power amplifier without the four-way waveguide power combiner.

bandpass filter. The second and third carrier contain medium-power MMIC amplifiers. The fourth carrier contains a 0.5 W MMIC power amplifier. The output of the 0.5 W MMIC power amplifier is connected to a microstrip four-way power divider.

7.9   INTEGRATED KU BAND AUTOMATIC TRACKING SYSTEM

Tracking communication systems use the mono-pulse tracking principle. The mono-pulse tracking principle is the most popular way to obtain accurate information about the target angular position in radar systems, see [1–12]. Tracking radars and scan radars systems use mono-pulse antennas in the accurate determination of angular deviation with respect to the antenna axis, off-boresight angle. Also radio communication systems that need to track a narrow beam antenna to the transmitter use mono-pulse tracking systems. Satellite and tracking communication systems use mono-pulse tracking principle to secure communication links with very narrow beam antennas. Military and commercial identification systems use this principle to obtain narrow beam information links.

A Ku-band two-axis automatic tracking system can be implemented by using a four-element mono-pulse antenna connected to a phase comparator network. The concept is widely used in the communication industry. The antenna can be a reflector antenna or an antenna array. The elements of the reflector feed can be placed at a distance of at least $\lambda/2$, a half wavelength apart each. When the target is located along the antenna boresight, each element is equidistant from the antenna elements and all signals are received in phase. However, when the target is off boresight, due to the difference in path length (L), a phase difference is introduced between the signals which is used to calculate the error angle (θ). The tracking system consists of antennas, a mono-pulse comparator, up and downcoverters a mono-pulse processor at baseband frequencies, and DC and control units, as shown in Figure 7.32. The

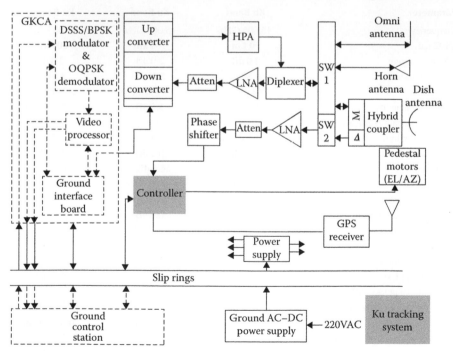

FIGURE 7.32   Ku band automatic tracking system block diagram.

development and design of the Ku band automatic tracking system is based on MIC, waveguide, and MMIC.

Technology. The power divider and combiners in the power amplifier module are waveguide power combiners to minimize losses in the transmitter. Packed MMIC components are used to minimize system volume and weight.

7.9.1 AUTOMATIC TRACKING SYSTEM LINK BUDGET CALCULATIONS

The downlink budget tracking system calculations are listed in Table 7.17 for three distances: 50 km, 100 km, and 200 km. The transmitting antenna gain is 20 dBi.

The transmitter power is 44 dBm. The receiving antenna gain is 45 dBi. The tracking system consists of three antennas: a reflector antenna, a horn antenna, and an omnidirectional antenna. The uplink tracking system budget calculations are listed in Table 7.18 for three distances: 50 km, 100 km, and 200 km. The transmitting antenna gain is 45 dBi. The transmitter power is 43 dBm. The receiving antenna gain is 20 dBi.

The downlink budget tracking system calculations for the dish to omnidirectional channel are listed in Table 7.19 for three distances: 70 km, 75 km, and 80 km. The transmitting antenna gain is 2.15 dBi. The transmitter power is 44 dBm. The receiving dish antenna gain is 45 dBi.

TABLE 7.17
Downlink (DNL) Budget Calculations

Parameter	Ku Band	Ku Band	Ku Band
Frequency	15.005 GHz	15.005 GHz	15.005 GHz
Distance	**50 km**	**100 km**	**200 km**
RX noise figure	2.0 dB	2.0 dB	2.0 db
IF bandwidth	8 MHz	8 MHz	8 MHz
TX power	44 dBm	44 dBm	44 dBm
TX component loss	5.5 dB	5.5 dB	5.5 dB
TX antenna gain (vertical)	20 dBi	20 dBi	20 dBi
TX pointing loss	1.5 dB	1.5 dB	1.5 dB
TX radom loss	0.5 dB	0.5 dB	0.5 dB
TX EIRP	56.5 dBm	56.5 dBm	56.5 dBm
Free space loss	150 dB	156 dB	162 dB
Atmospheric absorption	2.24 dB	4.49 dB	8.98 dB
Precipitation absorption	0.0 dB	0.0 dB	0.0 dB
Total propagation loss	152.24 dB	160.49 dB	170.98 dB
RX antenna gain	45 dBi	45 dBi	45 dBi
RX polarization loss	0.5 dB	0.5 dB	0.5 dB
RX pointing loss	1.0 dB	1.0 dB	1.0 dB
RX component loss (MP)	5.0 dB	5.0 dB	5.0 dB
Effective carrier power at RX input	**−57.24 dbm**	**−65.49 dBm**	**−75.98 dBm**
RX noise threshold	103.28 dBm	103.28 dBm	103.28 dBm
Calculated C/N @ RX input	46.04 dB	37.79 dB	27.3 dB
Required C/N @ RX input	5.2 dB	5.2 dB	5.2 dB
Calculated fade margin	**40.84 dB**	**32.59 dB**	**22.1 dB**

TABLE 7.18
Uplink (UPL) Budget Calculations

Parameter	Ku Band	Ku Band	Ku Band
Frequency	14.759 GHz	14.759 GHz	14.759 GHz
Distance	**50 km**	**100 km**	**200 km**
RX noise figure	3.0 dB	3.0 dB	3.0 dB
If bandwidth	16 MHz	16 MHz	16 MHz
TX power	43 dBm	43 dBm	43 dBm
TX component loss	6.0 dB	6.0 dB	6.0 dB
TX antenna gain	45 dBi	45 dBi	45 dBi
TX pointing loss	1.5 dB	1.5 dB	1.5 dB
TX radom loss	0.5 dB	0.5 dB	0.5 dB
TX EIRP	80 dBm	80 dBm	80 dBm
Free space loss	150 dB	156 dB	162 dB
Atmospheric absorption	2.14 dB	4.27 dB	8.55 dB
Precipitation absorption	0.0 dB	0.0 dB	0.0 dB
Total propagation loss	152.14 dB	160.77 dB	170.55 dB
RX antenna gain (vertical)	20 dBi	20 dBi	20 dBi
RX polarization loss	0.5 dB	0.5 dB	0.5 dB
RX pointing loss	0.5 dB	0.5 dB	0.5 dB
RX component loss	8.3 dB	8.3 dB	8.3 dB
RX PG	16.9 dB	16.9 dB	16.9 dB
Effective carrier power at RX input	**−44.54 dBm**	**−53.17 dBm**	**−62.95 dBm**
Rx noise threshold	99.28 dBm	99.28 dBm	99.28 dBm
Calculated C/N @ RX input	54.74 dB	46.11 dB	36.33 dB
Required C/N @ RX input	8.5 dB	8.5 dB	8.5 dB
Calculated fade margin	**46.24 dB**	**37.61 dB**	**27.83 dB**

TABLE 7.19
Downlink (DNL) Budget Calculations: Dish-Omni

Parameter	Ku Band	Ku Band	Ku Band
Frequency	15.005 GHz	15.005 GHz	15.005 GHz
Distance	**70 km**	**75 km**	**80 km**
RX noise figure	2.0 dB	2.0 dB	2.0 dB
IF bandwidth	8 MHz	8 MHz	8 MHz
TX power	44 dBm	44 dBm	44 dBm
TX component loss	5.5 dB	5.5 dB	5.5 db
TX antenna gain (vertical)	2.15 dBi	2.15 dBi	2.15 dBi
TX pointing loss	0.0 dB	0.0 dB	0.0 dB
TX radom loss	0.0 dB	0.0 dB	0.0 dB
TX EIRP	40.65 dBm	40.65 dBm	40.65 dBm
Free space loss	152.9 dB	153.5 dB	154.0 db
Atmospheric absorption	2.07 dB	2.22 dB	2.37 dB

(Continued)

TABLE 7.19 (*Continued*)
Downlink (DNL) Budget Calculations: Dish-Omni

Parameter	Ku Band	Ku Band	Ku Band
Precipitation absorption	0.0 dB	0.0 dB	0.0 dB
Total propagation loss	154.97 dB	155.72 dB	156.37 dB
RX antenna gain	45 dBi	45 dBi	45 dBi
RX polarization loss	0.5 dB	0.5 dB	0.5 dB
RX pointing loss	1.0 dB	1.0 dB	1.0 dB
RX component loss (MP)	5.0 dB	5.0 dB	5.0 dB
Effective carrier power at RX input	**−75.82 dBm**	**−76.57 dBm**	**−77.22 dBm**
RX noise threshold	103.28 dBm	103.28 dBm	103.28 dBm
Calculated C/N @ RX input	27.46 dB	26.71 dB	26.06 dB
Required C/N @ RX input	5.2 dB	5.2 dB	5.2 dB
Calculated fade margin	**22.26 dB**	**21.51 dB**	**20.86 dB**

The downlink budge tracking system calculations for the horn to omnidirectional channel are listed in Table 7.20 for three distances: 2 km, 5 km, and 10 km. The transmitting omnidirectional antenna gain is 2.15 dBi. The transmitter power is 44 dBm. The receiving horn antenna gain is 14 dBi.

The downlink budget and tracking system calculations for the omnidirectional to omnidirectional channel are listed in Table 7.21 for three distances: 1 km, 2 km, and 3 km. The transmitting omnidirectional antenna gain is 2.15 dBi. The transmitter power is 44 dBm. The receiving omnidirectional antenna gain is 2.15 dBi.

TABLE 7.20
Downlink (DNL) Budget Calculations: Dish-Omni

Parameter	Ku Band	Ku Band	u Band
Frequency	15.005 GHz	15.005 GHz	15.005 GHz
Distance	**3 km**	**5 km**	**10 km**
RX noise figure	2.0 db	2.0 dB	2.0 dB
IF bandwidth	8 MHz	8 MHz	8 MHz
TX power	44 dBm	44 dBm	44 dBm
TX component loss	5.5 dB	5.5 dB	5.5 dB
TX antenna gain (vertical)	2.15 dBi	2.15 dBi	2.15 dBi
TX pointing loss	0.0 dB	0.0 dB	0.0 dB
TX radom loss	0.0 dB	0.0 dB	0.0 dB
TX eirp	40.65 dBm	40.65 dBm	40.65 dBm
Free space loss	125.5 dB	129.9 dB	136.0 dB
Atmospheric absorption	0.13 dB	0.22 dB	0.45 dB
Precipitation absorption	0.0 dB	0.0 dB	0.0 dB
Total propagation loss	125.63 dB	130.12 dB	136.45 dB
RX antenna gain (1)	14 dBi	14 dBi	14 dBi

TABLE 7.20 (*Continued*)
Downlink (DNL) Budget Calculations: Dish-Omni

Parameter	Ku Band	Ku Band	u Band
RX polarization loss	0.5 dB	0.5 dB	0.5 dB
RX pointing loss	0.5 dB	0.5 dB	0.5 dB
RX component loss (MP)	5.0 dB	5.0 dB	5.0 dB
Effective carrier power at RX input	**−76.98 dBm**	**−81.47 dBm**	**−87.8 dBm**
RX noise threshold	103.28 dBm	103.28 dBm	103.28 dBm
Calculated C/N @ RX input	26.3 dB	21.81 dB	15.48 dB
Required C/N @ RX input	5.2 dB	5.2 dB	5.2 dB
Calculated fade margin	**21.1 dB**	**16.61 dB**	**10.28 dB**

TABLE 7.21
Downlink (DNL) Budget Calculations: Omni-Omni

Parameter	Ku Band	Ku Band	Ku Band
Frequency	15.005 GHz	15.005 GHz	15.005 GHz
Distance	**1 km**	**2 km**	**3 km**
RX noise figure	2.0 dB	2.0 dB	2.0 dB
If bandwidth	8 MHz	8 MHz	8 MHz
TX power	44 dBm	44 dbm	44 dBm
TX component loss	5.5 dB	5.5 dB	5.5 dB
TX antenna gain (vertical)	2.15 dBi	2.15 dBi	2.15 dBi
TX pointing loss	0.0 dB	0.0 dB	0.0 dB
TX radom loss	0.0 dB	0.0 dB	0.0 dB
TX EIRP	40.65 dBm	40.65 dBm	40.65 dBm
Free space loss	115.964 dB	122.0 dB	125.5 dB
Atmospheric absorption	0.0449 dB	0.09 dB	0.13 dB
Precipitation absorption	0.0 dB	0.0 dB	0.0 dB
Total propagation loss	116.0 dB	122.09 dB	125.63 dB
RX antenna gain	2.15 dBi	2.15 dBi	2.15 dBi
RX polarization loss	0.5 dB	0.5 dB	0.5 dB
RX pointing loss	0.0 dB	0.0 dB	0.0 dB
RX component loss (MP)	5.0 dB	5.0 dB	5.0 dB
Effective carrier power at RX input	**−78.7 dBm**	**−84.79 dBm**	**−88.33 dBm**
RX noise threshold	103.28 dBm	103.28 dBm	103.28 dBm
Calculated C/N @ RX input	24.58 dB	18.49 dB	14.95 dB
Required C/N @ RX input	5.2 dB	5.2 dB	5.2 dB
Calculated fade margin	**19.38 dB**	**13.29 dB**	**9.75 dB**

7.9.2   Ku Band Tracking System Antennas

7.9.2.1   Mono-Pulse Parabolic Reflector Antenna

The parabolic reflector antenna [1] consists of a radiating feed that is used to illuminate a reflector that is curved in the form of an accurate parabolic with diameter D as presented in Figure 7.32. This shape enables a very beam to be obtained. To provide the optimum illumination of the reflecting surface, the level of the parabola illumination should be greater by 10 dB in the center than at the parabola edges. The parabolic reflector antenna gain can be calculated by using Equation 7.66. α is the parabolic reflector antenna efficiency.

Parabolic reflector antenna gain

$$G \cong 10\log_{10}\left(\alpha\frac{(\pi D)^2}{\lambda^2}\right) \tag{7.66}$$

Reflector antenna specifications
Frequency: 14.5–15.3 GHz
Gain: 45 dBi
Beam width: 0.8° to 0.9°
Dish diameter: 1.6 m

Mono-pulse comparator, rat-race coupler

A rat-race coupler is shown in Figure 7.33. The rat-race circumference is 1.5 wavelengths. The distance from A to Δ port is $3\lambda\backslash4$. The distance from A to Σ port is $\lambda\backslash4$. For an equal-split rat-race coupler, the impedance of the entire ring is fixed at $1.41 \times Z_0$, or 70.7 Ω for $Z_0 = 50$ Ω. For an input signal V, the outputs at ports 2 and 4 are equal in magnitude, but 180 degrees out of phase.

Figure 7.34 presents the orientation between the mono-pulse antenna and the target. The distance between the two elements is d. A wavefront is incident at an angle θ. The phase difference between the two antennas is $\Delta\Phi$. The angle θ can be calculated by using Equation 7.67.

$$\theta = \sin^{-1}\left(\frac{\lambda\Delta\Phi}{2\pi d}\right) \tag{7.67}$$

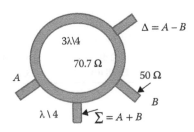

FIGURE 7.33   Rat-race coupler.

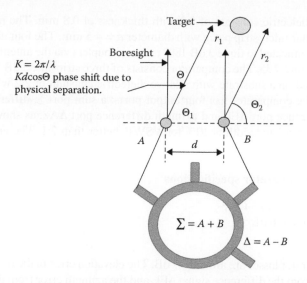

FIGURE 7.34 Orientation between the nonopulse antenna and the target.

Ku Band Mono-Pulse reflector antenna feed

A mono-pulse double-layer antenna was designed at 15 GHz. The mono-pulse double-layer antenna consists of four circular patch antennas as shown in Figure 7.35. The resonator and the feed network was printed on a substrate with relative dielectric constant of 2.5 with thickness of 0.8 mm. The resonator is a circular microstrip resonator with diameter $a = 4.2$ mm. The radiating element was printed on a substrate

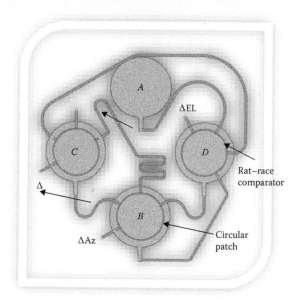

FIGURE 7.35 A microstrip stacked mono-pulse antenna and mono-pulse comparator.

with relative dielectric constant of 2.2 with thickness of 0.8 mm. The radiating element is a circular microstrip patch with diameter $a = 4.5$ mm. The four circular patch antennas are connected to three 3 dB 180° rat-race couplers via the antenna feed lines, as shown in Figure 7.35. The comparator consists of three strip-line 3 dB 180° rat-race couplers printed on a substrate with relative dielectric constant of 2.2 with thickness of 0.8 mm. The comparator has four output ports: a sum port Σ, difference port Δ, elevation difference port ΔEl, and azimuth difference port ΔAz, as shown in Figure 7.35. The antenna bandwidth is 10% for VSWR better than 2:1. The antenna beam width is around 36°. The measured antenna gain is around 10 dBi.

Mono-pulse comparator specifications

Frequency: 14.5–15.3 GHz
Insertion loss: 0.6 dB
VSWR: 1.3:1

The comparator losses are around 0.7 dB. The elevation error in the tracking system is calculated from the difference signal ΔEL and the azimuth error from the difference signal ΔAz. The resulting local minimum in the Δ port at the center of the boresight is very deep, more than –20 dB, as shown in Figure 7.36. A high angular accuracy in the tracking process is achieved by comparing the sum and difference signals. A unique tracking algorithm is implemented inside the mono-pulse processor.

Reflector antenna performance

Frequency: 14.5–15.3 GHz

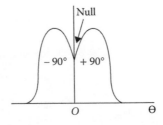

FIGURE 7.36   Mono-pulse antenna radiation pattern at the Δ port.

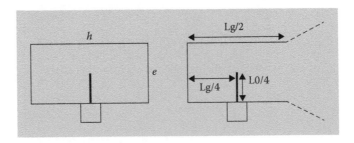

FIGURE 7.37   Ku band horn antenna feed.

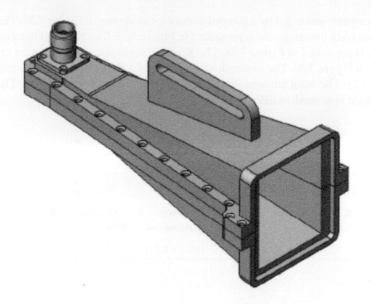

FIGURE 7.38   Ku band horn antenna assembly.

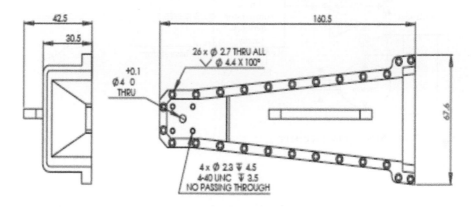

FIGURE 7.39   Ku band horn antenna fabrication drawing.

Gain: 45 dBi
Beam width: −0.9°
Dish diameter: −1.6 m

7.9.2.2   *Horn Antenna*
Horn antenna specifications

Frequency: 14.5–15.3 GHz
Gain: 14 dBi
Dimensions: 160.5 × 67.6 × 42.5 mm

The horn antenna is fed by a coaxial connector as shown in Figure 7.37. The transition from coax to waveguide is presented in Figure 7.37. The Ku band horn antenna assembly is presented in Figure 7.38. The Ku band horn antenna fabrication drawing is shown in Figure 7.39. The dimensions in inches of a Ku band waveguide are listed in Table 7.22. The horn antenna dimensions are $160.5 \times 67.6 \times 42.5$ mm. The horn antenna gain is around 14 dBi.

TABLE 7.22
Ku Band Waveguide Dimensions in Inches

WR Size	AMC Model	Frequency GHz	Material Type	Inside Dimensions	Outside Dimensions	Wall Size	Cover Flange
62	207	12.4 - 18.0	6061 Al.	0.622×0.311	0.702×0.391	.040	UG1665/U

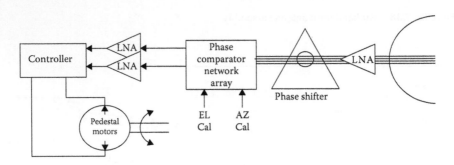

FIGURE 7.40   Mono-pulse processor.

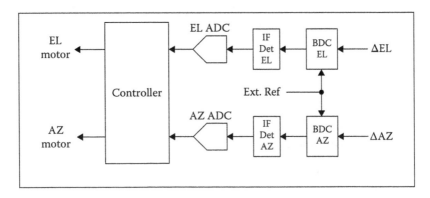

FIGURE 7.41   Tracking system controller.

7.9.2.3 Omnidirectional Antenna

The omni antenna is a quarter-wave length monopole antenna. The antenna length is around 5 mm. The monopole ground plane diameter is 120 mm.

Omnidirectional antenna specifications

Frequency: 14.5–15.3 GHz
Gain: 2 dBi
Dimensions: Ø 12 mm × 120 mm

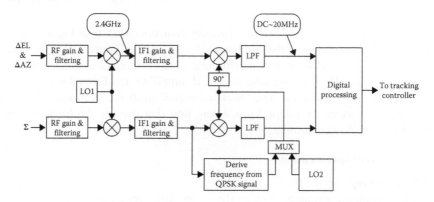

FIGURE 7.42   Mono-pulse tracking unit.

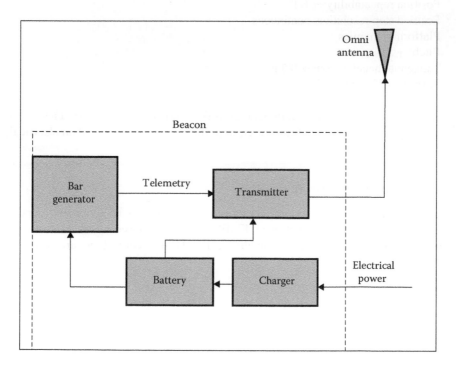

FIGURE 7.43   Omnidirectional link.

7.9.3 Mono-Pulse Processor

A block diagram of the tracking mono-pulse system is shown in Figure 7.40.

The tracking mono-pulse system consists of antennas, a low noise amplifier (LNA) phase comparator array, and a controller. The block diagram of the tracking controller system is shown in Figure 7.41. A detailed block diagram of the mono-pulse tracking unit is shown in Figure 7.42. The sum, elevation difference, and azimuth difference signals are amplified by an LNA and down converted by a mixer to 2.4 GHz. The signals are amplified and downconverted to DC and up to 20 MHz. The downconverted signal is fed to a digital processing unit. The digital processing unit supplies the tracking data to the tracking controller shown in Figure 7.41. A block diagram of the mono-pulse tracking unit is shown in Figure 7.42. The mono-pulse tracking unit consists of sum and difference channels. Each channel consists of an amplifier, filter, IF downconverter mixer, IF amplifier and filter, downconverter mixer to baseband, and filter. The baseband signal from the sum and difference channels is connected to a digital processing unit that provide the tracking commands to the tracking controller.

Pointing system specifications

Elevation range: 0° to 50°
Azimuth range: continuous in either direction, 360° continuous
Accuracy: ± 0.1° azimuth, elevation
Position repeatability: ± 0.1°
Position step resolution: continuous
Platform dynamics
Pitch: ± 5°/s
Tangential acceleration: ± 0.5 g
Turning: 45°/s and 3°/s²

A block diagram of the omnidirectional link is shown in Figure 7.43. The omnidirectional link consists of a transmitter, omnidirectional antenna, and an electrical power supply unit.

7.9.4 High Power Amplifier

The design of RF amplifiers and components is presented in books and papers [13–16]. The desired output power of 47 dBm can be achieved by combining nine 6.5-watt packed MMIC amplifier modules. The HPA specifications are listed in Table 7.23.

TABLE 7.23
HPA Specifications

Parameter	Value	Tolerance
TX frequency	14.5 GHz to 14.8 GHz	
1 db compression point	47 dBm	Min under all conditions
TX gain	80 dBm	Min under all conditions
TX gain adjustment range	+6.0 dB to –20 dB	
TX level flatness	+/–0.8 dB	Over any 36 MHz BW
TX gain stability	+/–0.8 dB	Over all temperature and frequency
TX linearity	–53 dbc	2 carriers @ 6 dB back-off
Input impedance	50 Ω	
Input connector	SMA	
Input VSWR	01:01.2	Nominal
Input N.F.	6 dB	Maximum
Output impedance	50 Ω	
Output connector	WR75	W/Gasket
Output VSWR	01:01.2	Nominal
Output port protection	Open/short internally protected	–
Visual indicators	Green LED: Power ON Red LED: Summary alarm	–
BIT indications	FWD VSWR REV VSWR HI VOLTAGE LOW VOLTAGE AGC SAT (low RF) HI TEMP	–
POWER	28VDC / TDB Amp	Not to exceed
Temperature	Operational: –40°C + 55°C Storage: –60°C + 75°C	–
ODU	IP65	–
Vibration	1 g random	Operational
Shock	10 g	Operational
Weight	5 kg	–

7.9.4.1   HPA Design Based on a 6.5 W Ku Band Power Amplifier
Basic power amplifier module performance

6.5-watt Ku band power amplifier
Frequency range: 13–16 GHz
38 dBm nominal psat
24 dB nominal gain

14 dB nominal return loss
0.25-um PHEMT. MMIC technology
10 lead flange package
Bias conditions: 8 V @ 2.6 A Idq.
Package dimension: 0.45 × 0.68 × 0.12 in.

HPA DC power

DC voltage: 8V
Current: 35 A
Total power: 300W max.

The power amplifier block diagram with nine 6.5 W power modules is presented in Figure 7.44. The –20 dBm input power is amplified around 50 dB by a medium power module to 27 dBm. The output of the 27 dBm amplifier is connected to a printed nine-way power divider. The output ports of the power divider are connected to nine 6.5 W modules with 23 dB gain. The output power of each 6.5 W module is around 38 dBm.

The nine 6.5 W modules are combined by a waveguide combiner. The output power of the HPA is 47 dBm. The transmitter gain and power budget is listed in Table 7.24.

A packed MMIC 6.5 W power module is shown in Figure 7.45. The HPA DC power tree is shown in Figure 7.46. The expected results of the 1:9 waveguide power combiner are listed in Table 7.25.

7.9.4.2   HPA Design with 41.5 dBm Power Modules

The desired output power of 47 dBm can be achieved by combining four 14-watt MMIC power amplifiers modules. The HPA specifications are listed in Table 7.23.

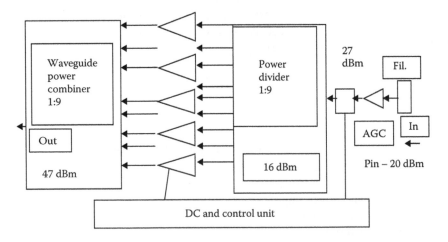

FIGURE 7.44   Power amplifier block diagram, 9 × 6.5 W power modules.

TABLE 7.24

Transmitter Gain and Power Budget

Component	Gain/Loss (dB)	Pout (dBm) Amp.
Input power min.	–	−20
Amplifier	19–24	−1
Filter	−1	−2
Amplifier	20	18
Amplifier	9	27
9-way power divider	−10.5	16.5
Amplifier	23	38
1:9 power combiner	10	47
Total with AGC	70–76	–

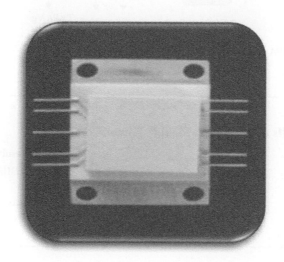

FIGURE 7.45 Packed MMIC 6.5 W power module.

Basic 42 dBm power amplifier module performance

f = 13.75–14.5 GHz
Output power at 1 dB gain compression point: P1 dB 41.5–42.0 dBm
Power gain at 1 dB gain compression point: G1 dB 5.0–6.0 dB
Drain current IDS1: 5.5–6.0A
Power added efficiency had VDS = 9V IDSQ = 4.4A 28%
Third-order intermodulation distortion: IM3 dBc −25

The power amplifier block diagram with four 14 W power modules is presented in Figure 7.47. The −20 dBm input power is amplified around 50 dB by a medium

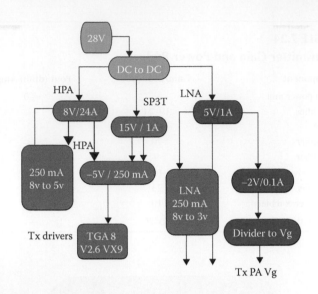

FIGURE 7.46   HPA DC power tree, 9 × 6.5 W modules.

TABLE 7.25
Expected Results of the 1:9 Waveguide Power Combiner

Parameter	Measured Results
Frequency range	14.5–15.3 GHz
Insertion loss	0.8 dB
Amplitude balance	0.4 dB max.
Phase balance	+5° max.
VSWR (input/output)	1.5:1

power module to 27 dBm. The output of the 27 dBm amplifier is connected to a printed four-way power divider. The output ports of the power divider are connected to four 6.5 W modules with 23 dB gain. The output power of each 6.5 W module is around 38 dBm.

The four 6.5 W modules are combined to four 14 W power modules. The four 14 W modules are combined by a waveguide combiner. The output power of the HPA is 47 dBm. The transmitter gain and power budget is listed in Table 7.10. The HPA DC power tree of the 4 × 14 W modules is presented in Figure 7.48.

HPA DC Power

DC voltage: 9 V
Current: 35 A
Total power: 315 W max.

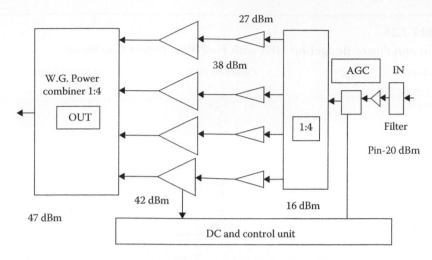

FIGURE 7.47 Power amplifier block diagram, 4 × 14 W power modules.

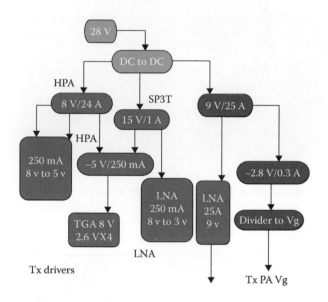

FIGURE 7.48 HPA DC power tree, 4 × 14 W modules.

The transmitter gain and power budget is listed in Table 7.26. The waveguide power divider and combiner of the power amplifier with 9 × 6.5 W power modules is shown in Figure 7.49.

The waveguide power divider and combiner of the power amplifier with 4 × 14 W power modules is shown in Figure 7.50.

TABLE 7.26
Gain and Power Budget for HPA with Four-Way Power Combiner

Component	Gain/Loss (dB)	Pout (dBm) Amp.
Input power min.		−20
Amplifier	19–24	−1
Filter	−1	−2
Amplifier	20	18
Amplifier	9	27
4-way power divider	−7	20
Amplifier	23	38
Amplifier	5	43
4-way power combiner	5	48
Total with AGC	70–76	

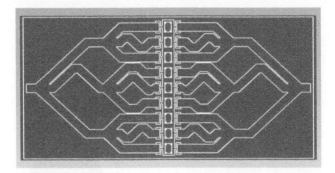

FIGURE 7.49 Power amplifier with 9 × 6.5 W power modules.

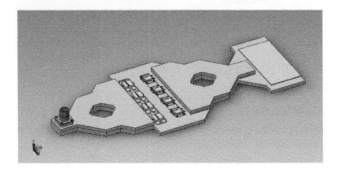

FIGURE 7.50 Power amplifier with 4 × 14 W power modules.

7.9.5   TRACKING SYSTEM DOWN- AND UPCONVERTERS

The design of the down- and upconverter unit is presented in this section.

7.9.5.1   Tracking System Upconverter Design

The upconverter consists of an RF amp with moderate NF to provide low overall system NF, a high IP3 double balanced mixer with 20 dBm local oscillator drive to provide linearity, medium power amplifiers, a 2 W power amplifier with high linearity, and band-pass filters. The block diagram of the upconverter is shown in Figure 7.51.

The upconverter specifications are listed in Table 7.27.

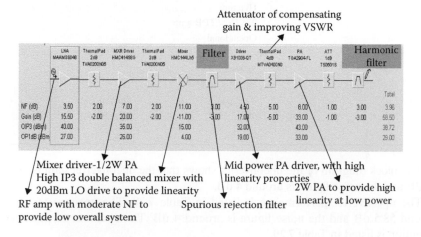

FIGURE 7.51   Block diagram of the upconverter.

TABLE 7.27
Upconverter Specifications

Parameter	Value	Tolerance
IF input frequency	2.38 GHz, 2.48 GHz	
RF output frequency	14.5 GHz, 14.8 GHz	
1 dB compression point	21 dBm	Min under all conditions
BUC gain	54 dBm	Min under all conditions
BUC level flatness	+/−0.8 dB	Over any 36 MHz BW
BUC gain stability	+/−0.8 dB	All temperature and frequency
BUC linearity	−53 dBc	2 carriers 300K apart @ 6 dB back-off
Input impedance	50 Ω	
Input connector	SMA	
Input VSWR	01:01.2	Nominal
Input N.F.	3 dB	Maximum
Output impedance	50 ohms	
Output connector	SMA	W/Gasket

(Continued)

TABLE 7.27 (Continued)
Upconverter Specifications

Parameter	Value	Tolerance
Output VSWR	01:01.2	Nominal
Visual indicators	Green LED: Power ON	–
	Red LED: Summary alarm	
BIT indications	Hi voltage	–
	Low voltage	
	AGC SAT (low RF)	
	Hi temp	
Power	28VDC / TDB amp	–
Temperature	Operational:	–
	–40°C + 55°C	
	Storage:	
	–60°C + 75°C	
Vibration	1 g random	Operational
Shock	10 g	Operational
Weight	0.85 kg	–

The block diagram of the upconverter shows that the upconverter gain is around 58 dB and the noise figure is around 4 dB.

The upconverter performance is listed in Table 7.28. The upconverter gain is around 58.5 dB and the noise figure is around 4 dB. The upconverter power consumption is listed in Table 7.29.

7.9.5.2 Tracking System Downconverter Design

The downconverter consists of an RF amplifier with moderate NF to provide low overall system NF, a high IP3 double balanced image reject mixer with 20 dBm local oscillator drive to provide linearity, a medium power amplifier with high linearity, and band-pass filters. A block diagram of the down converter is shown in Figure 7.52.

The downconverter specifications are listed in Table 7.30.

The block diagram of the downconverter shows that the downconverter gain is around 61 dB and the noise figure is around 2 dB. The downconverter performance is listed in Table 7.31. The downconverter gain is around 61 dB and the noise figure is around 2 dB. Downconverter power consumption is listed in Table 7.32.

TABLE 7.28
Upconverter Performance

Parameter	Nominal	Delta
Gain dB	58.5	±4.5
NF dB	4	±0.8
OP1 dBm	29	±1.1
ORR3@-41 dBm input (dBc)	42.5	–

TABLE 7.29
Upconverter Power Consumption

Component	Voltage [V]	Current [mA]	Power [W]
IF LNA	5	180	0.9
Mixer driver	5	500	2.5
PA driver	5	100	0.5
PA driver	−0.5	10	0.005
PA	7	700	4.9
PA	−0.57	50	0.0285
Total		1540	8.8335

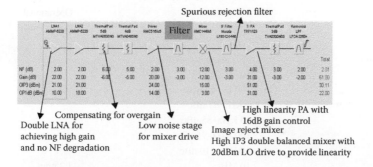

FIGURE 7.52   Block diagram of the downconverter.

TABLE 7.30
Downconverter Specifications

Parameter	Value	Tolerance
IF output frequency	2.38 GHz, 2.48 GHz	
RF input frequency	15 GHz, 15.3 GHz	
1 dB compression point	2 dBm	Min under all conditions
BDC gain	58 dBm	Min under all conditions
BDC level flatness	+/−0.8 dB	Over any 36 MHz BW
BDC gain stability	+/−0.8 dB	Over all temperature and frequency
BDC linearity	−53 dBc	2 carriers 300K apart @ 6 dB back-off
Input impedance	50 Ω	–
Input connector	SMA	–
Input VSWR	01:01.2	Nominal
Input N.F.	2.4 dB	Maximum
Output impedance	50 Ω	–
Output connector	SMA	W/Gasket

(Continued)

TABLE 7.30
Downconverter Specifications

Parameter	Value	Tolerance
Output VSWR	01:01.2	Nominal
Visual indicators	Green LED: Power ON	–
	Red LED.	
BIT indications	Hi voltage	–
	Low voltage	
	AGC SAT (low RF)	
Power	28VDC / TDB Amp	Not to exceed
Temperature	Operational: –40°C + 55°C	–
	Storage: –60°C + 75°C	
Vibration	1 g random	Operational
Shock	10 g	Operational
Weight	0.45 kg	–
LO phase noise	SSB phase noise offset:	–
	10 Hz–35 dBc	
	100 Hz–65 dBc	
	1 KHz–77 dBc	
	10 KHz–85 dBc	
	100 KHz–95 dBc	
	1 MHz–110 dBc	
Reference	10 MHz	1.2 ppm
	Internal	TCXO

TABLE 7.31
Downconverter Performance

Parameter	Nominal	Delta
Gain dB	61	±3.7
NF dB	2	±0.6
OP1 dBm	22	±2
ORR3@ – 62 dBm input (dBc)	62.53	–

TABLE 7.32
Downconverter Power Consumption

Component	Voltage [V]	Current [mA]	Power [W]
LNA1	3	55	0.165
LNA2	3	55	0.165
MXR driver	3	65	0.195
IF PA	7	600	4.2
IF PA	5	25	0.125
IF PA	–5	15	0.075
Total		815	4.925

7.9.6 TRACKING SYSTEM INTERFACE

The tracking system interface block diagram is shown in Figure 7.53. The HPA interface block diagram is shown in Figure 7.54. The Ku band automatic tracking system assembly is shown in Figure 7.55.

Control

LO frequency set – SPI or RS-232 (both available)
SPI standard protocol
RS-232 standard protocol
Indications (via RS-232):
Overvoltage

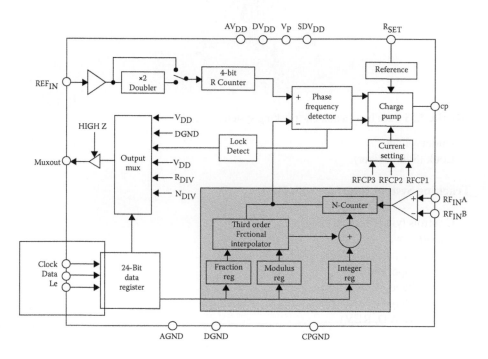

FIGURE 7.53 Tracking system interface block diagram.

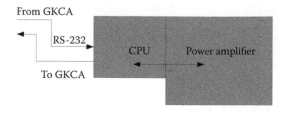

FIGURE 7.54 HPA interface block diagram.

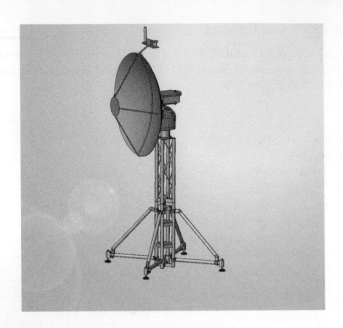

FIGURE 7.55   Ku band automatic tracking system.

Undervoltage
Lock (Synthesizer)

Tracking System Interface with HPA

Controls (via RS-232):
On/off power
Indications (via RS-232):
High temperature
Overvoltage
Undervoltage
VSWR (FWD, REV)
AGC status

REFERENCES

1. C. A. Balanis, *Antenna Theory: Analysis and Design*, 2nd Edition. Hoboken, NJ: Wiley, 1996.
2. L. C. Godara, Editor, *Handbook of Antennas in Wireless Communications*, Boca Raton, FL: CRC Press LLC, 2002.
3. J. D. Kraus and R. J. Marhefka, *Antennas for All Applications*, 3rd Edition, McGraw Hill, 2002.
4. J. R. James, P. S. Hall and C. Wood, *Microstrip Antenna Theory and Design*, London: Institution of Engineering and Technology, 1981.

5. A. Sabban and K. C. Gupta, Characterization of radiation loss from microstrip discontinuities using a multiport network modeling approach, *IEEE Transaction on Microwave Theory and Techniques*, vol. 39, no. 4, 705–712, April 1991.
6. A. Sabban, PhD Thesis, Multiport network model for evaluating radiation loss and coupling among discontinuities in microstrip circuits, University of Colorado at Boulder, CO, January 1991.
7. A. Sabban, *Microstrip Antenna Arrays, Microstrip Antennas*, N. Nasimuddin (Ed.), ISBN: 978-953-307-247-0, Croatia: InTech, pp. 361–384, 2011.
8. A. Sabban, A new wideband stacked microstrip antenna, IEEE Antenna and Propagation Symposium, Houston, TX, June 1983.
9. A. Sabban, *Low Visibility Antennas for Communication Systems*, Taylor & Francis Group, 2015.
10. A. Sabban, Wideband microstrip antenna arrays, IEEE Antenna and Propagation Symposium MELCOM, Tel-Aviv, Israel, June 1981.
11. A. Sabban, *RF Engineering, Microwave and Antennas*, Israel: Saar Publications, 2014.
12. K. Fujimoto and J. R. James, Editors, *Mobile Antenna Systems Handbook*, Boston, MA: Artech House, 1994.
13. J. Rogers and C. Plett, *Radio Frequency Integrated Circuit Design*, Norwood, MA: Artech House, 2003.
14. N. Malufa and K. Williams, *An Introduction to Microelectromechanical System Engineering*, Norwood, MA: Artech House, 2004.
15. S. A. Mass, *Nonlinear Microwave and RF Circuits*, Norwood, MA: Artech House, 1997.
16. A. Sabban, *Wideband RF Technologies and Antenna in Microwave Frequencies*, Hoboken, NJ: Wiley Sons, July 2016.

8 Novel Wearable Antennas for Wireless Communication Systems

Low-profile small antennas are crucial in the development of commercial compact systems. Small printed antennas suffer from low efficiency.

8.1 WIDEBAND WEARABLE METAMATERIAL ANTENNAS FOR COMMUNICATION APPLICATIONS

Metamaterial technology is used to design small wideband wearable antennas with high efficiency. Design considerations and computed and measured results of printed metamaterial antennas with high efficiency are presented in this chapter. The proposed antenna may be used in communication and medical systems. The antenna S_{11} results for different positions on the human body are presented in this chapter. The gain and directivity of the patch antenna with SRR is higher by 2.5 dB than the patch antenna without SRR. The resonant frequency of the antenna with SRR on the human body is shifted by 3%.

8.1.1 INTRODUCTION

Microstrip antennas are widely used in communication systems. Microstrip antennas have several advantages such as low profile, flexibility, light weight, small volume, and low production cost. Compact printed antennas have been presented in journals and books, see [1–4]. However, small printed antennas suffer from low efficiency. Meta-material technology is used to design small printed antennas with high efficiency. Printed wearable antennas were presented in [5]. Artificial media with negative dielectric permittivity were presented in [6]. Periodic SRR and metallic posts structures may be used to design materials with dielectric constant and permeability less than 1 as presented in [6–14]. In this chapter metamaterial technology is used to develop small antennas with high efficiency. The RF transmission properties of human tissues have been investigated in several papers such as [15,16]. Several wearable antennas have been presented in papers in recent years, see [17–24]. New wearable printed metamaterials antennas with high efficiency are presented in this chapter. The bandwidth of the metamaterial antenna with SRR and metallic strips is around 50% for VSWR better than 2.3:1. Computed and measured results of metamaterial antennas on the human body are discussed in this paper.

8.1.2 Printed Antennas with Split Ring Resonators

A microstrip dipole antenna with split ring resonators (SRR) is shown in Figure 8.1. The microstrip loaded dipole antenna with SRR provides horizontal polarization. The slot antenna provides vertical polarization. The resonant frequency of the antenna with SRR is 400 MHz. The resonant frequency of the antenna without SRR is 10% higher. The antennas shown in Figure 8.1 consist of two layers. The dipole feed network is printed on the first layer. The radiating dipole with SRR is printed on the second layer. The thickness of each layer is 0.8 mm. The dipole and the slot antenna create a dual polarized antenna. The computed S_{11} parameters are presented in Figure 8.2.

The length of the dual polarized antenna with SRR shown in Figure 8.1 is 19.8 cm. The length of the dual polarized antenna without SRR shown in Figure 8.3 is 21 cm. The ring width is 1.4 mm the spacing between the rings is 1.4 mm. The antennas have been analyzed by using Agilent ADS software. The matching stub locations and dimensions have been optimized to get the best VSWR results. The length of the stub L in Figures 8.1 and 8.3 is 10 mm. The locations and number of the coupling stubs may vary the antenna axial ratio from 0 dB to 30 dB. The number of coupling stubs may be minimized. The number of coupling stubs in Figure 8.1 is three. The antenna axial ratio value may be adjusted also by varying the slot feed location. The dimensions of the antenna shown in Figure 8.3 are presented in [5].

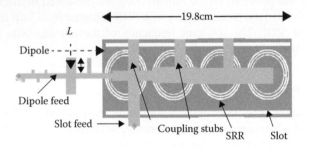

FIGURE 8.1   Printed antenna with split ring resonators.

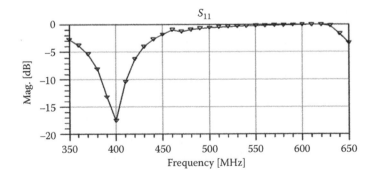

FIGURE 8.2   Computed S_{11} for antenna with split ring resonators.

The bandwidth of the antenna shown in Figure 8.3 is around 10% for VSWR better than 2:1. The antenna beam width is 100°. The antenna gain is around 2 dBi. The computed S_{11} parameters are presented in Figure 8.4. Figure 8.5 presents the measured S_{11} parameters for the antenna. There is a good agreement between measured and computed results. The antenna presented in Figure 8.1 has been modified as shown in Figure 8.6. The location and the dimension of the coupling stubs have been modified to get two resonant frequencies. The first resonant frequency is 370 MHz and is lower by 20% than the resonant frequency of the antenna without the SRR (Figure 8.7).

Metallic strips have been added to the antenna with SRR as presented in Figure 8.8. The computed S_{11} parameter of the antenna with metallic strips is presented in Figure 8.9. The antenna bandwidth is around 50% for VSWR better than 3:1. The computed radiation pattern is shown in Figure 8.10. The 3D computed radiation pattern is shown in Figure 8.11. The directivity and gain of the antenna with SRR is around 5 dBi, see Figure 8.12. The directivity of the antenna without SRR is around 2 dBi. The length of the antennas with SRR is smaller by 5% than the antennas without SRR. Moreover, the resonant frequency of the antennas with SRR is lower by 5% to 10%.

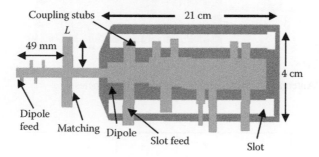

FIGURE 8.3 Dual polarized microstrip antenna.

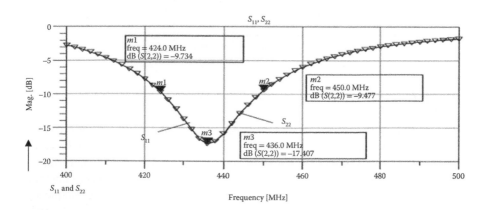

FIGURE 8.4 Computed S_{11} and S_{22} results for antenna without SRR.

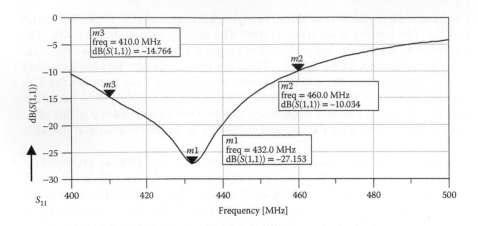

FIGURE 8.5 Measured S_{11} of the antenna without SRR.

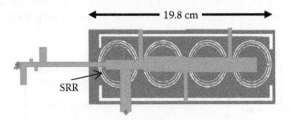

FIGURE 8.6 Antenna with SRR with two resonant frequencies.

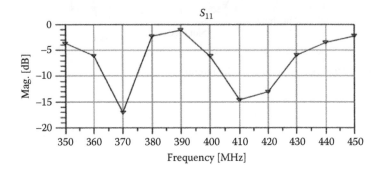

FIGURE 8.7 S_{11} for antenna with two resonant frequencies.

The feed network of the antenna presented in Figure 8.8 has been optimized to yield VSWR better than 2:1 in the frequency range of 250 MHz to 440 MHz. Optimization of the number of coupling stubs and the distance between the coupling stubs may be used to tune the antenna resonant frequency. An optimized antenna with two coupling stubs has two resonant frequencies. The first resonant frequency is 370 MHz and the second resonant frequency is 420 MHz. An antenna with SRR with two coupling stubs is presented in Figure 8.13.

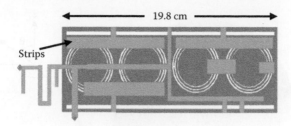

FIGURE 8.8   Antenna with SRR and metallic strips.

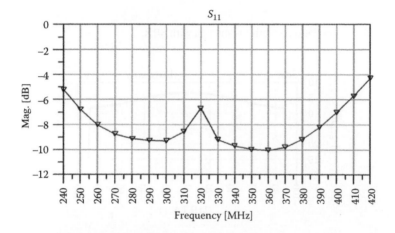

FIGURE 8.9 S_{11} for antenna with SRR and metallic strips.

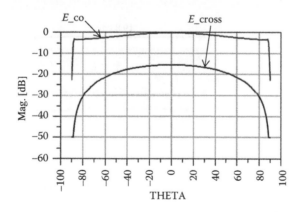

FIGURE 8.10   Radiation pattern for antenna with SRR.

The computed S_{11} parameter of the antenna with two coupling stubs is presented in Figure 8.14. The 3D radiation pattern for the antenna with SRR and two coupling stubs is shown in Figure 8.15.

The antenna with metallic strips has been optimized to yield wider bandwidth as shown in Figure 8.16. The computed S_{11} parameter of the modified antenna with

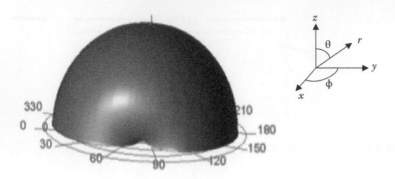

FIGURE 8.11   3D radiation pattern for antenna with SRR.

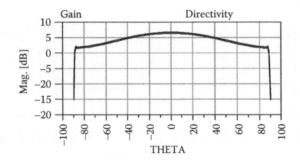

FIGURE 8.12   Directivity of the antenna with SRR.

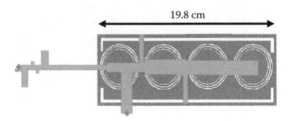

FIGURE 8.13   Antenna with SRR with two coupling stubs.

metallic strips is presented in Figure 8.17. The antenna bandwidth is around 50% for VSWR better than 2.3:1.

8.1.3   Folded Dipole Metamaterial Antenna with SRR

The length of the antenna shown in Figure 8.3 may be reduced from 21 cm to 7 cm by folding the printed dipole as shown in Figure 8.18. Tuning bars are located along the feed line to tune the antenna to the desired frequency. The antenna bandwidth is around 10% for VSWR better than 2:1 as shown in Figure 8.19. The antenna beam

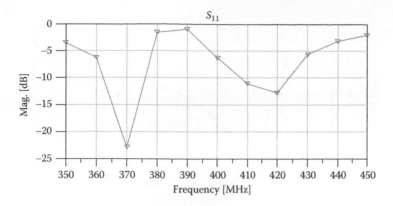

FIGURE 8.14 S_{11} for antenna with SRR with two coupling stubs.

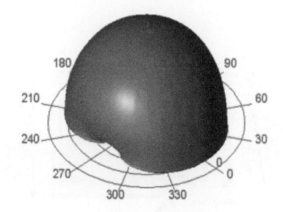

FIGURE 8.15 3D radiation pattern for antenna with SRR and two coupling stubs.

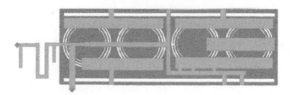

FIGURE 8.16 Wideband antenna with SRR and metallic strips.

width is around 100°. The antenna gain is around 2 dBi. The size of the antenna with SRR shown in Figure 8.6 may be reduced by folding the printed dipole as shown in Figure 8.20. The dimensions of the folded dual polarized antenna with SRR presented in Figure 8.20 are 11 × 11 × 0.16 cm. Figure 8.21 presents the computed S_{11} parameters for the antenna. The antenna bandwidth is 10% for VSWR better than 2:1. The computed radiation pattern of the folded antenna with SRR is shown in Figure 8.22.

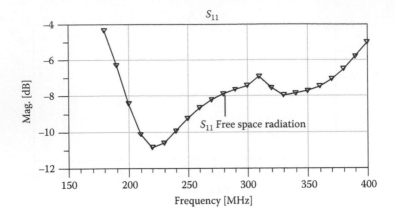

FIGURE 8.17 S_{11} for antenna with SRR and metallic strips.

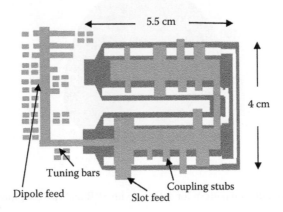

FIGURE 8.18 Folded dipole antenna, $7 \times 5 \times 0.16$ cm.

8.2 STACKED PATCH ANTENNA LOADED WITH SRR

First, a microstrip stacked patch antenna [1–3] was designed. The second step was to design the same antenna with SRR. The antenna consists of two layers. The first layer consists of FR4 dielectric substrate with dielectric constant of 4 that is 1.6 mm thick. The second layer consists of RT-DUROID 5880 dielectric substrate with dielectric constant of 2.2 that is 1.6 mm thick. The dimensions of the microstrip stacked patch antenna shown in Figure 8.23 are $33 \times 20 \times 3.2$ mm. The antenna has been analyzed by using Agilent ADS software. The antenna bandwidth is around 5% for VSWR better than 2.5:1. The antenna beam width is around 72°. The antenna gain is around 7 dBi. The computed S_{11} parameters are presented in Figure 8.24. The radiation pattern of the microstrip stacked patch is shown in Figure 8.25. The antenna with SRR is shown in Figure 8.26. This antenna has the same structure as the antenna

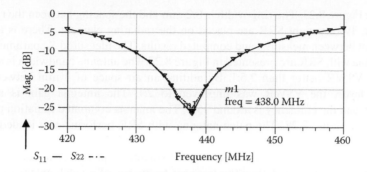

FIGURE 8.19 Folded antenna computed S_{11} and S_{22} results.

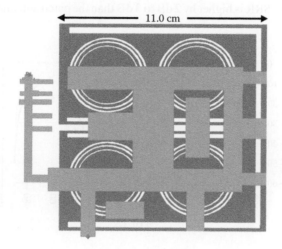

FIGURE 8.20 Folded dual polarized antenna with SRR.

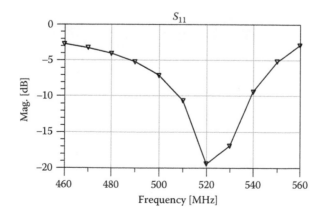

FIGURE 8.21 Computed S_{11} for folded antenna with SRR.

shown in Figure 8.23. The ring width is 0.2 mm and the spacing between the rings is 0.25 mm. Twenty-eight SRR are placed on the radiating element. There is a good agreement between measured and computed results. The measured S_{11} parameters of the antenna with SRR are presented in Figure 8.27. The antenna bandwidth is around 12% for VSWR better than 2.5:1. By adding an air space of 4 mm between the antenna layers the VSWR was improved to 2:1. The antenna gain is around 9–10 dBi, and the efficiency is around 95%. The antenna computed radiation pattern is shown in Figure 8.28. The patch antenna with SRR performs as a loaded patch antenna. The effective area of a patch antenna with SRR is higher than the effective area of a patch antenna without SRR. The resonant frequency of a patch antenna with SRR is lower by 10% than the resonant frequency of a patch antenna without SRR.

The antenna beam width is around 70°. The gain and directivity of the stacked patch antenna with SRR is higher by 2 dB to 3 dB than the patch antenna without SRR.

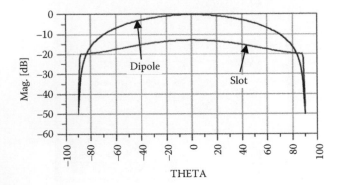

FIGURE 8.22   Radiation pattern of the folded antenna with SRR.

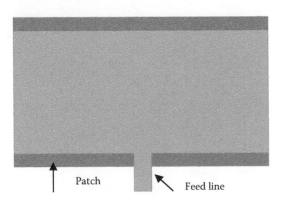

FIGURE 8.23   A microstrip stacked patch antenna.

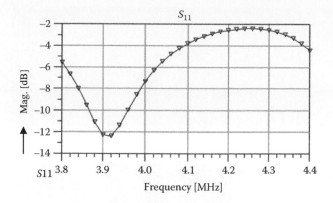

FIGURE 8.24 Computed S_{11} of the microstrip stacked patch.

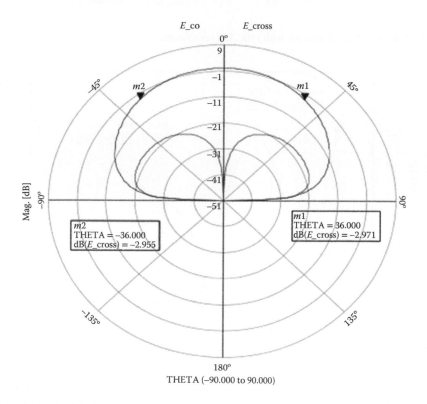

FIGURE 8.25 Radiation pattern of the microstrip stacked patch.

8.3 PATCH ANTENNA LOADED WITH SPLIT RING RESONATORS

A patch antenna with split ring resonators has been designed. The antenna is printed on RT-DUROID 5880 dielectric substrate with dielectric constant of 2.2 that is 1.6 mm thick. The dimensions of the microstrip patch antenna shown in Figure 8.29 are

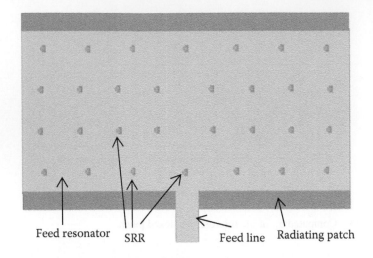

Feed resonator   SRR   Feed line   Radiating patch

FIGURE 8.26   Printed antenna with split ring resonators.

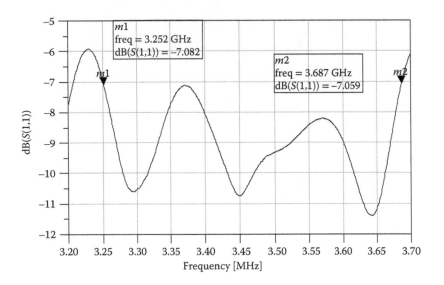

FIGURE 8.27   Measured S_{11} for patch with split ring resonators.

36 × 20 × 1.6 mm. The antenna bandwidth is around 5% for S_{11} lower than −9.5 dB. However, the antenna bandwidth is around 10% for VSWR better than 3:1. The antenna beam width is around 72°. The antenna gain is around 7.8 dBi. The directivity of the antenna is 8. The antenna gain is 6.03. The antenna efficiency is 77.25%. The measured S_{11} parameters are presented in Figure 8.30. The gain and directivity of the patch antenna with SRR is higher by 2.5 dB than the patch antenna without SRR.

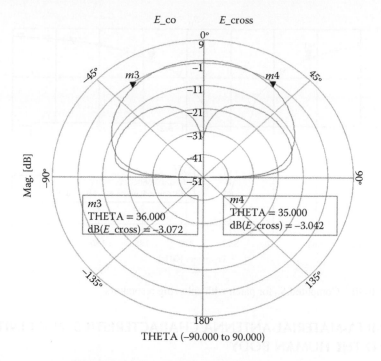

FIGURE 8.28   Radiation pattern for patch with SRR.

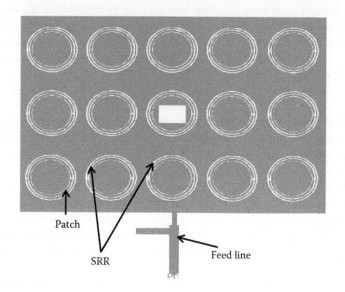

FIGURE 8.29   Patch antenna with split ring resonators.

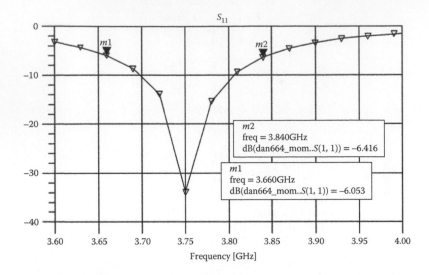

FIGURE 8.30 Computed S_{11} for patch with split ring resonators.

8.4 META-MATERIAL ANTENNA CHARACTERISTICS IN VICINITY TO THE HUMAN BODY

The antenna's input impedance variation as a function of distance from the human body had been computed by using the structure presented in Figure 8.31. Electrical properties of human body tissues are listed in Table 8.1; see [15]. The antenna location on the human body may be taken into account by calculating S_{11} for different dielectric constants of the body. The variation of the dielectric constant of the body from 43 at the stomach to 63 at the colon zone shifts the antenna resonant frequency by 2%. The antenna was placed inside a belt with thickness between 1 and 4 mm with dielectric constant from 2 to 4.

The air spacing between the belt and the patient shirt is varied from 0 mm to 8 mm. The dielectric constant of the patient shirt was varied from 2 to 4.

Figure 8.32 presents S_{11} results of the antenna with SRR shown in Figure 8.13 on the human body. The antenna resonant frequency is shifted by 3%. Figure 8.33 presents S_{11} results of the antenna with SRR and metallic strips, shown in Figure 8.16, on the human body. The antenna resonant frequency is shifted by 1%.

Figure 8.34 presents S_{11} results (of the antenna shown in Figure 8.3) for different air spacing between the antennas and human body, belt thicknesses, shirt thicknesses. Results presented in Figure 8.33 indicate that the antenna has VSWR better than 2.5:1 for air spacing up to 8 mm between the antennas and the body. Figure 8.35 presents S_{11} results for different positions relative to the human body of the folded antenna shown in Figure 8.6. The explanation of Figure 8.35 is given in Table 8.2. If the air spacing between the antennas and the human body is increased from 0 mm to 5 mm, the antenna resonant frequency is shifted by 5%. A tunable wearable antenna may be used to control the antenna resonant frequency at different positions on the human body, see [25].

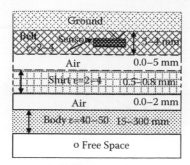

FIGURE 8.31   Wearable antenna environment.

TABLE 8.1
Summary of Electrical Properties of Human Body Tissues

Tissue	Property	434 MHz	600 MHz
Prostate	σ	0. 75	0.90
	ε	50.53	47.4
Skin	σ	0.57	0.6
	ε	41.6	40.43
Stomach	σ	0.67	0.73
	ε	42.9	41.41
Colon, Muscle	σ	0.98	1.06
	ε	63.6	61.9
Lung	σ	0.27	0.27
	ε	38.4	38.4

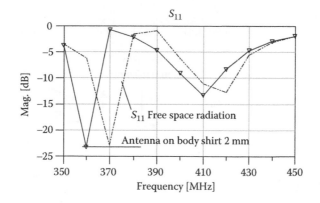

FIGURE 8.32 S_{11} of the antenna with SRR on the human body.

Figure 8.36 presents S_{11} results of the folded antenna with SRR shown in Figure 8.8 on the human body. The antenna resonant frequency is shifted by 2%. The radiation pattern of the folded antenna with SRR on the human body is presented in Figure 8.37.

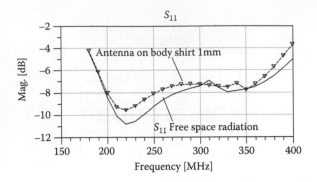

FIGURE 8.33 Antenna with SRR S_{11} results on the human body.

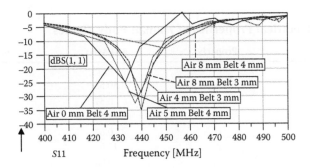

FIGURE 8.34 S_{11} results of the antenna shown in Figure 8.3 on the human body.

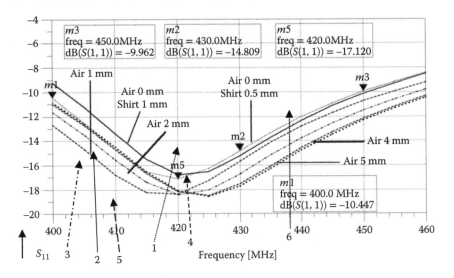

FIGURE 8.35 S_{11} results for different locations relative to the human body for the antenna shown in Figure 8.6.

TABLE 8.2

Explanation of Figure 8.35

Picture #	Line Type	Sensor Position
1	Dot	Shirt thickness 0.5 mm
2	Line	Shirt thickness 1 mm
3	Dash dot	Air spacing 2 mm
4	Dash	Air spacing 4 mm
5	Long dash	Air spacing 1 mm
6	Big dots	Air spacing 5 mm

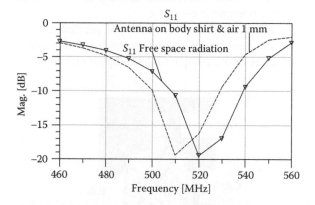

FIGURE 8.36 Folded antenna with SRR S_{11} results on the body.

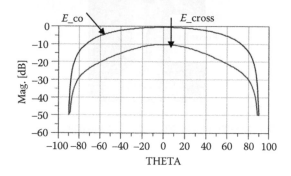

FIGURE 8.37 Radiation pattern of the folded antenna with SRR on human body.

8.5 METAMATERIAL WEARABLE ANTENNAS

The proposed wearable metamaterials antennas may be placed inside a belt as shown in Figure 8.38. Three to four antennas may be placed in a belt and attached to the patient's stomach. More antennas may be attached to the patient's back to improve the level of the received signal from different locations in the human body. The cable from each antenna is connected to a recorder. The received signal is transferred via an SP8T switch to the receiver. The antennas receive a signal that is transmitted from various positions in the human body. The medical system selects the signal with the highest power.

In several systems the distance separating the transmitting and receiving antennas is in the near-field zone. In these cases the electric field intensity decays rapidly with distance. The near fields only transfer energy to close distances from the antenna and do not radiate energy to far distances. The radiated power is trapped in the region near to the antenna. In the near-field zone the receiving and transmitting antennas are magnetically coupled. The inductive coupling value between two antennas is measured by their mutual inductance. In these systems we have to consider only the near-field electromagnetic coupling.

In Figures 8.39 through 8.42 several photos of printed antennas for medical applications are shown. The dimensions of the folded dipole antenna are $7 \times 6 \times 0.16$ cm. The dimensions of the compact folded dipole presented in [5] and shown

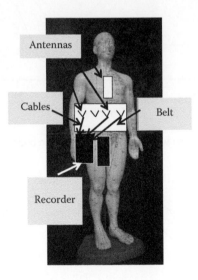

FIGURE 8.38 Medical system with printed wearable antenna.

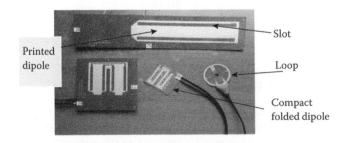

FIGURE 8.39 Microstrip antennas for medical applications.

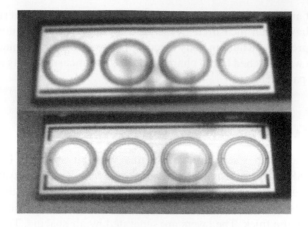

FIGURE 8.40   Metamaterial antennas for medical applications.

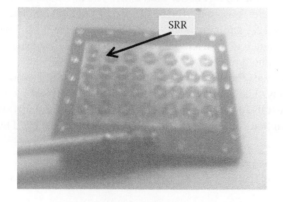

FIGURE 8.41   Metamaterial patch antenna with SRR.

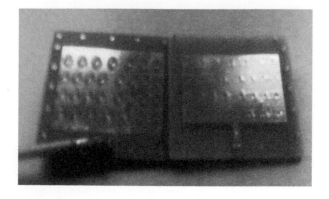

FIGURE 8.42   Metamaterial stacked patch antenna with SRR.

in Figure 8.39 are 5 × 5 × 0.5 cm. The antenna's electrical characteristics on the human body have been measured by using a phantom. The phantom has been designed to represent the human body electrical properties as presented in [5]. The tested antenna was attached to the phantom during the measurements of the antenna's electrical parameters.

8.6 WIDEBAND STACKED PATCH WITH SRR

A wideband microstrip stacked patch antenna with air spacing [1–3] has been designed with SRR. The antenna consists of two layers. The first layer consists of FR4 dielectric substrate with dielectric constant of 4 that is 1.6 mm thick. The second layer consists of RT-DUROID 5880 dielectric substrate with dielectric constant of 2.2 that is 1.6 mm thick. The layers are separated by air spacing. The dimensions of the microstrip stacked patch antenna shown in Figure 8.43 are 33 × 20 × 3.2 mm. The antenna has been analyzed using Agilent ADS software. The antenna bandwidth is around 10% for VSWR better than 2.0:1. The antenna beam width is around 72°. The antenna gain is around 90 dBi–10 dBi. The antenna efficiency is around 95%. The computed S_{11} parameters are presented in Figure 8.44. The radiation pattern of the stacked patch is shown in Figure 8.45. There is a good agreement between measured and computed results.

Figure 8.32 presents the S_{11} results of the antenna with SRR shown in Figure 8.13 on the human body. The antenna resonant frequency is shifted by 3%. Figure 8.33 presents the S_{11} results of the antenna with SRR and metallic strips shown in Figure 8.16 on the human body. The antenna resonant frequency is shifted by 1%.

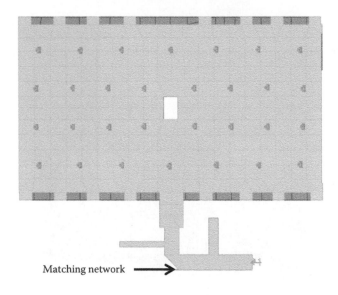

Matching network ⟶

FIGURE 8.43 Wideband stacked patch antenna with SRR.

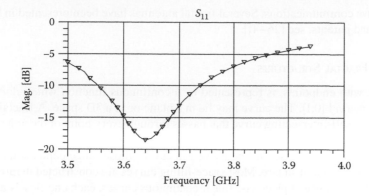

FIGURE 8.44 Wideband stacked antenna with SRR, S_{11} results.

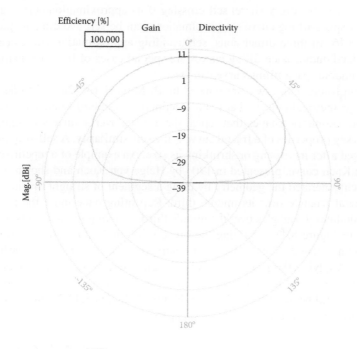

FIGURE 8.45 Radiation pattern of the stacked antenna with SRR.

8.7 FRACTAL PRINTED ANTENNAS

8.7.1 INTRODUCTION

A **fractal antenna** is an antenna that uses antenna design with similar fractal segments to maximize the antenna effective area. Fractal antennas are also referred as a multilevel structure with space filling curves. The key aspect lies in a repetition of a motif over two or more scale sizes or "iterations," Fractal antennas are very compact, multiband or wideband, and have useful applications in cellular telephone and microwave communications. Several fractal antennas have been presented in books, papers, and patents, see [26–41].

8.7.2 Fractal Structures

A curve, with endpoints, is represented by a continuous function whose domain is the unit interval [0,1]. The curve may lie in a plane or in a 3D space. A fractal curve is a densely self-intersecting curve that passes through every point of the unit square. A fractal curve is a continuous mapping from the unit interval to the unit square.

In mathematics, a space-filling curve is a curve whose range contains the entire two-dimensional unit square. Most space-filling curves are constructed iteratively as a limit of a sequence of piecewise linear continuous curves, each one closely approximating the space-filling limit. Where two sub-curves intersect (in the technical sense) in space-filling curves, there is self-contact without self-crossing. A space-filling curve can be (everywhere) self-crossing if its approximation curves are self-crossing. A space-filling curve's approximations can be self-avoiding, as presented in Figure 8.46. In three dimensions, self-avoiding approximation curves can even contain joined ends. Space-filling curves are special cases of fractal constructions. No differentiable space-filling curve can exist.

The term fractal curve was introduced by B. Mandelbrot [26–27] to describe a family of geometrical objects that are not defined in standard Euclidean geometry. Fractals are geometric shapes that repeat themselves over a variety of scale sizes. One of the key properties of a fractal curve is the self-similarity. A self-similar object is unchanged after increasing or shrinking its size. An example of a repetitive geometry is the Koch curve, presented in 1904 by Helge von Koch and shown in Figure 8.46b. Koch generated the geometry by using a segment of straight line and raising an equilateral triangle over its middle third. Repeating once more the process of erecting equilateral triangles over the middle thirds of straight line results in what is presented in Figure 8.47a. Iterating the process infinitely many times results in a curve of infinite length. This geometry is continuous everywhere but is nowhere differentiable. Applying the Koch process to an equilateral triangle, after many iterations, converges to the Koch snowflake shown in Figure 8.47. This process can be applied to several geometries as shown in Figures 8.48 and 8.49. Many variations of these geometries are presented in several papers.

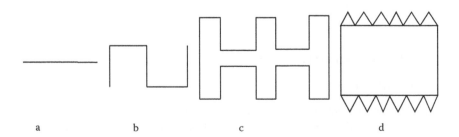

a   b   c   d

FIGURE 8.46   (a) Line. (b) Motif of bended line. (c) Bended line fractal structures. (d) Fractal structure.

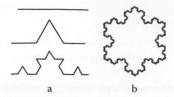

FIGURE 8.47 (a) Koch fractal structures. (b) Koch snowflakes.

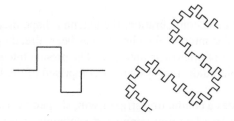

FIGURE 8.48 Folded fractal structures.

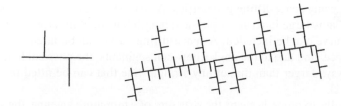

FIGURE 8.49 Variations of Koch fractal structures.

8.7.3 FRACTAL ANTENNAS

Fractal geometries may be applied to design antennas and antenna arrays. The advantages of printed circuit technology and printed antennas enhance the design of fractal printed antennas and microwave components. The effective area of a fractal antenna is significantly higher than the effective area of a regular printed antenna. A fractal antenna may operate with good performance at several different frequencies simultaneously. Fractal antennas are compact multiband antennas. The directivity of fractal antennas is usually higher than the directivity of a regular printed antenna. The number of elements in a fractal antenna array may be reduced by around a quarter of the number of elements in a regular array. A fractal antenna could be considered a nonuniform distribution of radiating elements. Each of the elements contributes to the total radiated power density at a given point with a given amplitude and phase. By spatially superposing these line radiators we can study the properties of a fractal antenna array.

The small antenna features are:

- A large input reactance (either capacitive or inductive) that usually has to be compensated with an external matching network.

- A small radiating resistance.
- Small bandwidth and low efficiency.
- This means that it is highly challenging to design a resonant antenna in a small space in terms of the wavelength at resonance.

The use of microstrip antennas is well known in mobile telephony handsets [30]. The PIFA (planar inverted F antenna) configuration is popular in mobile communication systems. The advantages of PIFAs are their low profile, their low fabrication costs < and easy integration within the system structure. One of the miniaturization techniques used in this antenna system is based on space-filling curves. In some particular cases of antenna configuration, the antenna shape may be described as a multi-level structure. The multilevel technique has been already proposed to reduce the physical dimensions of microstrip antennas. The present integrated multi-service antenna system for communication systems is comprised of the following parts and features.

The antenna includes a conducting strip or wire shaped by a space-filling curve, composed by at least two-hundred connected segments, forming a substantially right angle with each adjacent segment smaller than a hundredth of the free-space operating wavelength. The important reduction size of such antenna systems is obtained by using space-filling geometries. A space-filling curve can be described as a curve that is large in terms of physical length but small in terms of the area in which the curve can be included. A space-filling curve can be fitted over a flat or curved surface, and due to the angles between segments, the physical length of the curve is always larger than that of any straight line that can be fitted in the same area (surface).

Additionally, to properly shape the structure of a miniature antenna, the segments of the space-filling curves must be shorter than a tenth of the free-space operating wavelength. The antenna is fed with a two-conductor structure such as a coaxial cable, with one of the conductors connected to the lower tip of the multilevel structure and the other conductor connected to the metallic structure of the system which acts as a ground plane. This antenna type features a size reduction of 20% compared to the typical size of a conventional external quarter-wave whip antenna. This feature together with the small profile of the antenna, which can be printed on a low cost dielectric substrate, allows a simple and compact integration of the antenna structure.

Reducing the size of the radiating elements can be achieved by using a PIFA configuration, consisting of connecting two parallel conducting sheets, separated either by air or a dielectric, magnetic, or magneto-dielectric material. The sheets are connected through a conducting strip near one of the sheet's corners and orthogonally mounted to both sheets.

The antenna is fed through a coaxial cable, with its outer conductor connected to first sheet, and the second sheet coupled either by direct contact or capacitive to inner conductor of the coaxial cable.

In Figures 8.50a and 8.50b are presented two examples of a space-filling perimeter of the conducting sheet to achieve an optimized miniaturization of the antenna.

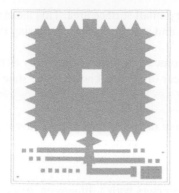 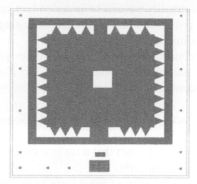

FIGURE 8.50   (a) Patch with space-filling perimeter of the conducting sheet. (b) Microstrip patch with space-filling perimeter of the conducting sheet.

8.8   ANTI-RADAR FRACTALS AND/OR MULTILEVEL CHAFF DISPERSERS

8.8.1   DEFINITION OF CHAFF

Chaff was one of the forms of countermeasure employed against radar. It usually consists of a large number of electromagnetic dispersers and reflectors, normally arranged in the form of strips of metal foil packed in a bundle. Chaff is usually employed to foil or to confuse surveillance and tracking radar.

Geometry of dispersers

In [31] new geometry for the dispersers or reflectors which improve the properties of radar chaff is presented. Some of the geometries presented here of the dispersers or reflectors are related with some forms for antennas. Multilevel and fractal structures antennas are distinguished as being of reduced size and exhibiting multiband behavior, as has been expounded already in patent publications [32].

The main electrical characteristic of a radar chaff disperser is:

Its radar cross-section (RCS), which is related to the reflective capability of the disperser.

A fractal curve for a chaff disperser is defined as a curve comprising at least ten segments which are connected so that each element forms an angle with its neighbors; no pair of these segments defines a longer straight segment, and these segments and smaller than a tenth part of the resonant wavelength in free space of the entire structure of the dispenser.

In many of the configurations presented, the size of the entire disperser is smaller than a quarter of the lowest operating wavelength.

The space-filling curves (or fractal curves) can be characterized by:

1. They are long in terms of physical length but small in terms of area in which the curve can be included. The dispersers with a fractal form are long

electrically but can be included in a very small surface area. This means it is possible to obtain smaller packaging and a denser chaff cloud using this technique.

2. Frequency response: Their complex geometry provides a spectrally richer signature when compared with rectilinear dispersers known in the state of the art.

The fractal structure properties of dispersers not only introduce an advantage in terms of reflected radar signal response, but also in terms of aerodynamic profile of dispersers. It is known that a surface offers greater resistance to air than a line or a one-dimensional form.

Therefore, giving a fractal form to the dispersers with a dimension greater than unity (D>1) increases resistance to the air and improves the time of suspension.

8.9 DEFINITION OF MULTILEVEL FRACTAL STRUCTURE

Multilevel structures are a geometry related with fractal structures. In the case of radar chaff, a multilevel structure is defined as a structure which includes a set of polygons, which are characterized as having the same number of sides, wherein these polygons are electromagnetically coupled either by means of capacitive coupling, or by means of an ohmic contact. The region of contact between the directly connected polygons is smaller than 50% of the perimeter of the polygons mentioned in at least 75% of the polygons that constitute the defined multilevel structure.

A multilevel structure provides both:

- A reduction in the size of dispensers and an enhancement of their frequency response.
- Can resonate in a non-harmonic way, and can even cover simultaneously and with the same relative bandwidth at least a portion of numerous bands.

The fractal structure (SFC) is preferred when a reduction in size is required, while multilevel structures are preferred when it is required that the most important considerations be given to the spectral response of radar chaff.

The main advantages for configuring the form of the chaff dispersers are:

1. The dispersers are small; consequently more dispersers can be encapsulated in the same cartridge, rocket, or launch vehicle.
2. The dispersers are also lighter, therefore they can spend more time floating in the air than the conventional chaff.
3. Due to the smaller size of the chaff dispersers, the launching devices (cartridges, rockets, etc.) can be smaller with regard to chaff systems in the state of the art providing the same RCS.

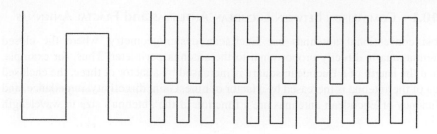

FIGURE 8.51   Fractal curves which can be used to configure a chaff disperser.

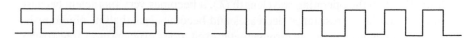

FIGURE 8.52   Hilbert fractal curves.

4. Due to the lighter weight of the chaff dispersers, the launching devices can shoot the packages of chaff farther from the launching devices and locations.
5. Chaff constituted by multilevel and fractal structures provides larger RCS at longer wavelengths than conventional chaff dispersers of the same size.
6. The dispersers with long wavelengths can be configured and printed on light dielectric supports having a non-aerodynamic form and a greater resistance to the air, thereby allowing for a longer suspension time.
7. The dispersers provide a better frequency response with regard to dispersers of the state of the art. In Figure 8.51 such size compression structures based on fractal curves are presented.

Figure 8.52 shows several examples of Hilbert fractal curves (with increasing iteration order) which can be used to configure the chaff disperser.

8.10   ADVANCED ANTENNA SYSTEM

The main advantage of an advanced antenna system lies in the multiband and multi-service performance of the antenna. This enables convenient and easy connection of a simple antenna for most communication systems and applications. The main advantages addressed by advanced antennas featured similar parameters (input impedance, radiation pattern) at several bands maintaining their performance, compared with conventional antennas. Fractal shapes permit achivement of a compact antenna of reduced dimensions compared to other conventional antennas. Multilevel antennas introduced a higher flexibility to design multiservice antennas for real applications, extending the theoretical capabilities of ideal fractal antennas to practical, commercial antennas.

8.10.1   Comparison between Euclidean Antennas and Fractal Antennas

Most conventional antennas use Euclidean design/geometry, where the closed antenna area is directly proportional to the antenna perimeter. Thus, for example, when the length of a Euclidean square is increased by a factor of three, the enclosed area of the antenna is increased by a factor of nine. Gain, directivity, impedance, and efficiency of Euclidean antennas are a function of the antenna's size to wavelength ratio.

Euclidean antennas are typically desired to operate within a narrow range (e.g., 10–40%) around a central frequency f_c which in turn dictates the size of the antenna (e.g., half or quarter wavelength). When the size of a Euclidean antenna is made much smaller than the operating wavelength (λ), it becomes very inefficient because the antenna's radiation resistance decreases and becomes less than its ohmic resistance (i.e., it does not couple electromagnetic excitations efficiently to free space). Instead, it stores energy reactively within its vicinity (reactive impedance X_c). These aspects of Euclidean antennas work together to make it difficult for small Euclidean antennas to couple or match to feeding or excitation circuitry, and cause them to have a high Q factor (lower bandwidth). The Q (quality) factor may be defined as approximately the ratio of input reactance X_{in} to radiation resistance R_r, $Q = {X_{in}}/{R_r}$.

The Q factor may also be defined as the ratio of average stored electric energy (or magnetic energy stored) to the average radiated power. Q can be shown to be inversely proportional to bandwidth.

Thus, small Euclidean antennas have very small bandwidth, which is of course undesirable (a matching network may be needed). Many known Euclidean antennas are based upon closed-loop shapes.

Unfortunately, when small in size, such loop-shaped antennas are undesirable because, as discussed above, the radiation resistance decreases significantly when the antenna size is decreased. This is because the physical area (A) contained within the loop-shaped antenna's contour is related to the loop perimeter.

Radiation resistance R_r of a circular loop-shaped Euclidean antenna is defined by R_r, as given in Equation 8.1; K is a constant.

$$R_r = \eta \pi (2/3)(KA/\lambda)^2 = 20\pi^2 \left({C}/{\lambda}\right) \tag{8.1}$$

Since the resistance R_c is only proportional to the perimeter (C), then for $C<1$, the resistance R_c is greater than the radiation resistance R_r and the antenna is highly inefficient. This is generally true for any small circular Euclidean antenna. A small-sized antenna will exhibit a relatively large ohmic resistance and a relatively small radiation resistance R_r. This low efficiency limits the use of the small antennas.

Fractal geometry is a non-Euclidean geometry which can be used to overcome the problems with small Euclidean antennas. Radiation resistance R_r of a fractal antenna decreases as a small power of the perimeter (C) compression, with a fractal loop or island always having a substantially higher radiation resistance than a small Euclidean loop antenna of equal size. Fractal geometry may be grouped into:

- Random fractals, which may be called chaotic or Brownian fractals.
- Deterministic or exact fractals. In deterministic fractal geometry, a self-similar structure results from the repetition of a design or motif (generator) with self-similarity and structure at all scales. In deterministic or exact self-similarity, fractal antennas may be constructed through recursive or iterative means. In other words, fractals are often composed of many copies of themselves at different scales, thereby allowing them to defy the classical antenna performance constraint which is size to wavelength ratio.

8.10.2   MULTILEVEL AND SPACE-FILLING GROUND PLANES FOR MINIATURE AND MULTIBAND ANTENNAS

A new family of antenna ground planes of reduced size and enhanced performance is based on an innovative set of geometries.

These new geometries are known as multilevel and space-filling structures, which had been previously used in the design of multiband and miniature antennas.

One of the key issues of the present antenna system is considering the ground plane of an antenna as an integral part of the antenna that mainly contributes to its radiation and impedance performance (impedance level, resonant frequency, and bandwidth).

The multilevel and space-filling structures are used in the ground plane of the antenna, obtaining a better return loss or VSWR, a better bandwidth, multiband behavior, or a combination of all these effects. The technique can be seen as well as a means of reducing the size of the ground plane and therefore the size of the overall antenna. The key point of the present antenna system is shaping the ground plane of an antenna in such a way that the combined effect of the ground plane and the radiating element enhances the performance and characteristics of the whole antenna device, either in terms of bandwidth, VSWR, multiband, efficiency, size, or gain.

Multilevel geometry

The resulting geometry is no longer a solid, conventional ground plane, but a ground plane with a multilevel or space-filling geometry, at least in a portion of ground plane.

A multilevel geometry for a ground plane consists of a conducting structure including a set of polygons, featuring the same number of sides, electromagnetically coupled either by means of a capacitive coupling or ohmic contact. The contact region between directly connected polygons is narrower than 50% of the perimeter of polygons in at least 75% of polygons defining conducting ground-plane. In this definition of multilevel geometry, circles and ellipses are included as well, since they can be understood as polygons with infinite number of sides.

Space-filling curve

A Space filling curve (hereafter SFC) is a curve that is large in terms of physical length but small in terms of the area in which the curve can be included.

A curve composed by at least ten segments which are connected in such a way that each segment forms an angle with their neighbors, that is, no pair of adjacent segments define a larger straight segment, and wherein the curve can be optionally periodic along a fixed straight direction of space if, and only if, the period is defined by a non-periodic curve composed by at least ten connected segments and no pair of adjacent and connected segments defines a straight longer segment.

A space-filling curve can be fitted over a flat or curved surface, and due to the angles between segments, the physical length of the curve is always larger than that of any straight line that can be fitted in the same area (surface).

Additionally, to properly shape the ground plane, the segments of the SFCs included in the ground plane must be shorter than a tenth of the free-space operating wavelength.

Figure 8.53 shows several examples of fractal geometries which can be used as Space-filling curves. Figure 8.54 shows several examples of Hilbert fractal curves which can be used as Space-filling curves.

The curves shown in the Figure 8.53 are some examples of such SFCs. Due to the special geometry of the multilevel and space-filling structure, the current distributes over the ground plane in such a way that it enhances the antenna performance and features in terms of:

- Reduced size compared to antennas with a solid ground plane
- Enhanced bandwidth compared to antennas with a solid ground plane
- Multi-frequency performance
- Better VSWR features at the operating band or bands
- Better radiation efficiency
- Enhanced gain

Figure 8.55a shows a patch antenna above a particular example of a new ground-plane structure formed by both multilevel and space-filling geometries. Figure 8.55b shows a monopole antenna above a ground-plane structure formed by both multilevel and space-filling geometries.

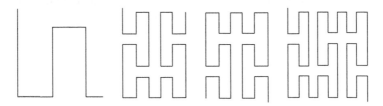

FIGURE 8.53   Fractal curves which can be used as space-filling curves.

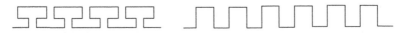

FIGURE 8.54   Hilbert fractal curves which can be used as space-filling curves.

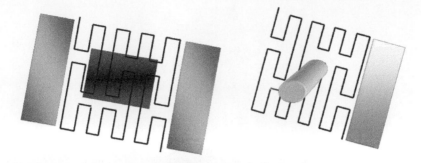

FIGURE 8.55   (a) Patch antenna above a new ground-plane structure. (b) Monopole antenna above a ground-plane structure formed by both multilevel and space-filling geometries.

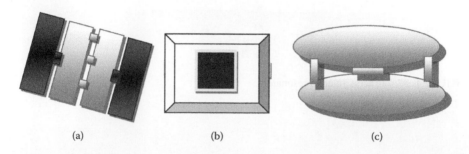

| (a) | (b) | (c) |

FIGURE 8.56   Examples of different contour shaped multilevel ground planes (a) Rectangular ground planes (b) Multilevel rectangular ground plane (c) Circular ground planes.

Figure 8.56 shows several examples of different contour shapes for multilevel ground planes, such as rectangular (Figure 8.56a and b) and circular (Figure 8.56c).

8.11   APPLICATIONS OF FRACTAL PRINTED ANTENNAS

In this chapter several designs of fractal printed antennas are presented for communication applications. These fractal antennas are compact and efficient. The antenna gain is around 8 dBi with 90% efficiency.

8.11.1   New 2.5 GHz Fractal Antenna with Space-Filling Perimeter on the Radiator

A new fractal microstrip antenna was designed as presented in Figure 8.57. The antenna was printed on Duroid substrate 0.8 mm thick with a dielectric constant of 2.2. The antenna dimensions are 5.2 × 48.8 × 0.08 cm. The antenna was designed using ADS software.

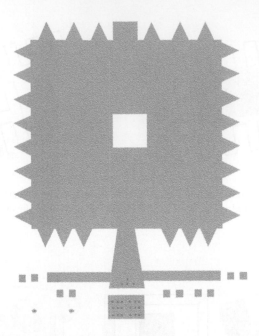

FIGURE 8.57　Fractal antenna resonators.

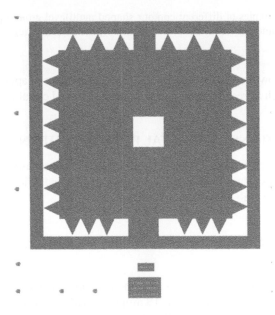

FIGURE 8.58　Fractal antenna patch radiator.

The antenna bandwidth is around 2% around 2.5 GHz for VSWR better than 3:1. The antenna bandwidth may be improved to 5%, for VSWR better than 2:1, by adding a second layer above the resonator. A patch radiator is printed on the second layer as presented in Figure 8.58. The radiator was printed on FR4 substrate 0.8 mm thick with a dielectric constant of 4.5. The electromagnetic fields radiated by the resonator are electromagnetically coupled to the patch radiator. The patch radiator dimensions are $45.2 \times 48.8 \times 0.08$ cm. The stacked fractal antenna structure is shown in Figure 8.59. The spacing between the two layers may be varied to get wider bandwidth. The S_{11} parameter for the fractal stacked patch with 8 mm air spacing between the layers is presented in Figure 8.60. The S_{11} parameter of the fractal stacked patch

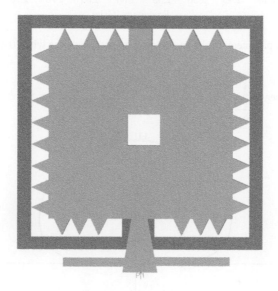

FIGURE 8.59 Fractal stacked patch antenna structure.

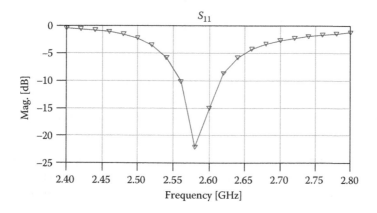

FIGURE 8.60 S_{11} parameter of the fractal stacked patch antenna with 8 mm air spacing.

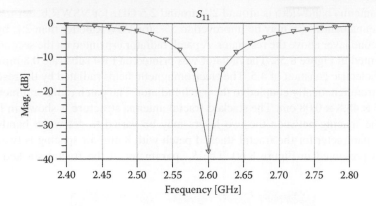

FIGURE 8.61 S_{11} parameter of the fractal stacked patch antenna with 10 mm air spacing.

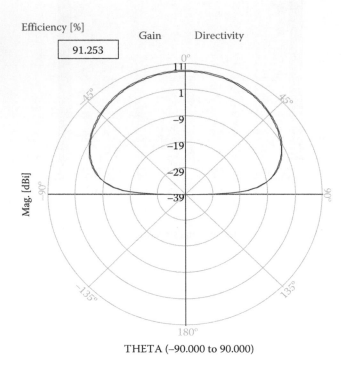

FIGURE 8.62   Fractal stacked patch antenna radiation pattern with 10 mm air spacing.

antenna with 10 mm air spacing is given in Figure 8.61. The antenna bandwidth is improved to 5% for VSWR better than 2:1. The fractal stacked patch antenna radiation pattern is shown in Figure 8.62. The antenna beam width is around 76°, with 8 dBi gain and 91% efficiency.

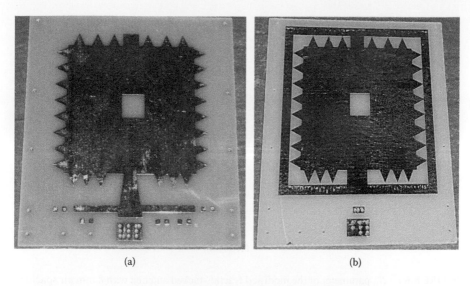

(a)   (b)

FIGURE 8.63 Fractal stacked patch antenna: (a) resonator, (b) radiator.

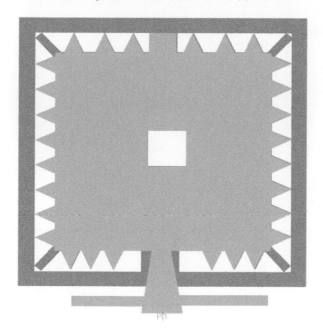

FIGURE 8.64 A modified fractal stacked patch antenna structure.

A photo of the stacked fractal patch antenna is shown in Figure 8.63. The antenna resonator is shown in Figure 8.63a. The antenna radiator is shown in Figure 8.63b. A modified version of the antenna is shown in Figure 8.64. The S_{11} parameter of the modified fractal stacked patch antenna with 8 mm air spacing is given in Figure 8.65.

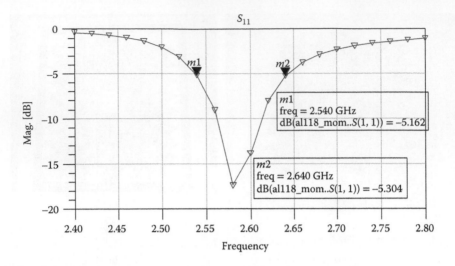

FIGURE 8.65 S_{11} parameter of the modified fractal stacked antenna with 8 mm air spacing.

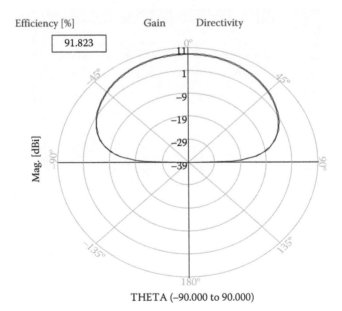

FIGURE 8.66 Fractal stacked patch antenna radiation pattern with 8 mm air spacing.

The antenna bandwidth is around 10% for VSWR better than 3:1. The fractal stacked patch antenna radiation pattern is shown in Figure 8.66. The antenna beam width is around 76, with 8 dBi gain and 91.82% efficiency.

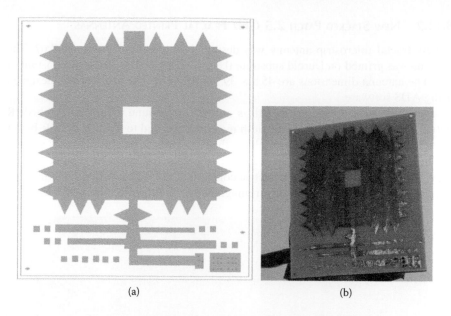

FIGURE 8.67 Resonator of a fractal stacked patch antenna: (a) layout, (b) resonator photo.

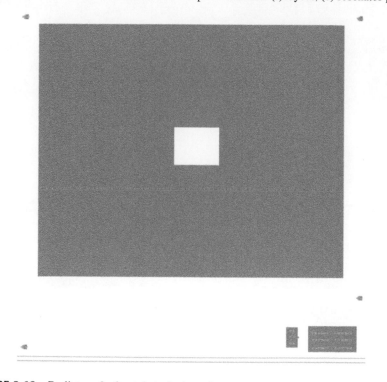

FIGURE 8.68 Radiator of a fractal stacked patch antenna.

8.11.2 New Stacked Patch 2.5 GHz Fractal Printed Antennas

A new fractal microstrip antenna was designed as presented in Figure 8.67. The antenna was printed on Duroid substrate 0.8 mm thick with a dielectric constant of 2.2. The antenna dimensions are 45.8 × 39.1 × 0.08 cm. The antenna was designed using ADS software.

The antenna resonator bandwidth is around 2% around 2.52 GHz for VSWR better than 3:1. The antenna bandwidth may be improved to 6%, for VSWR better than 3:1, by adding a second layer above the resonator. A patch radiator is printed on the second layer as presented in Figure 8.68. The radiator was printed on FR4 substrate 0.8 mm thick with a dielectric constant of 4.5. The electromagnetic fields radiated by the resonator are electromagnetically coupled to the patch radiator.

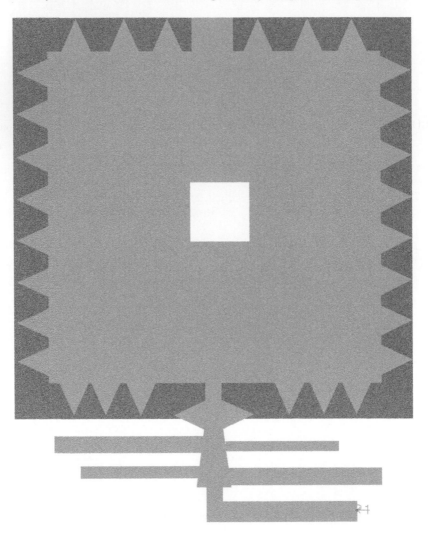

FIGURE 8.69   Layout of the fractal stacked patch antenna.

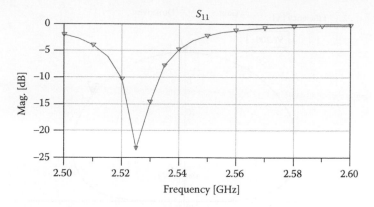

FIGURE 8.70 Computed S_{11} parameter of the single-layer fractal antenna.

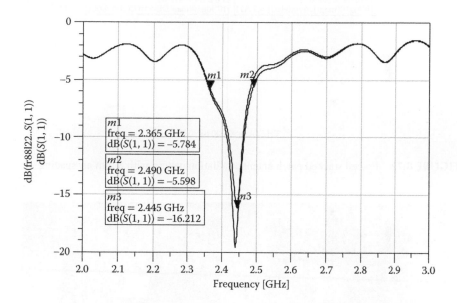

FIGURE 8.71 Measured and computed S_{11} parameter of the fractal stacked patch antenna with no air spacing between the layers.

The patch radiator dimensions are $45.8 \times 39.1 \times 0.08$ cm. The stacked fractal antenna structure is shown in Figure 8.69. The spacing between the two layers may be varied to get wider bandwidth. The single-layer fractal antenna S_{11} parameter is presented in Figure 8.70.

A comparison of the computed and measured S_{11} parameter of the fractal stacked patch antenna with no air spacing is given in Figure 8.71. There is a good agreement of measured and computed results. The fractal stacked patch antenna radiation pattern is shown in Figure 8.72. The antenna beam width is around 82°, with 7.5 dBi

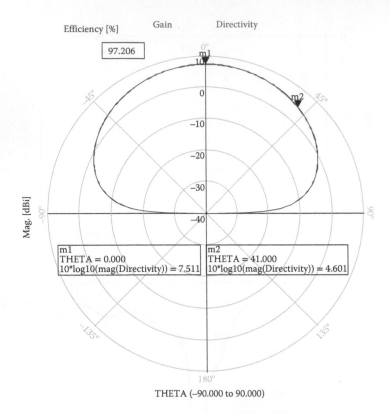

FIGURE 8.72   Fractal stacked patch antenna radiation pattern with 8 mm air spacing.

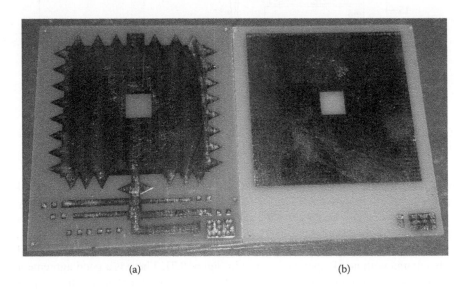

FIGURE 8.73   Fractal stacked patch antenna; (a) resonator. (b) radiator.

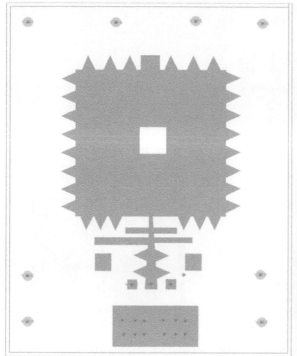
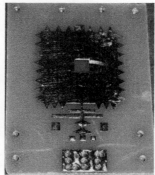

FIGURE 8.74   (a) Resonator of the 8 GHz fractal stacked patch antenna. (b) 8 GHz fractal resonator photo.

gain and 97.2% efficiency. A photo of the fractal stacked patch antenna is shown in Figure 8.73. The antenna resonator is shown in Figure 8.74a. The antenna radiator is shown in Figure 8.74b.

8.11.3 New 8 GHz Fractal Printed Antennas with Space-Filling Perimeter of the Conducting Sheet

A new fractal microstrip antenna was designed as presented in Figure 8.74. The antenna was printed on Duroid substrate 0.8 mm thick with a dielectric constant of 2.2. The antenna dimensions are $17.2 \times 21.8 \times 0.08$ cm. The antenna was designed using ADS software.

The antenna resonator bandwidth is around 3% around 7. 2 GHz for VSWR better than 2:1. The antenna bandwidth is improved to 22% for VSWR better than 3:1, by adding a second layer above the resonator. A patch radiator is printed on the second layer as presented in Figure 8.75. The radiator was printed on FR4 substrate 0.8 mm thick with a dielectric constant of 4.5. The electromagnetic fields radiated by the resonator are electromagnetically coupled to the patch radiator. The patch radiator dimensions are $17.2 \times 21.8 \times 0.08$ cm. The stacked fractal antenna structure is shown in Figure 8.76. The spacing between the two layers may be varied to

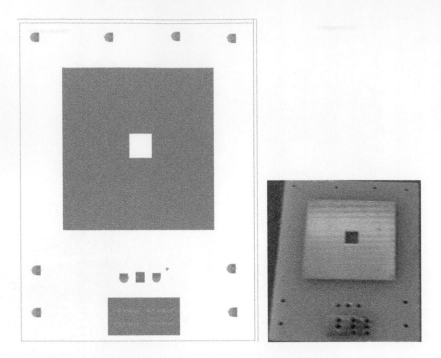

FIGURE 8.75   (a) Radiator of the 8 GHz fractal stacked patch antenna. (b) Radiator photo.

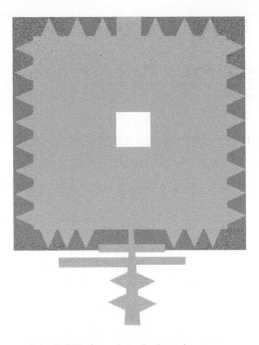

FIGURE 8.76   Layout of the 8 GHz fractal stacked patch antenna.

get wider bandwidth. The single-layer fractal antenna S_{11} parameter is presented in Figure 8.77. The computed S_{11} parameter of the fractal stacked patch antenna with 2 mm air spacing is given in Figure 8.78. The fractal stacked patch antenna radiation pattern at 7.5 GHz is shown in Figure 8.79. The antenna beam width is around 82°, with 7.8 dBi gain and 82.2% efficiency. The fractal stacked patch antenna radiation pattern at 8 GHz is shown in Figure 8.80. The antenna beam width is around 82°, with 7.5 dBi gain and 95.3% efficiency. A photo of the fractal stacked patch antenna is shown in Figure 8.81. The antenna resonator is shown in Figure 8.81a. The antenna radiator is shown in Figure 8.81b.

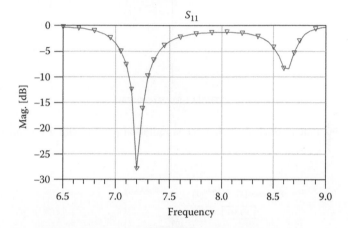

FIGURE 8.77   Computed S_{11} of the 8 GHz fractal stacked patch antenna.

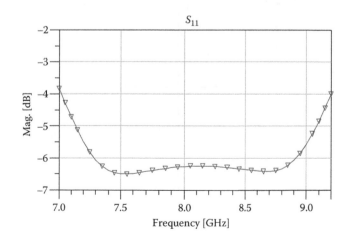

FIGURE 8.78   Computed S_{11} of the 8 GHz fractal stacked patch antenna with 2 mm air spacing.

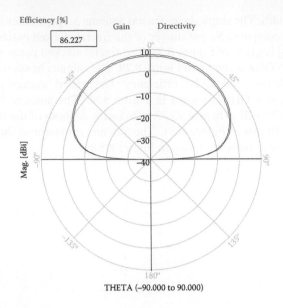

FIGURE 8.79 Fractal stacked patch antenna radiation pattern with 2 mm air spacing at 7.5 GHz.

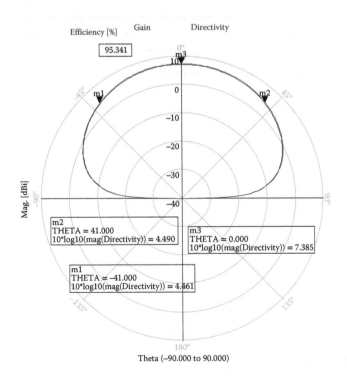

FIGURE 8.80 Fractal stacked patch antenna radiation pattern with 2 mm air spacing at 8 GHz.

8.11.4 New Stacked Patch 7.4 GHz Fractal Printed Antennas

A new fractal microstrip antenna was designed as presented in Figure 8.82. The antenna was printed on Duroid substrate 0.8 mm thick with a dielectric constant of 2.2. The antenna dimensions are $18 \times 12 \times 0.08$ cm. The antenna was designed using ADS software.

The antenna resonator bandwidth is around 2% around 7. 4 GHz for VSWR better than 2:1. The antenna bandwidth is improved to 10%, for VSWR better than 3:1, by adding a second layer above the resonator. A patch radiator is printed on the second layer as presented in Figure 8.83. The radiator was printed on FR4 substrate 0.8 mm thick with a~ dielectric constant of 4.5. The electromagnetic fields radiated by the resonator are electromagnetically coupled to the patch radiator. The fractal stacked patch dimensions are $18 \times 12 \times 0.08$ cm. The stacked fractal antenna structure is shown in Figure 8.84. The spacing between the two layers may be varied to get wider bandwidth. The computed S_{11} parameter of the fractal stacked patch antenna with 3 mm air spacing is given in Figure 8.85. The fractal stacked patch antenna radiation pattern at 7.5 GHz is shown in Figure 8.86. The antenna beam width is around 86°, with 7.9 dBi gain and 89.7% efficiency.

A modified antenna structure is presented in Figure 8.87. The antenna matching network has been modified and S_{11} at 7.45 GHz is −23.5 dB as shown in Figure 8.88. The computed S_{11} parameter of the fractal stacked patch antenna with 3 mm air spacing is given in Figure 8.88. The fractal stacked patch antenna bandwidth is around 9% for VSWR better than 3:1. The fractal stacked patch antenna radiation pattern at 7.5 GHz is shown in Figure 8.89. The antenna beam width is around 85°, with 7.8 dBi gain and 86.2% efficiency.

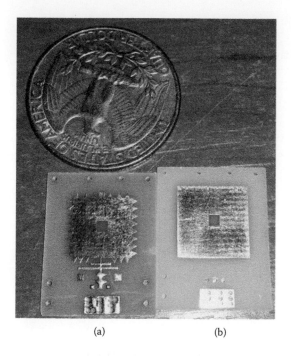

(a)   (b)

FIGURE 8.81 A photo of the fractal stacked patch antenna: (a) resonator, (b) radiator.

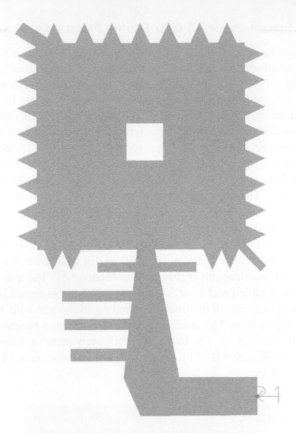

FIGURE 8.82 Layout of the 7.4 GHz fractal resonator.

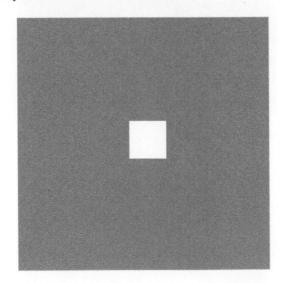

FIGURE 8.83 Radiator of a 7.4 GHz fractal stacked patch antenna.

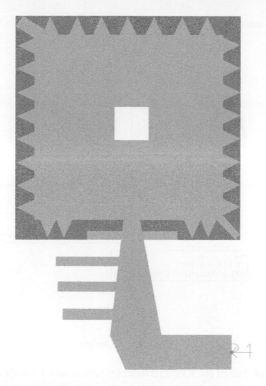

FIGURE 8.84 Layout of the 8 GHz fractal stacked patch antenna.

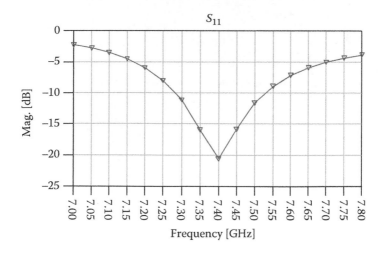

FIGURE 8.85 Computed S_{11} of the 7.4 GHz modified fractal antenna with 3 mm air spacing.

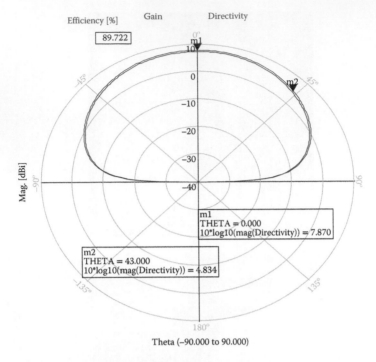

FIGURE 8.86   Fractal stacked patch antenna radiation pattern with 3 mm air spacing at 7.5 GHz.

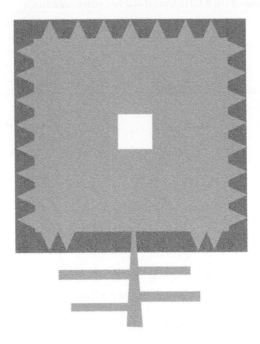

FIGURE 8.87   Layout of the modified 7.4 GHz fractal stacked patch antenna.

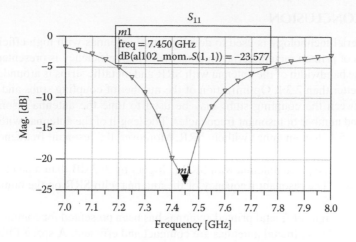

FIGURE 8.88 Computed S_{11} of the 7.4 GHz modified fractal antenna with 3 mm air spacing.

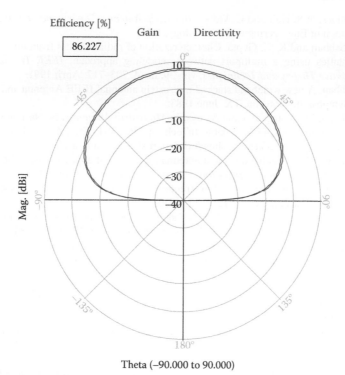

Theta (−90.000 to 90.000)

FIGURE 8.89 Modified fractal patch antenna radiation pattern with 3 mm air spacing at 7.5 GHz.

8.12 CONCLUSION

Metamaterial technology is used to develop small antennas with high efficiency. A new class of printed metamaterial antennas with high efficiency is presented in this paper. The bandwidth of the antenna with SRR and metallic strips is around 50% for VSWR better than 2.3:1. Optimization of the number of coupling stubs and the distance between the coupling stubs may be used to tune the antenna resonant frequency and number of resonant frequencies. The length of the antennas with SRR is smaller by 5% than antennas without SRR. Moreover, the resonant frequency of the antennas with SRR is lower by 5% to 10% than antennas without SRR. The gain and directivity of the patch antenna with SRR is higher by 2–3 dB than a patch antenna without SRR. The resonant frequency of the antenna with SRR on the human body is shifted by 3%.

Several designs of fractal printed antennas has been presented for communication applications. These fractal antennas are compact and efficient. A space-filling technique and Hilbert curves were employed to design the fractal antennas. The antenna bandwidth is around 10% with VSWR better than 3:1. The antenna gain is around 8 dBi with 90% efficiency.

REFERENCES

1. J.R. James, P. S. Hall and C. Wood *Microstrip Antenna Theory and Design*, London: Institution of Engineering and Technology, 1981.
2. J. A. Sabban and K. C. Gupta, Characterization of radiation loss from microstrip discontinuities using a multiport network modeling approach, *IEEE Transaction on Microwave Theory and Techniques*, vol. 39, no. 4, 705–712, April 1991.
3. A. Sabban, A new wideband stacked microstrip antenna, IEEE Antenna and Propagation Symposium, Houston, TX, June 1983.
4. A. Sabban, Microstrip antenna Arrays, in *Microstrip Antennas*, N. Nasimuddin (Ed.), ISBN: 978-953-307-247-0, Croatia: InTech, pp. 361–384, 2011, Available from: http://www.intechopen.com/articles/show/title/microstrip-antenna-arrays.
5. A. Sabban, New wideband printed antennas for medical applications, *IEEE Transactions on Antennas and Propagation*, vol. 61, no. 1, 84–91, January 2013.
6. J. B. Pendry et al., Extremely low frequency plasmons in metallic mesostructures. *Physical Review Letters*, vol. 76, 4773–4776, 1996.
7. J. B. Pendry et al., Magnetism from conductors and enhanced nonlinear phenomena, *IEEE Transactions on Microwave Theory Techniques*, vol. 47, 2075–2084, 1999.
8. R. Marqués et al., Comparative analysis of edge and broadside coupled split ring resonators for metamaterial design. Theory and experiment, *IEEE Transactions on Antennas Propagation*, vol. 51, 2572–2581, 2003.
9. R. Marqués et al., Novel small resonant electromagnetic particles for metamaterial and filter design. Proceedings of International Conference Electromagnetics in Advanced Applications' 03, Torino, Italy, 2003, pp. 439–442.
10. R. Marqués et al., Left-handed-media simulation and transmission of EM waves in subwavelength split-ring-resonator-loaded metallic waveguides. *Physical Review Letters*, vol. 89, 183901, 2002.
11. J. D. Baena et al., Experimental results on metamaterial simulation using SRR-loaded waveguides. Proceedings of IEEE-AP/S International Symposium on Antennas and Propagation, Ohio, June 2003, pp. 106–109.

12. R. Marqués et al., A new 2-D isotropic lefthanded metamaterial design: Theory and experiment, *Microwave and Optical Technology Letters*, vol. 35, 405–408, 2002.

13. R. A. Shelby et al., Microwave transmission through a two-dimensional, isotropic, left-handed metamaterial. *Applied Physics Letters*, vol. 78, 489–491, 2001.

14. J. Zhu and G. V. Eleftheriades, A compact transmission-line metamaterial antenna with extended bandwidth, *IEEE Antennas and Wireless Propagation Letters*, vol. 8, 295–298, 2009.

15. L. C. Chirwa et al., Electromagnetic radiation from ingested sources in the human intestine between 150 MHz and 1.2 GHz, *IEEE Transaction on Biomedical Engineering*, vol. 50, no. 4, 484–492, April 2003.

16. D. Werber, A. Schwentner, E. M. Biebl, Investigation of RF transmission properties of human tissues, *Advances in Radio Science*, vol. 4, 357–360, 2006.

17. B. Gupta, S. Sankaralingam and S. Dhar, Development of wearable and implantable antennas in the last decade, Mediterranean Microwave Symposium (MMS), Cyprus, 2010, pp 251–267.

18. T. Thalmann et al., Investigation and design of a multi-band wearable antenna, 3rd European Conference on Antennas and Propagation (EuCAP), Berlin, Germany, 2009, pp. 462–465.

19. P. Salonen, Y. Rahmat-Samii and M. Kivikoski, Wearable antennas in the vicinity of human body, IEEE Antennas and Propagation Society International Symposium, Monterey, CA, vol. 1, 2004, pp. 467–470.

20. T. Kellomaki, J. Heikkinen and M. Kivikoski, Wearable antennas for FM reception, First European Conference on Antennas and Propagation (EuCAP), Nice, France, November 2006, pp. 1–6.

21. A. Sabban, Wideband printed antennas for medical applications, Asia Pacific Microwave Conference (APMC), Singapore, December 2009.

22. A. Alomainy et al., Transient characteristics of wearable antennas and radio propagation channels for ultrawideband body-centric wireless communication, *IEEE Transactions on Antennas and Propagation*, vol. 57, no. 4, 875–884, April 2009.

23. M. Klemm and G. Troester, Textile UWB antenna for wireless body area networks, *IEEE Transactions on Antennas and Propagation*, vol. 54, no. 11, 3192–3197, November 2006.

24. P. M. Izdebski, H. Rajagoplan and Y. Rahmat-Sami, Conformal ingestible capsule antenna: A novel chandelier meandered design, *IEEE Transactions on Antennas and Propagation*, vol. 57, no. 4, 900–909, April 2009.

25. A. Sabban, Wideband tunable printed antennas for medical applications, *IEEE Antenna and Propagation Symposium*, Chicago, IL, July 2012.

26. B. B. Mandelbrot, The Fractal Geometry of Nature, New York: W.H. Freeman and Company, 1983.

27. B. B. Mandelbrot, How long is the coast of Britain? Statistical self-similarity and fractional dimension, *Science*, vol. 156, 636–638, 1967.

28. F. J. Falkoner, *The Geometry of Fractal Sets*, Cambridge: Cambridge University Press, 1990.

29. C. A. Balanis, *Antenna Theory Analysis and Design*, 2nd Edition, Hoboken, NJ: John Wiley & Sons, 1997.

30. K. Virga and Y. Rahmat-Samii, Low-profile enhanced-bandwidth PIFA antennas for wireless communications packaging, *IEEE Transactions on Microwave Theory and Techniques*, vol. 45 no. 10, 1879–1888, October 1997.

31. M. I. Skolnik, *Introduction to Radar Systems*, London: McGraw-Hill, 1981.

32. US Patent 5087515 A, Ward C. Stevens, Edward A. Sturm, Bruce C. Roma, Chaff fiber comprising insulative coating thereon, and having an evanescent radar reflectance characteristic, and method of making the same, 1992, USA.

33. Baliarda C. P. European Patent Application EP 1317018 A2. Anti-radar space-filling and/or multilevel chaff dispersers. 27.11.2002

34. T. Chiou, K. Wong, Design of compact microstrip antennas with a slotted ground plane, IEEE-Antennas and Propagation Society International Symposium (APS), Boston, MA, July 8–12, 2001.

35. R. C. Hansen, Fundamental limitations on Antennas, *Proceedings of the IEEE*, vol. 69, no. 2, 170–182, February 1981.

36. D. Pozar, *The Analysis and Design of Microstrip Antennas and Arrays*, Piscataway, NJ: IEEE Press, 1995, 08855–1331

37. J. F. Zurcher and F. E. Gardiol, *Broadband Patch Antennas*, Norwood, MA: Artech House, 1995.

38. I. Minin, Microwave and millimeter wave technologies from photonic bandgap devices to antenna and applications, Chap. 16, *Fractal Antenna Applications*, M. V. Rusu and R. Baican (Eds.), Intech, ISBN 978-953-7619-66-4, pp. 351–382, March 2010.

39. M. V. Rusu et al., Minkowski fractal microstrip antenna for RFID tags, Proceedings of EuMW2008 Symposium, Amsterdam, October, 2008.

40. H. Rahimi et al., Small patch antenna based on fractal design for wireless sensors, MME07, 18th Workshop on Micromachining, Micromechanics, and Microsystems, Portugal, September 16–18, 2007.

41. A. Sabban. *Low Visibility Antennas for Communication Systems*, New York: Taylor & Francis Group, 2015.

9 Active Wearable Printed Antennas for Medical Applications

Low profile compact active and tunable antennas are needed in several communication systems. Printed antennas possess attractive features such as low profile, flexibility , light weight, small volume, and low production cost. The resonant frequency of microstrip antennas is altered due to environmental conditions, different antenna locations, and different modes of operation. Wearable printed active and tunable antennas are not widely presented in the literature. However, microstrip antennas have been widely presented in books and papers in the last decade [1–7]. A new class of wideband active and tunable wearable antennas for medical applications is presented in this chapter. For example, the antenna VSWR is better than 2:1 at 434 MHz ±5%. The antenna beam width is around 100°. The antenna gain is around 0–2 dBi. A voltage-controlled varactor is used to control the antenna resonant frequency at different locations on the human body. Amplifiers may be connected to the wearable antenna feed line to increase the system dynamic range.

9.1 TUNABLE PRINTED ANTENNAS

The communication and biomedical industry has undergone continuous growth in the last decade. Low profile compact tunable antennas are crucial in the development of wearable human biomedical systems. Tunable antennas consist of a radiating element and of a voltage-controlled diode, a varactor. Varactor diodes are semiconductor devices that allow for voltage-controlled variable capacitance. The radiating element may be a microstrip patch antenna, dipole, or loop antenna. The antenna resonant frequency may be tuned using a varactor to compensate for variations in antenna resonant frequency at different locations.

9.2 VARACTOR THEORY

Varactor diodes are semiconductor devices that are used in many microwave systems where a voltage-controlled variable capacitance is required.

PN junction diodes exhibit a variable capacitance effect and PN diodes can be used for voltage-controlled variable capacitance. However, special PN diodes are optimized and fabricated to give the required capacitance values. Varactor diodes normally enable much higher ranges of capacitance change to be achieved as a result of the PN diodes' optimized design. Varactor diodes are widely used in RF devices. The circuit capacitance is varied by applying a controlled voltage. Varactor diodes are used in voltage-controlled oscillators (VCOs). Varactor diodes are also used in tunable filters and antennas.

269

9.2.1   VARACTOR DIODE BASICS

The varactor diode consists of a standard PN junction, see Figure 9.1. The diode is operated under reverse bias conditions; this gives rise to three regions and there is no conduction. The left and right ends of the diode are P and N regions, where current can be conducted. However, around the junction is the depletion region where no current carriers are available. As a result, current can be carried in the P and N regions, but the depletion region is an insulator. This is similar to a capacitor structure. It has conductive plates separated by an insulating dielectric. The capacitance of a capacitor depends on the plate area, the dielectric constant of the insulator between the plates, and the distance between the two plates. In the case of the varactor diode, it is possible to increase and decrease the width of the depletion region by changing the level of the reverse bias. This has the effect of changing the distance between the plates of the capacitor. However to be able to use varactor diodes to their best advantage it is necessary to understand features of varactor diodes including the capacitance ratio, Q, gamma, reverse voltage, and the like.

A varactor provides electrically controllable capacitance, which can be used in tuned circuits. It is small and inexpensive. Its disadvantages compared to a manually controlled variable capacitor are a lower Q, nonlinearity, lower voltage rating, and a more limited range.

Any PN junction has a junction capacitance that is a function of the voltage across the junction. The electric field in the depletion layer that is set up by the ionized donors and acceptors is responsible for the voltage difference that balances the applied voltage. A higher reverse bias widens the depletion layer, uncovering more fixed charge and raising the junction potential. The capacitance of the junction is $C = Q (V)/V$, and the *incremental capacitance* is $c = \Delta Q (V)/\Delta V$. The capacitance to be used in the formula for the resonant frequency is the incremental capacitance, where it is assumed that the incremental voltage ΔV is small compared to V. Finite voltages give rise to nonlinearities. The capacitance decreases as the reverse bias increases, according to the relation $C = C_0/(1 + V/V_0)^n$, where C_0 and V_0 are constants. The diode forward voltage is approximately V_0. The exponent n depends on how the doping density of the semiconductors depends on distance away from the junction. For a graded junction (linear variation), $n = 0.33$. For an abrupt junction (constant doping density), $n = 0.5$. If the density jumps abruptly at the junction, then decreases (called hyperabrupt), n can be made as high as $n = 2$. The varactor capacitance is given in Equation 9.1. The circuit frequency f_r may be calculated by using Equation 9.2.

$$C = \frac{A\varepsilon}{d} \qquad (9.1)$$

where C is capacitance, A *is plate area*, and d *is* diode thickness (Figure 9.2).

$$f_r = \frac{1}{2\pi\sqrt{LC}} \qquad (9.2)$$

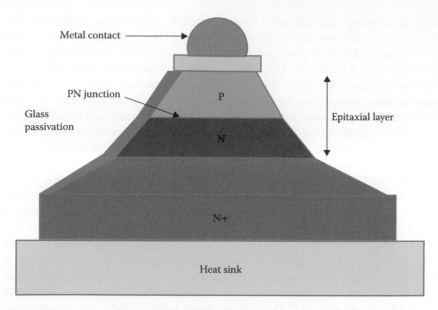

FIGURE 9.1　Internal structure of a varactor.

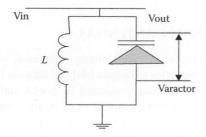

FIGURE 9.2　Varactor example.

9.2.2 Types of Varactors

Abrupt and hyperabrupt type: When the changeover PN junction is abrupt then it is called an abrupt varactor. When change is very abrupt, it is called a hyperabrupt varactor. Varactors are used in oscillators to sweep for different frequencies.

Gallium-arsenide varactor diodes: The semiconductor material used is gallium arsenide. They are used for frequencies from 18 GHz up to and beyond 600 GHz.

9.3　DUALLY POLARIZED TUNABLE PRINTED ANTENNA

A compact tunable microstrip dipole antenna has been designed to provide horizontal polarization. The antenna consists of two layers. The first layer consists of RO3035 0.8 mm dielectric substrate. The second layer consists of RT-Duroid 5880 0.8 mm dielectric substrate. The substrate thickness affects the antenna bandwidth. The printed slot antenna provides vertical polarization. The printed dipole and the slot antenna provide dual orthogonal polarizations. The dimensions of the dual polarized antenna are $26 \times 6 \times 0.16$ cm. Also, tunable compact folded dual polarized antennas have been designed. The dimensions of the compact antennas are $5 \times 5 \times 0.05$ cm. Varactors are connected to the antenna feed lines as shown in Figure 9.3. The voltage- controlled varactors are used to control the antenna resonant frequency. The varactor bias voltage may be varied automatically to set the antenna resonant frequency at different locations on the human body. The antenna may be used as a wearable antenna on a human body. It may be attached to the patient's shirt in the stomach or back zone of the patient. The antenna has been analyzed using Agilent ADS software. There is a good agreement between measured and computed results. The antenna bandwidth is around 10% for VSWR better than 2:1. The antenna beam width is around 100°. The antenna gain is around 2 dBi.

Figure 9.4 presents the antenna's measured S_{11} parameter without a varactor. Figure 9.5 presents the antenna's S_{11} parameter as a function of different varactor capacitances. Figure 9.6 presents the tunable antenna resonant frequency as a function of the varactor capacitance. The antenna resonant frequency varies around 5% for capacitances up to 2.5 pF. The antenna beam width is 100°. The antenna cross polarized field strength may be adjusted by varying the slot feed location.

9.4 WEARABLE TUNABLE ANTENNAS

As presented in Chapter 6, the antenna's input impedance varies as a function of distance from the body. Properties of human body tissues are listed in Table 6.2, see [8,9]. Wearable antennas have been presented in books and papers over the last decade [10–17]. Wearable antenna electrical performance was computed by using ADS software [18]. The analyzed structure is presented in Figure 6.14. Wearable tunable antennas are not widely presented. In this section, several wearable tunable antennas are presented. Figure 9.7 presents S_{11} results for different belt and shirt

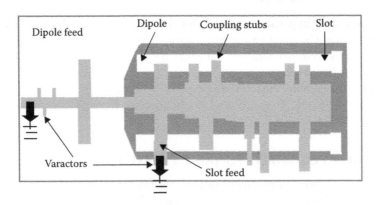

FIGURE 9.3   Dual polarized tunable antenna, $26 \times 6 \times 0.16$ cm.

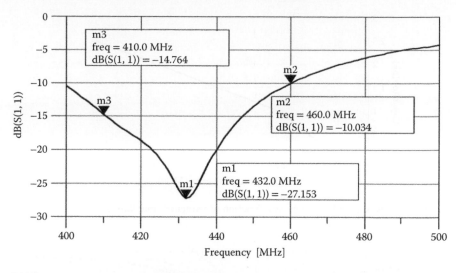

FIGURE 9.4 Measured S_{11} on human body.

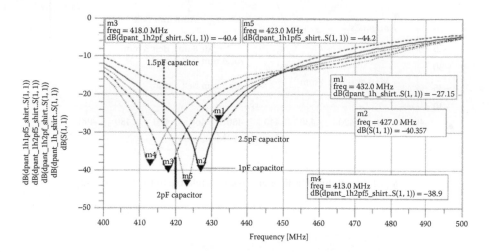

FIGURE 9.5 The tunable S_{11} parameter as a function of varactor capacitance.

thicknesses and different air spacings between the antennas and the human body. When the antenna resonant frequency is shifted the voltage across the varactor is varied to tune the antenna resonant frequency.

If the air spacing between the sensors and the human body is increased from 0 mm to 5 mm the antenna resonant frequency is shifted by 5%. A voltage-controlled varactor is used to tune the antenna resonant frequency due to different antenna locations on a human body. Figure 9.8 presents several compact tunable antennas for medical applications. A voltage-controlled varactor may be used also to tune the loop antenna resonant frequency at different antenna locations on the body.

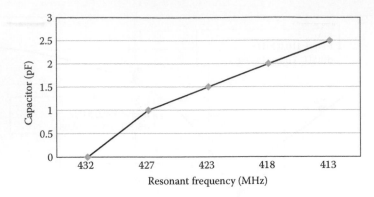

FIGURE 9.6   Resonant frequency as a function of varactor capacitance.

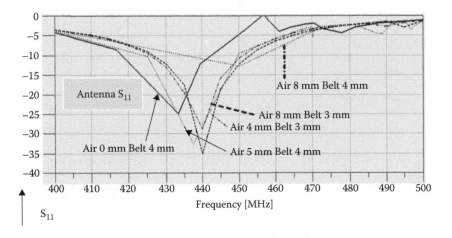

FIGURE 9.7 S_{11} of the antenna for different spacings relative to the human body.

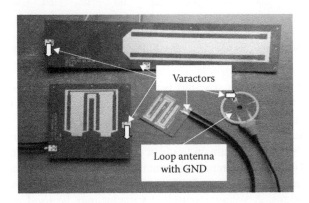

FIGURE 9.8   Tunable antennas for medical applications.

9.5 VARACTORS

Tuning varactors are voltage-variable capacitors designed to provide electronic tuning of microwave components. Varactors are manufactured on silicon and gallium arsenide substrates. Gallium arsenide varactors offer higher Q and may be used at higher frequencies than silicon varactors. Hyperabrupt varactors provide nearly linear variation of frequency with applied control voltage. However abrupt varactors provide inverse fourth root frequency dependence. MACOM offers several gallium arsenide hyperabrupt varactors such as the MA46 series. Figure 9.9 presents the $C-V$ curves of varactors MA46505 to MA46506. Figure 9.10 presents the $C-V$ curves of varactors MA46 H070 to MA46 H074.

9.6 MEASUREMENTS OF TUNABLE ANTENNAS

Figure 9.11 presents a compact tunable antenna with a varactor. A varactor was connected to the antenna feed line. The varactor bias voltage was varied from 0 V to 9 V. Figure 9.12 presents the measured S_{11} as a function of varactor bias voltage. The antenna resonant frequency was shifted by 5% for bias voltage between 7 V and 9 V. We may conclude that varactors may be used to compensate variations in the antenna resonant frequency at different locations on the human body.

9.7 FOLDED DUAL POLARIZED TUNABLE ANTENNA

The dimensions of the folded dual polarized antenna presented in Figure 9.6 are $7 \times 5 \times 0.16$ cm. The length and width of the coupling stubs in Figure 9.13 are 12 mm by 9 mm. Small tuning bars are located along the feed line to tune the antenna to the desired resonant frequency.

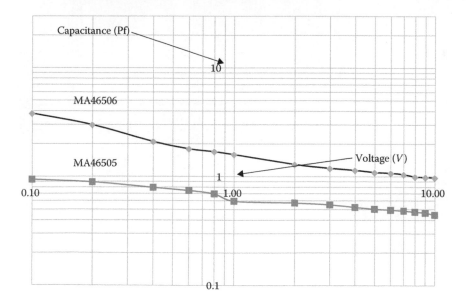

FIGURE 9.9 Varactor capacitance as a function of bias voltage.

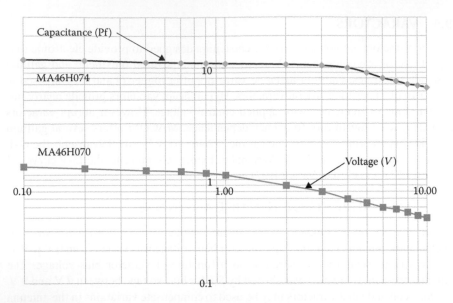

FIGURE 9.10   *C–V* curves of varactors MA46 H070 to MA46 H074.

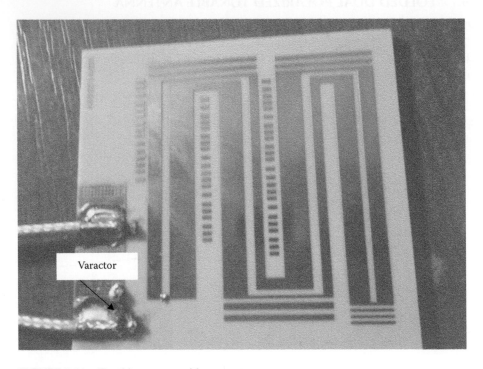

FIGURE 9.11   Tunable antenna with a varactor.

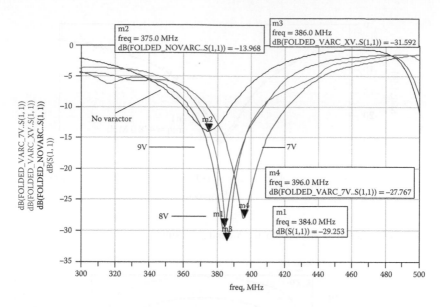

FIGURE 9.12 Measured S_{11} as a function of varactor bias voltage.

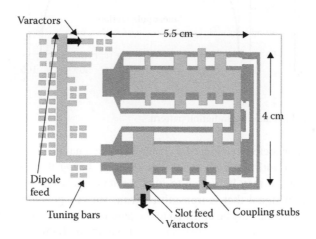

FIGURE 9.13 Tunable folded dual polarized antenna.

Figure 9.14 presents computed S_{11} and S_{22} parameters for the antenna. The computed radiation pattern of the folded dipole is shown in Figure 9.15.

9.8 MEDICAL APPLICATIONS FOR TUNABLE ANTENNAS

Three to four tunable folded dipole or tunable loop antennas may be assembled in a belt and attached to the patient's stomach or back, as shown in Figure 9.16. The bias voltage to the varactors is supplied by a recorder battery. The RF and DC cables from

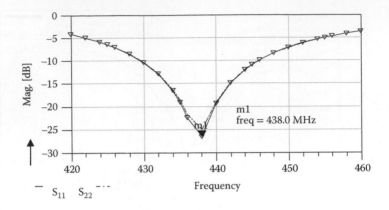

FIGURE 9.14   Folded antenna computed S_{11} and S_{22} results.

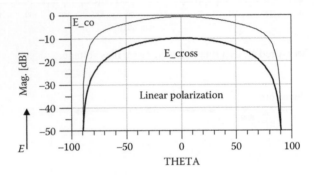

FIGURE 9.15   Folded antenna radiation pattern.

each antenna is connected to a recorder. The received signal is routed to a switching matrix. The signal with the highest level is selected during the medical test. The varactors bias voltage may be varied to tune the antenna resonant frequency. The antennas receive a signal that is transmitted from various positions in the human body. A tunable antenna may be attached to the patient's back in order to improve the level of the received signal from different locations in the human body. In several applications the distance separating the transmitting and receiving antennas is less than the far field distance, $2D^2/\lambda$, where D is the largest dimension of the source of the radiation, and λ is the wavelength. In these applications the amplitude of the electromagnetic field close to the antenna fall off rapidly with distance from the antenna. The electromagnetic fields do not radiate energy to infinite distances, but instead their energies remain trapped in the antenna near zone. The near fields transfer energy only to close distances from the receivers. In these applications, we have to refer to the near field and not to the far field radiation. The receiving and transmitting antennas are magnetically coupled. Change in current flow through one wire induces a voltage across the ends of the other wire through electromagnetic induction. The proposed tunable wearable antennas may be placed on the patient body as

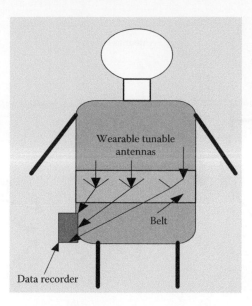

FIGURE 9.16 Tunable wearable antenna.

shown in Figure 9.17a. The patient in Figure 9.17b is wearing a wearable antenna. The antennas belt is attached to the front or back of the patient's body. Figure 9.18 presents several compact tunable antennas for medical applications. A voltage-controlled varactor may be used also to tune the wearable antenna resonant frequency at different antenna locations on the body.

9.9 ACTIVE WEARABLE ANTENNAS

Active wearable antennas may be used in receiving or transmitting channels. In transmitting channels, a power amplifier is connected to the antenna. In receiving channels, a low noise amplifier (LNA) is connected to the receiving antenna.

9.9.1 BASIC CONCEPT OF ACTIVE ANTENNAS

Active antennas (AAs) are devices combining a radiating element with active components. The radiating element is designed to provide the optimal load to the active elements. The integration of the antenna and the active components drastically reduces the complexity of the matching network. In the last decade, active antennas have been employed in wireless and in medical communication systems [19–27]. The current major applications of active antennas are large electronically scanned arrays, known as phased arrays. Indeed arrays of active antennas, or active arrays, are well suited for mobile terminals requiring dynamic satellite tracking. The most common approach toward achieving fast-beam scanning is through the integration of monolithic microwave integrated circuit (MMIC) phase shifters, LNAs, and solid state power amplifiers with the antenna elements. In some cases, hybrid electro/

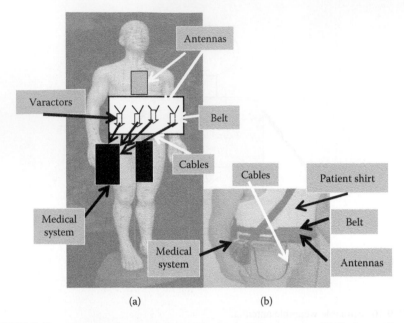

FIGURE 9.17 (a) Medical system with printed wearable antennas. (b) Patient with printed wearable antenna.

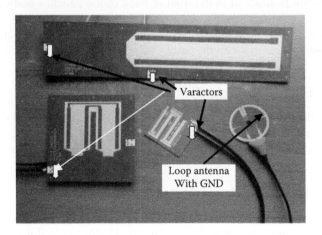

FIGURE 9.18 Tunable antennas for medical applications.

mechanical arrays combining mechanical steering with electrical steering/shaping are considered. This architecture is often used to reduce the number of active control elements by limiting the electrical scanning in only one plane. This is often the case for mobile user terminals where azimuth scanning is performed by mechanical rotation and elevation agility is realized by a linear phased array. In the last decade, printed transmission lines and antennas replaced coaxial transmission lines and metallic radiators in phased array systems. Developments in MMIC technology and other fabrication processes allowed automated low-cost production process of phased arrays with a high integration level.

Phased arrays emerged as a new promising technology for radar and communication systems around 1970. Phased arrays replace mechanically scanned antennas. They are much faster for beam switching than mechanically scanned antennas, and reduce significantly the size, weight, and power associated with a gimbal. Early phased array antennas were passive antennas. The front end of the antenna was composed of array elements with phase shifters. A passive manifold was employed for RF combining to form a single beam. At the output of the manifold was a switch with an LNA (receive channel) and power amplifier (transmit channel). Solid-state electronic device capability was not developed enough to include active amplifiers at the front end of the array for each array element. With the LNA and amplifier behind the manifold, the amount of RF loss was quite large causing inefficiency on transmit (power aperture) and limitations on sensitivity of the receiving. With the great progress of GaAs MMIC technology in the last twenty years, solid state device dimensions have been minimized to the size of the array elements, enabling distributed phased array architectures. High power amplifiers (HPAs) and LNAs could be placed close to the front end and connected to each radiating element. This resulted in drastic power efficiency improvement and much higher receive sensitivity, since the only loss before the first LNA was the radiating element and a radome. The amplifiers were packaged in transmit/receive (T/R) modules with phase shifter and attenuator. This phased array architecture was called an "active" phased array.

9.9.2 Active Wearable Receiving Loop Antenna

Figure 9.19 presents a basic receiver block diagram with an active antenna. In Figure 9.19, the LNA is an integral part of the antenna.

An E PHEMT LNA was connected to a loop antenna. The active antenna layout is shown in Figure 9.20.

A receiving active antenna block diagram is presented in Figure 9.21. The radiating element is connected to the LNA via an input matching network. An output matching network connects the amplifier port to the receiver. A DC bias network supplies the required voltages to the amplifiers. The amplifier specification is listed in Table 9.1. The amplifier complex S parameters are listed in Table 9.2. The amplifier noise parameters are listed in Table 9.3. The loop antenna S_{11} parameter on the human body is presented in Figure 9.22. A textile sleeve covers the loop antenna to

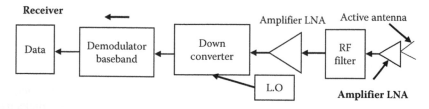

FIGURE 9.19 Receiver block diagram with active receiving antenna.

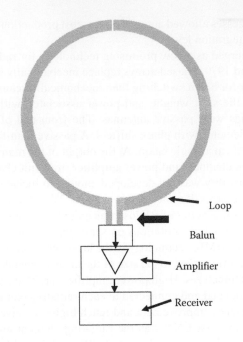

FIGURE 9.20   Active printed loop antenna layout.

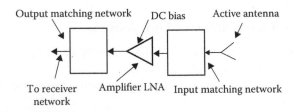

FIGURE 9.21   Receiving active antenna block diagram.

match the loop to the antenna environment. The radiating loop antenna and the textile sleeve are attached to the human body.

The antenna bandwidth is around 20% for VSWR better than 3:1. The active loop antenna S_{21} parameter, gain, on the human body is presented in Figure 9.23. The active antenna gain is 25±2.5 dB for frequencies ranging from 350 MHz to 580 MHz. The active loop antenna noise figure is presented in Figure 9.24. The active loop antenna noise figure is 0.7±0.2 dB for frequencies ranging from 400 MHz to 900 MHz.

9.9.3   COMPACT DUAL POLARIZED RECEIVING ACTIVE ANTENNA

A printed compact dual polarized antenna is shown in Figure 9.25. The compact antenna consists of two layers. The first layer consists of FR4 0.25 mm dielectric substrate. The second layer consists of Kapton 0.25 mm dielectric substrate. In

TABLE 9.1

LNA Amplifier Specification

Parameter	Specification	Remarks
Frequency range	0.4–3 GHz	–
Gain	26 dB @ 0.4 GHz	Vds = 3V; Ids = 60 mA
	18 dB @ 2 GHz	
NF	0.4 dB @ 0.4 GHz	Vds = 3V; Ids = 60 mA
	0.5 dB @ 2 GHz	
P1 dB	18.9 dBm @ 0.4 GHz	Vds = 3V; Ids = 60 mA
	19.1 dBm @ 2 GHz	
OIP3	32.1 dBm @ 0.4 GHz	Vds = 3V; Ids = 60 mA
	33.6 dBm @ 2 GHz	
Max. input power	17 dBm	–
Vgs	0.48V	Vds = 3V; Ids = 60 mA
Vds	3V	–
Ids	60 mA	–
Supply voltage	±5V	–
Package	Surface Mount	–
Operating temperature	–40°C–80°C	–
Storage temperature	–50°C–8100°C	–

TABLE 9.2

LNA Amplifier S Parameters

F-GHz	S_{11}	$S_{11}°$	S_{21}	$S_{21}°$	S_{12}	$S_{12}°$	S_{22}	$S_{22}°$
0.10	0.986	–17.17	25.43	168.9	0.008	88.22	0.55	–14.38
0.19	–31.76	0.964	24.13	158.9	0.016	74.88	0.54	–22.98
0.279	0.93	–45.77	22.97	149.5	0.021	65.77	0.51	–33.65
0.323	0.92	–53.39	22.45	145.3	0.026	62.38	0.49	–39.2
0.413	0.89	–65.72	20.98	137.27	0.03	57.9	0.46	–49.3
0.50	0.87	–77.1	19.54	130.3	0.034	53.03	0.43	–57.5
0.59	0.83	–87.12	18.08	124.14	0.038	48.18	0.40	–64.12
0.726	0.8	–100.8	16.22	115.7	0.042	42.06	0.36	–74.86
0.816	0.77	–108.8	15.07	110.75	0.044	39.53	0.34	–80.87
1.04	0.74	–126.2	12.74	100.13	0.049	33.69	0.29	–94.96
1.21	0.71	–137.6	11.25	92.91	0.051	30.05	0.26	–104
1.53	0.687	–154.2	9.29	82.06	0.055	26.08	0.22	–119
1.75	0.67	–164.1	8.24	75.31	0.058	23.14	0.20	–128.4
2.02	0.67	–174.6	7.27	67.82	0.06	20.88	0.18	–138.8

Figure 9.26, the LNA, presented in Section 9.9.2, is an integral part of the dual polarized receiving antenna. The active dual polarized antenna S_{21} parameter, gain, on the human body is presented in Figure 9.27. The active antenna gain is 25±3 dB for frequencies ranging from 400 MHz to 650 MHz. There is a good match between the

TABLE 9.3
Noise Parameters

F-GHz	NFMIN	N11X	N11Y	rn
0.5	0.079	0.3284	24.56	0.056
0.7	0.112	0.334	36.08	0.05
0.9	0.144	0.3396	47.4	0.045
1	0.16	0.3424	52.98	0.042
1.9	0.306	0.3682	100.93	0.029
2	0.322	0.3711	106.01	0.029
2.4	0.387	0.3829	125.79	0.029
3	0.484	0.401	153.93	0.036
3.9	0.629	0.429	−167.3	0.059
5	0.808	0.4645	−125.53	0.11
5.8	0.937	0.4912	−99.03	0.162
6	0.969	0.498	−92.92	0.177

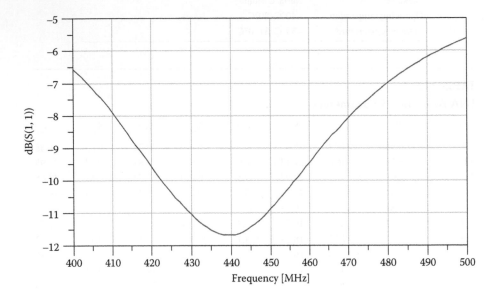

FIGURE 9.22   Loop antenna S_{11} parameter on the human body.

gains of the vertical and horizontal antennas. The gain difference between the gains of the vertical and horizontal antennas is around ±0.5 dB. The active dual polarized antenna noise figure is presented in Figure 9.28. The active loop antenna noise figure is 0.8±0.4 dB for frequencies ranging from 400 MHz to 900 MHz.

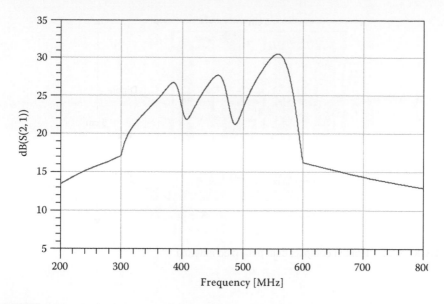

FIGURE 9.23 Active loop antenna S_{21} parameter, gain, on the human body.

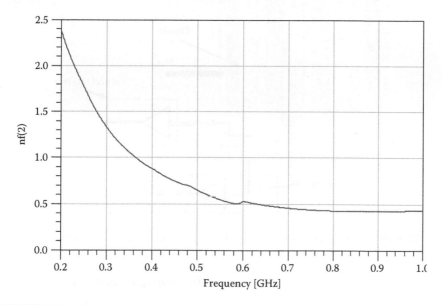

FIGURE 9.24 Active loop antenna noise figure.

9.10   ACTIVE TRANSMITTING ANTENNA

Figure 9.29 presents a basic transmitter block diagram with an active antenna. The HPA is an integral part of the antenna.

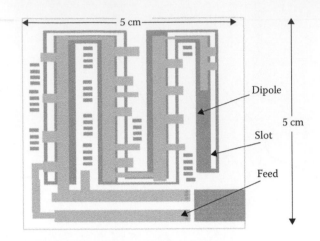

FIGURE 9.25   Printed compact dual polarized antenna.

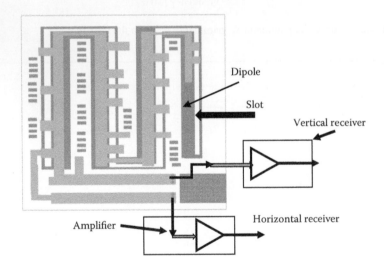

FIGURE 9.26   Active printed compact dual polarized receiving antenna layout.

9.10.1 COMPACT DUAL POLARIZED ACTIVE TRANSMITTING ANTENNA

A printed compact dual polarized transmitting antenna is shown in Figure 9.30. The antenna dimensions are $5 \times 5 \times 0.05$ cm.

The active transmitting dual polarized antenna layout is shown in Figure 9.30. In Figure 9.31, the HPA is an integral part of the antenna and is connected to the transmitting antenna. The HPA is a MMIC GaAs MESFET. The transmitting active antenna block diagram is presented in Figure 9.31. The radiating element is connected to the HPA via an output HPA matching network. An HPA input matching network connects the amplifier port to the transmitter.

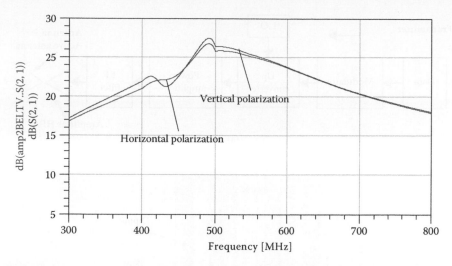

FIGURE 9.27 Active dual polarized antenna S_{21} parameter, gain, on the human body.

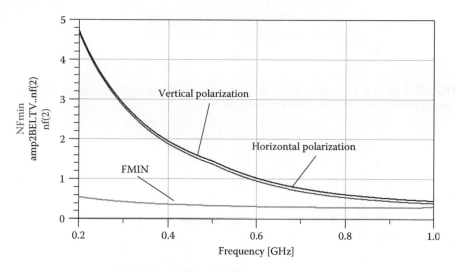

FIGURE 9.28 Active dual polarized antenna noise figure.

The amplifier specification is listed in Table 9.4. The amplifier pin description is given and presented in Figure 9.32.

Pin	Function
1	DC bias
3	RF in
6	RF out
2,4,5,7,8	Ground. Via Holes.

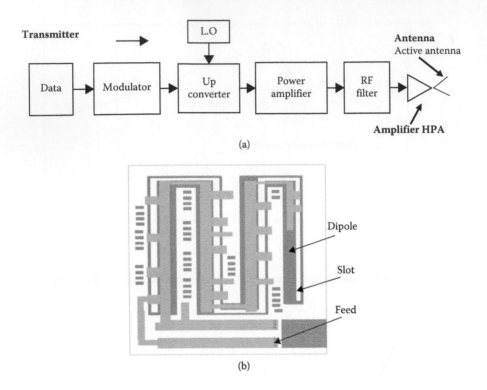

FIGURE 9.29 (a) Transmitter block diagram with active transmitting antenna. (b) Transmitting printed compact dual polarized antenna.

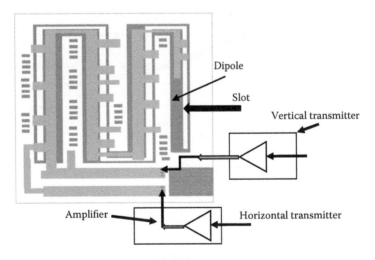

FIGURE 9.30 Transmitting active printed dual polarized antenna layout.

The HPA complex S parameters are listed in Table 9.5.

The active transmitting dual polarized antenna S_{11} parameter on the human body is presented in Figure 9.33. The active transmitting dual polarized antenna S_{21} parameter,

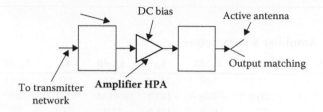

FIGURE 9.31   Transmitting active antenna block diagram.

TABLE 9.4
HPA Amplifier Specification

Parameter	Specification	Remarks
Frequency range	0.4–2.5 GHz	–
Gain	15 dB @ 0.4 GHz	Vds = 5V; Ids = 85 mA
	17.8 dB @ 2 GHz	
NF	5.5 dB @ 0.4 GHz	Vds = 5V; Ids = 85 mA
	5.5 dB @ 2 GHz	
P1 dB	18.0 dBm @ 0.4 GHz	Vds = 5V; Ids = 85 mA
	18.0 dBm @ 2 GHz	
OIP3	29 dBm @ 0.4 GHz	Vds = 5V; Ids = 85 mA
	29 dBm @ 2 GHz	
Max. input power	10 dBm	
Vgs	0.48 V	Vds = 5V; Ids = 85 mA
Vds	5 V	–
Ids	85 mA	–
Supply voltage	+ 5V	–
Package	Surface Mount	–
Operating temperature	−40°c–80°c	–
Storage temperature	−50°c–100°c	–

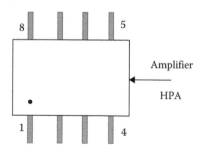

FIGURE 9.32   Amplifier pin description.

gain, on the human body is presented in Figure 9.34. The active dual polarized antenna gain is 14±3 dB for frequencies ranging from 380 MHz to 600 MHz. The active transmitting dual polarized antenna output power is around 18 dBm.

TABLE 9.5

High Power Amplifier S Parameters

F-GHz	S_{11} dB	S_{11}	S_{21} dB	S_{21}	S_{12} dB	S_{12}	S_{22} dB	S_{22}
0.20	0.065	−38.75	−3.09	−139.2	−47.56	157.63	−1.03	−74.66
0.28	−0.14	−60.8	7.46	163.7	−40.45	114	−3.6	−109.3
0.344	−1.1	−77	11.8	118.7	−37.9	78.4	−7.2	−131.6
0.4	−2.2	−88.5	13.8	85.24	−36.9	52.76	−11	−143.5
0.48	−3.7	−101.8	15.35	46.5	−36.6	25.4	−17	−143.1
0.52	−4.44	−107.5	15.8	30.2	−36.7	14.1	−19.4	−132.5
0.56	−5.1	−112.7	16.2	15.3	−36.8	3.64	−20.5	−118.9
0.64	−6.4	−122	16.8	−11.4	−37.2	−12.6	−19.2	−100.3
0.712	−7.4	−100.8	17.13	−32.7	−37.5	−25.4	−17.7	−100.6
0.8	−8.45	−137.6	17.5	−56.8	−38.1	−37.8	−16.3	−108.8
0.88	−9.2	−144.6	17.72	−77.1	−38.5	−49.4	−15.7	−119.7
1.04	−10.4	−158.6	18.1	−115.1	−39.6	−67.5	−15.3	−144.5
1.12	−10.8	−166.2	18.23	−133.3	−40.3	−75.8	−15.35	−157.5
1.24	−11.3	−178.7	18.37	−159.7	−41.3	−86.9	−15.9	−178.7
1.36	−11.8	167.4	18.4	174.4	−42.4	−91.4	−16.5	159.2
1.48	−12.2	151.2	18.4	149	−43.6	−94.9	−17.5	136.8
1.6	−12.8	134.3	18.3	123.3	−44.2	−93.4	−18.9	113.7
1.8	−14.3	101.2	17.9	83	−43	−86.3	−22	69.5
2	−16.5	61.8	17.3	43.5	−40.4	94.6	−27	6.42
2.16	−18.5	22.1	16.8	12.9	−38.	−105.5	−27.8	−70.2
2.28	−19.6	−14.9	16.3	−9.6	−37.2	−116.2	−25.1	−113.2
2.4	−19.4	−53.9	15.7	−31.8	−36	−128	−22.2	−147.2
2.56	−17.7	99.7	15	−60	−34.6	−145.6	−19.3	−179.4
2.7	−15.7	131	14.3	−84.3	−33.8	−160.3	−17.5	158.1
2.86	−13.7	159	13.5	−111.1	−33	−177.7	−16	134.7
3	−12.2	179.1	12.7	−134.1	−32.4	167.4	15.2	116.3

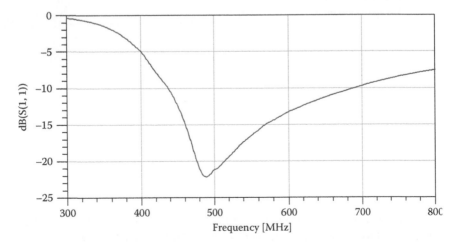

FIGURE 9.33 Active dual polarized antenna S_{11} parameter.

9.10.2 Active Transmitting Loop Antenna

The printed loop antenna is shown in Figure 9.35. The antenna dimensions are 5 × 5 × 0.05 cm. In Figure 9.35, the HPA is an integral part of the antenna. The HPA is a MMIC GaAs MESFET.

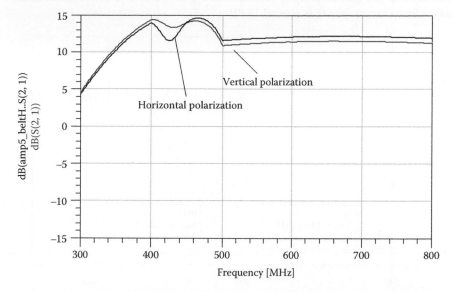

FIGURE 9.34   Active dual polarized antenna S_{21} parameter, gain, on the human body.

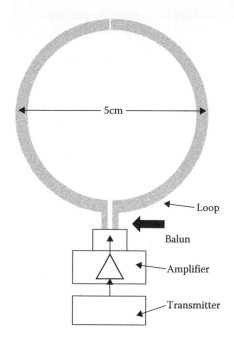

FIGURE 9.35   Active transmitting printed loop antenna layout.

The active transmitting loop antenna S_{21} parameter, gain, on the human body is presented in Figure 9.36. The active antenna gain is 14±3 dB for frequencies ranging from 400 MHz to 600 MHz. The active transmitting loop antenna S_{11} parameter on the human body is presented in Figure 9.37. The active transmitting loop antenna S_{22} parameter on the human body is presented in Figure 9.38. The active transmitting loop antenna output power is around 18 dBm.

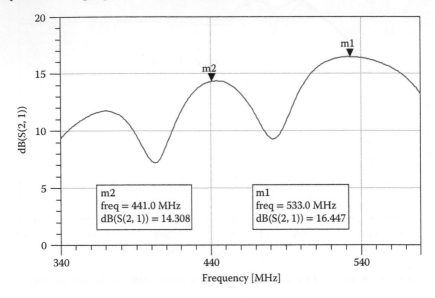

FIGURE 9.36 Active transmitting loop antenna S_{21} parameter.

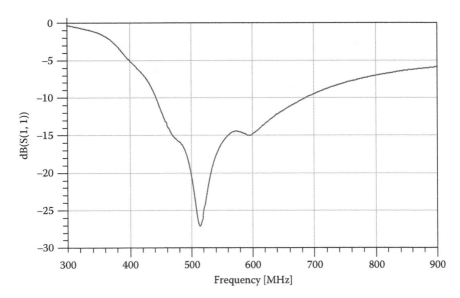

FIGURE 9.37 Active transmitting loop antenna S_{11} parameter.

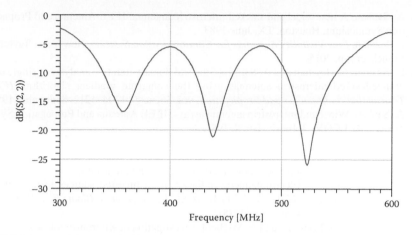

FIGURE 9.38 Active transmitting loop antenna S_{22} parameter.

9.11 CONCLUSIONS

This chapter presents wideband active printed antennas with high efficiency for commercial and medical applications. The antenna dimensions may vary from 26 cm by 6 cm by 0.16 cm to 5 cm by 5 cm by 0.05 cm according to the medical system specifications. The antenna's bandwidth is around 10% for VSWR better than 2:1. The antenna's beam width is around 100°. The tunable antenna's gain varies from 0 to 2 dBi. If the air spacing between the dual polarized antenna and the human body is increased from 0 mm to 5 mm the antenna resonant frequency is shifted by 5%. A varactor is employed to compensate for variations in the antenna resonant frequency at different locations on the human body.

Active wearable antennas may be used in receiving or transmitting channels. In transmitting channels a power amplifier is connected to the antenna. In receiving channels, a LNA is connected to the receiving antenna. The active loop antenna gain is 25±2.5 dB for frequencies ranging from 350 MHz to 580 MHz. The active loop antenna noise figure is 0.7±0.2 dB for frequencies ranging from 400 MHz to 900 MHz. The active dual polarized antenna gain is 25±3 dB for frequencies ranging from 400 MHz to 650 MHz. The gain difference between the gain of the vertical and horizontal antenna is around ±0.5 dB. The active dual polarized antenna noise figure is 0.8±0.4 dB for frequencies ranging from 400 MHz to 900 MHz. The active transmitting dual polarized antenna gain is 14±3 dB for frequencies ranging from 380 MHz to 600 MHz. The active transmitting dual polarized antenna output power is around 18 dBm.

REFERENCES

1. J. R. James, P. S. Hall and C. Wood, *Microstrip Antenna Theory and Design*, London: Institution of Engineering and Technology, 1981.
2. A. Sabban and K. C. Gupta, Characterization of radiation loss from microstrip discontinuities using a multiport network modeling approach, *IEEE Transaction on Microwave Theory and Techniques*, vol. 39, no. 4, 705–712, April 1991.

3. A. Sabban, A new wideband stacked microstrip antenna, IEEE Antenna and Propagation Symposium, Houston, TX, June 1983.

4. A. Sabban, *Low Visibility Antennas for Communication Systems*, New York: Taylor & Francis group, 2015.

5. R. Kastner, E. Heyman and A. Sabban, Spectral domain iterative analysis of single and double-layered microstrip antennas using the conjugate gradient algorithm, *IEEE Transaction on Antennas and Propagation*, vol. 36, no. 9, 1204–1212, September 1988.

6. A. Sabban, Wideband microstrip antenna arrays, IEEE Antenna and Propagation Symposium MELCOM, Tel-Aviv, Israel, 1981.

7. A. Sabban, Microstrip antenna arrays, in *Microstrip Antennas,* N. Nasimuddin (Ed.), ISBN: 978-953-307-247-0, Croatia: InTech, pp. 361–384 2011, Available from: http://www.intechopen.com/articles/show/title/microstrip-antenna-arrays.

8. L. C. Chirwa et al., Electromagnetic radiation from ingested sources in the human intestine between 150 MHz and 1.2 GHz, *IEEE Transaction on Biomedical Engineering*, vol. 50, no. 4, 484–492, April 2003.

9. D. Werber, A. Schwentner and E. M. Biebl, Investigation of RF transmission properties of human tissues, *Advances in Radio Science*, vol. 4, 357–360, 2006.

10. B. Gupta, S. Sankaralingam and S. Dhar, Development of wearable and implantable antennas in the last decade, Mediterranean Microwave Symposium (MMS), 2010, Guzelyurt, Turkey, pp. 251–267.

11. T. Thalmann et al., Investigation and Design of a Multi-Band Wearable Antenna, 3rd Edition, European Conference on Antennas and Propagation (EuCAP), 2009, Berlin, Germany, pp. 462–465.

12. P. Salonen, Y. Rahmat-Samii and M. Kivikoski, Wearable antennas in the vicinity of human body, IEEE Antennas and Propagation Society International Symposium, Monterey, CA, vol. 1, 467–470, 2004.

13. T. Kellomaki, J. Heikkinen and M. Kivikoski, Wearable antennas for FM reception, First European Conference on Antennas and Propagation (EuCAP), Nice, France, November 2006, pp. 1–6.

14. A. Sabban, Wideband printed antennas for medical applications, Asian Pacific Microwave Conference (APMC) 2009, Singapore, 12/2009.

15. Y. Lee, *Antenna Circuit Design for RFID Applications, Microchip Technology*, Microchip AN 710c.

16. A. Sabban, Inventor, *Microstrip antenna arrays*, U.S. Patent US 1986/4,623,893, 1986, USA.

17. A. Sabban, Inventor, *Dual polarized dipole wearable antenna*, U.S. Patent US 8203497, June 19, 2012, USA.

18. ADS software, Agilent, Available from: http://www.home.agilent.com/agilent/product.jspx?cc=IL&lc=eng&ckey=1297113&nid=-34346.0.00&id=1297113.

19. H. A. Wheeler, Small antennas, *IEEE Transactions on Antennas and Propagation*, vol. 23, no. 4, 462–469, 1975.

20. J. Lin and T. Itoh, Active integrated antennas, *IEEE Transactions on Microwave Theory and Techniques*, vol. 42, no. 12, 2186–2194, 1994.

21. A. Mortazwi, T. Itoh and J. Harvey, *Active Antennas and Quasi-Optical Arrays*, New York, NY: John Wiley & Sons, 1998.

22. S. Jacobsen and Ø. Klemetsen, Improved detectability in medical microwave radiothermometers as obtained by active antennas, *IEEE Transactions on Biomedical Engineering*, vol. 55, no. 12, 2778–2785, 2008.

23. S. Jacobsen and Ø. Klemetsen, Active antennas in medical microwave radiometry, *Electronics Letters*, vol. 43, no. 11, 606–608, 2007.

24. S. W. Ellingson, J. H. Simonetti and C. D. Patterson, Design and evaluation of an active antenna for a 29–47 MHz radio telescope array, *IEEE Transactions on Antennas and Propagation*, vol. 55, no. 3, 826–831, 2007.
25. D. Segovia-Vargas et al., Broadband active receiving patch with resistive equalization, *IEEE Transactions on Microwave Theory and Techniques*, vol. 56, no. 1, 56–64, 2008.
26. V. Rizzoli, A. Costanzo and P. Spadoni, Computer-aided design of ultra-wideband active antennas by means of a new figure of merit, *IEEE Microwave and Wireless Components Letters*, vol. 18, no. 4, 290–292, 2008.
27. G. Yun, Compact active integrated microstrip antennas with circular polarisation diversity, *IET Microwaves, Antennas and Propagation*, vol. 2, no. 1, 82–87, 2008.

10 New Wideband Passive and Active Wearable Slot and Notch Antennas for Wireless and Medical Communication Systems

Wideband wearable antennas for communication systems are crucial in novel wearable communication systems. Slot antennas are low profile and low cost and can be employed in wearable communication systems. The dynamic range and the efficiency of communication system can be improved by using active wearable antennas.

10.1 SLOT ANTENNAS

Slot antennas can be printed on a dielectric substrate or cut out of a surface they are to be mounted on [1–16]. Slot antennas can be excited by connecting a transmission line to the slot edges as shown in Figure 10.1a. Slot antennas can be excited by a microstip line as shown in Figure 10.1b. The radiation pattern of slot antennas is determined by the size and shape of the slot in a radiating surface. Slot antennas can be used at frequencies between 200 MHz and up to 40 GHz.

The feed transmission line excites the electric field distribution within the slot, and currents that travel around the slot perimeter. If we replace the slot with metal and the ground plane with air we get a dipole antenna. The slot antenna is dual to the dipole antenna as shown in Figure 10.1a. Babinet's principle [1] relates the electromagnetic fields of a slot antenna to its dual antenna, and relates the slot antenna to the dipole antenna. This principle states that the impedance of the slot antenna Z_s is related to the impedance of its dual antenna Z_d by Equation 10.1, Where η is the intrinsic impedance of free space and is equal to $120\pi\ \Omega$.

$$Z_s Z_d = \frac{\pi\eta^2}{4} \tag{10.1}$$

The impedance of a 0.5λ-long dipole is 73 Ω. By using Equation 10.1, the impedance of a 0.5λ-long slot antenna is around 486 Ω. The second major result of Babinet's principle is that the fields of the dual antenna are almost the same as the slot antenna (the fields components are interchanged, and called "duals"). That is, the

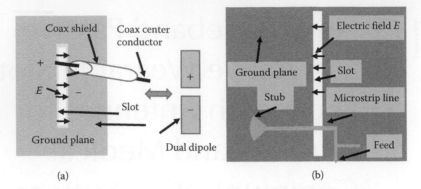

FIGURE 10.1 (a) Slot antenna and its dual dipole. (b) Printed slot antenna and microstrip line feed.

fields of the slot antenna (given with a subscript s) are related to the fields of its complement (given with a subscript d) as written in Equation 10.2.

$$E_{\theta s} = H_{\theta d}$$

$$E_{\phi s} = H_{\phi d}$$

$$H_{\theta s} = \frac{-E_{\theta d}}{\eta^2} \tag{10.2}$$

$$H_{\theta s} = \frac{-E_{\phi d}}{\eta^2}$$

The polarization of the dual antennas are reversed. The dipole antenna in Figure 10.1 is vertically polarized and the slot antenna will be horizontally polarized. In the far fields, the dipole electromagnetic fields vary as $1/r$ and $\sin\theta$ as written in Equation 10.3.

$$E_r = 0$$

$$E_\theta = j\eta_0 \frac{l\beta I_0 \sin\theta}{4\pi r} e^{j(\omega t - \beta r)} \tag{10.3}$$

$$H_\varphi = j\frac{l\beta I_0 \sin\theta}{4\pi r} e^{j(\omega t - \beta r)}$$

In the far fields, the slot electromagnetic fields vary as $1/r$ and $\sin\theta$ as written in Equation 10.4.

$$E_r = 0$$

$$H_{\theta s} = -j\frac{l\beta I_0 \sin\theta}{4\pi r\eta_0}e^{j(\omega t - \beta r)}$$

(10.4)

$$E_{\varphi s} = j\frac{l\beta I_0 \sin\theta}{4\pi r}e^{j(\omega t - \beta r)}$$

10.2 SLOT RADIATION PATTERN

The antenna radiation pattern represents the radiated fields in space at a point
$P(r, \theta, \varphi)$ as function of θ, φ. The antenna radiation pattern is three dimensional.
When φ is constant and θ vary we get the E-plane radiation pattern. When φ vary
and θ is constant, usually $\theta = \dfrac{\pi}{2}$, we get the H plane radiation pattern.

10.2.1 Slot E-Plane Radiation Pattern

The slot E-plane radiation pattern is given in Equation 10.5 and presented in
Figure 10.2.

$$\left|E_{\varphi s}\right| = j\frac{l\beta I_0 \sin\theta}{4\pi r} = A\sin\theta$$

(10.5)

At a given point $P(r, \theta, \varphi)$ the slot E-plane radiation pattern is given in
Equation 10.6.

$$\left|E_{\varphi s}\right| = j\frac{l\beta I_0 \left|\sin\theta\right|}{4\pi r} = A\left|\sin\theta\right|$$

Choose $A = 1$

(10.6)

$$\left|E_{\varphi s}\right| = \left|\sin\theta\right|$$

The slot E-plane radiation pattern in a spherical coordinate system is shown in
Figure 10.3.

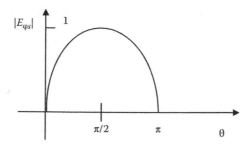

FIGURE 10.2 Slot E-plane radiation pattern.

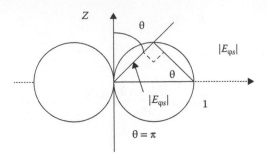

FIGURE 10.3   Slot E-plane radiation pattern in a spherical coordinate system.

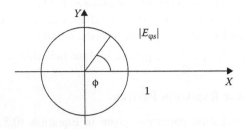

FIGURE 10.4   Slot H-plane radiation pattern for $\theta = \dfrac{\pi}{2}$.

10.2.2   SLOT H-plane RADIATION PATTERN

For $\theta = \dfrac{\pi}{2}$, the slot H-plane radiation pattern is given in Equation 10.7 and presented in Figure 10.4. At a given point $P(r, \theta, \varphi)$ the slot H-plane radiation pattern is given in Equation 10.7.

$$\left| E_{\varphi s} \right| = j \frac{l\beta I_0}{4\pi r} = A$$

Choose $A = 1$ (10.7)

$$\left| E_{\varphi s} \right| = 1$$

The slot H-plane radiation pattern in the xy plane is a circle with $r = 1$.

The radiation pattern of a vertical slot is omnidirectional. It radiates equal power in all azimuthal directions perpendicular to the axis of the antenna. The slot H-plane radiation pattern in a spherical coordinate system is shown in Figure 10.4.

10.3   SLOT ANTENNA IMPEDANCE

Antenna impedance determines the efficiency of transmitting and receiving energy in antennas. The dipole impedance is given in Equation 10.8. The slot impedance is given in Equation 10.9.

$$R_{\text{rad}} = \frac{2W_T}{I_0^2}$$

$$\text{For a dipole: } R_{\text{rad}} = \frac{80\pi^2 l^2}{\lambda^2} \tag{10.8}$$

$$Z_s = \frac{\pi\eta^2}{4Z_d} = \frac{\eta^2}{320\pi l^2} \tag{10.9}$$

By using Equation 10.9, the impedance of a 0.5λ-long slot antenna is around 565 Ω.

10.4 A WIDEBAND WEARABLE PRINTED SLOT ANTENNA

A wideband wearable printed slot antenna is shown in Figure 10.5. The slot antenna is printed on RT-DUROID 5880 dielectric substrate that is 1.2 mm thick with a dielectric constant of 2.2. The antenna electrical parameters were calculated and optimized by using ADS software. The dimensions of the slot antenna shown in Figure 10.5 are 66 × 60 × 1.2 mm. The slot antenna center frequency is 2.5 GHz. The computed S_{11} parameters are presented in Figure 10.6. The antenna bandwidth is around 50% for VSWR better than 2:1. The antenna bandwidth is around 70% for VSWR better than 3:1. The radiation pattern of the slot antenna is shown in Figure 10.7. The antenna beam width is around 90° at 2 GHz, as shown in Figure 10.7. The antenna gain is around 3 dBi. The slot antenna radiation pattern at 2.5 GHz is shown in Figure 10.8.

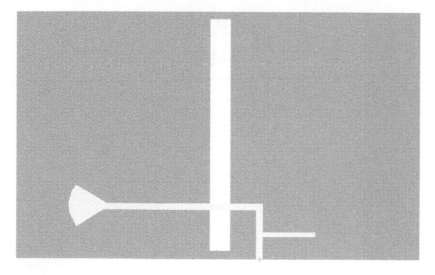

FIGURE 10.5 A wideband wearable printed slot antenna.

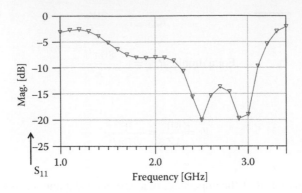

FIGURE 10.6 S_{11} of a wideband wearable printed slot antenna.

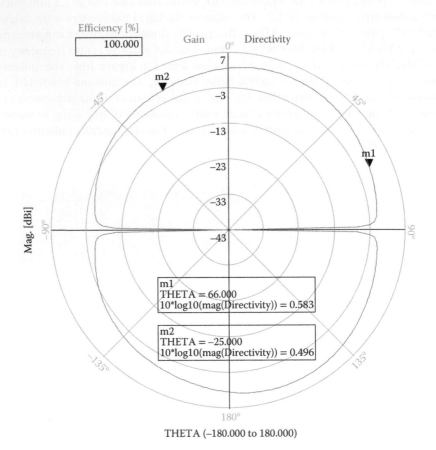

FIGURE 10.7   Radiation pattern of a wideband wearable printed slot antenna at 2 GHz.

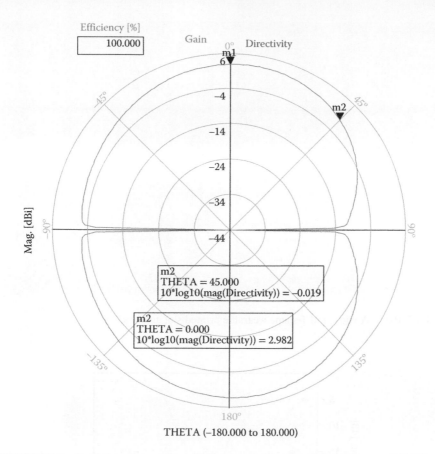

FIGURE 10.8 Radiation pattern of a wideband wearable printed slot antenna at 2.5 GHz.

10.5 A WIDEBAND T-SHAPE WEARABLE PRINTED SLOT ANTENNA

A wideband T-shape wearable printed slot antenna is shown in Figure 10.9. The slot antenna is printed on RT-DUROID 5880 dielectric substrate that is 1.2 mm thick with a dielectric constant of 2.2. The antenna electrical parameters were calculated and optimized by using ADS software. The dimensions of the slot antenna shown in Figure 10.9 are 66 × 60 × 1.2 mm. The slot antenna center frequency is around 2.25 GHz. The computed S_{11} parameters are presented in Figure 10.10. The antenna bandwidth is around 57% for VSWR better than 2:1. The antenna bandwidth is around 90% for VSWR better than 3:1. The radiation pattern of the T-shape slot antenna is shown in Figure 10.11. The antenna beam width is around 82° at 1.5 GHz, as shown in Figure 10.11. The antenna gain is around 3 dBi.

The computed S_{11} parameters of the T-shape slot on the human body are presented in Figure 10.12. The dielectric constant of human body tissue was taken as 45. The antenna was attached to a 1 mm thick shirt with a dielectric constant of 2.2. The antenna bandwidth is around 50% for VSWR better than 2:1. The antenna bandwidth

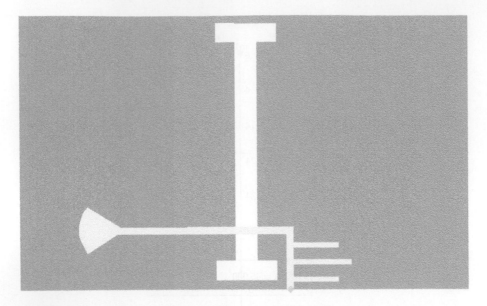

FIGURE 10.9   A wideband T-shape wearable printed slot antenna.

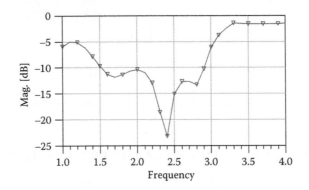

FIGURE 10.10 S_{11} of a wideband wearable printed slot antenna.

is around 57% for VSWR better than 3:1. The antenna center frequency is shifted by 10%. The feed network of the antenna shown in Figure 10.9 was optimized to match the antenna to the human body environment (see Figure 10.13). The computed S_{11} parameters of the modified T-shape slot on the human body are presented in 10.14. The modified antenna VSWR is better than 3:1 for frequencies ranging from 0.8 GHz to 3.9 GHz. The antenna gain at 1.5 GHz of the modified antenna is around 3 dBi (Figure 10.15). The radiation pattern of the modified T-shape slot antenna at 1.5 GHz is shown in Figure 10.16.

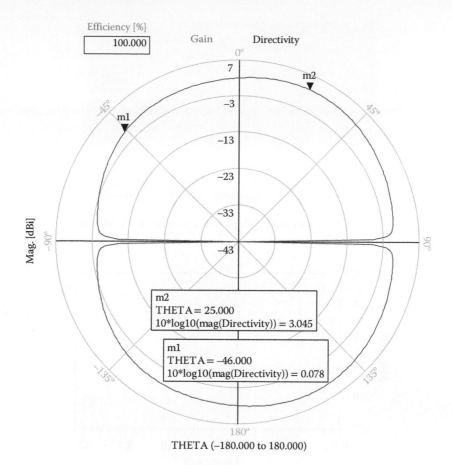

FIGURE 10.11   Radiation pattern of a wideband wearable printed slot antenna at 1.5 GHz.

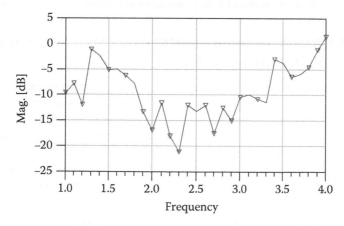

FIGURE 10.12 S_{11} of a wideband wearable printed slot antenna on the human body.

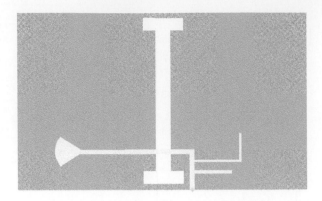

FIGURE 10.13   A modified wideband T-shape wearable printed slot antenna.

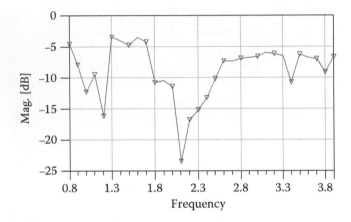

FIGURE 10.14 S_{11} of the modified T-shape wearable slot antenna on the human body.

10.6   WIDEBAND WEARABLE NOTCH ANTENNA FOR WIRELESS COMMUNICATION SYSTEMS

The wireless communication industry has been rapidly growth in recent years. Due to the huge progress in the development of communication systems in the last decade the development of wideband communication systems has seen continuous growth. However, development of wideband efficient antennas is one of the major challenges in the development of wideband wireless communication systems. Low-cost compact antennas are crucial in the development of communication systems. Printed notch antennas and miniaturization techniques are employed to develop efficient compact notch antennas.

10.6.1   WIDEBAND NOTCH ANTENNA 2.1 GHz–7.8 GHz

A wideband notch antenna has been designed. The antenna is printed on RT-DUROID 5880 dielectric substrate that is 1.2 mm thick with a dielectric

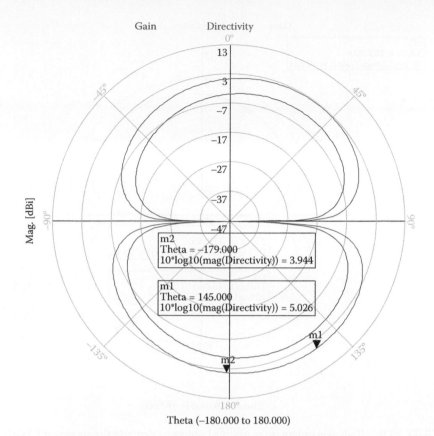

Gain   Directivity

m2
Theta = −179.000
10*log10(mag(Directivity)) = 3.944

m1
Theta = 145.000
10*log10(mag(Directivity)) = 5.026

Mag. [dBi]

Theta (−180.000 to 180.000)

FIGURE 10.15 Radiation pattern of the modified wideband wearable slot antenna at 1 GHz.

constant of 2.2. The notch antenna is shown in Figure 10.17. The notch antenna dimensions are 116.4 × 71.4 mm. The antenna center frequency is 5 GHz. The antenna bandwidth is around 100% for S_{11} lower than −6.5 dB, as presented in Figure 10.18. The notch antenna VSWR is better than 3:1 for frequencies from 2.1 GHz to 7.8 GHz. The antenna beam width is around 84°. The antenna gain is around 2.5 dBi. Figure 10.19 presents the radiation pattern of the wideband notch antenna at 3.5 GHz. Figure 10.20 presents the radiation pattern of the wideband notch antenna at 3 GHz.

10.7 WEARABLE TUNABLE SLOT ANTENNAS FOR WIRELESS COMMUNICATION SYSTEMS

A wideband wearable tunable slot antenna is shown in Figure 10.21. Tunable slot antennas consists of a slot antenna and a voltage-controlled diode, known as a varactor [17]. The antenna resonant frequency can be tuned by using a varactor to compensate for variations in antenna resonant frequency at different locations. The slot antenna is printed on RT-DUROID 5880 dielectric substrate that is 1.2 mm

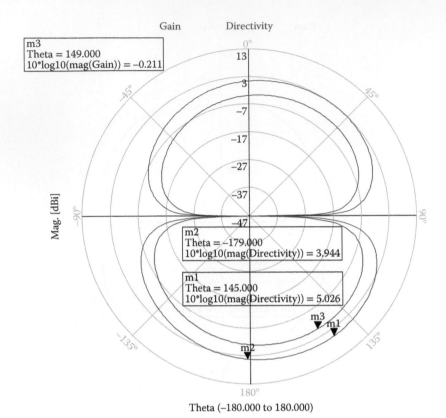

FIGURE 10.16   Radiation pattern of the modified wideband wearable slot antenna at 1.5 GHz.

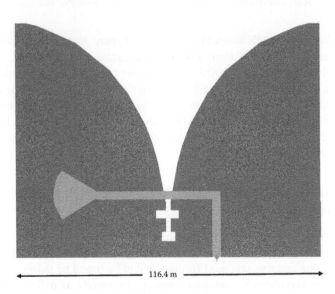

FIGURE 10.17   A wideband 2.1 GHz–7.8 GHz notch antenna.

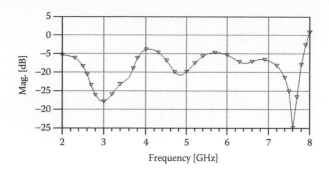

FIGURE 10.18 The computed S_{11} for a wideband 2.1 GHz–7.8 GHz notch antenna.

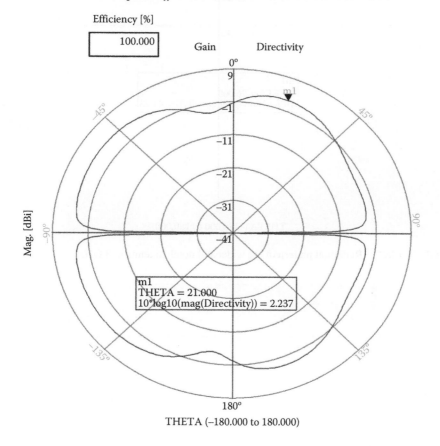

FIGURE 10.19 Radiation pattern of the wideband notch antenna at 3.5 GHz.

thick with a dielectric constant of 2.2. The antenna electrical parameters were calculated and optimized by using ADS software. The dimensions of the slot antenna shown in Figure 10.21 are 66 × 60 × 1.2 mm. A varactor is connected to the slot feed line. The varactor bias voltage can be varied automatically to set the

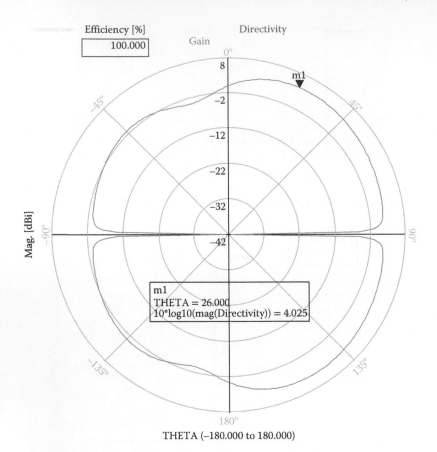

FIGURE 10.20 Radiation pattern of the wideband notch antenna at 3 GHz.

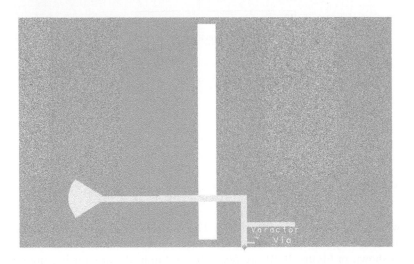

FIGURE 10.21 A wideband tunable wearable slot antenna.

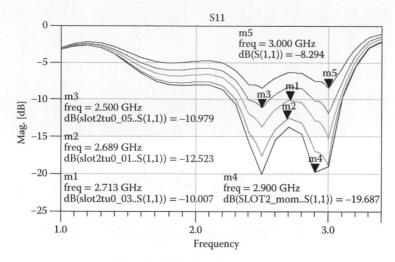

FIGURE 10.22 S_{11} of a wideband tunable wearable printed slot antenna.

antenna resonant frequency at different locations and environments. The slot antenna center frequency is 2.5 GHz. The S_{11} parameters for varactor capacitances ranging from 0.1pF to 1pF are presented in Figure 10.22. The antenna bandwidth is around 40% for VSWR better than 2:1. The antenna bandwidth is 60% for VSWR better than 3:1.

10.8 A WIDEBAND T-SHAPE TUNABLE WEARABLE PRINTED SLOT ANTENNA

A wideband T-shape wearable printed slot antenna is shown in Figure 10.23. The slot antenna is printed on RT-DUROID 5880 dielectric substrate that is 1.2 mm thick with a dielectric constant of 2.2. The antenna electrical parameters were calculated and optimized using ADS software. The dimensions of the slot antenna shown in Figure 10.23 are 66 × 60 × 1.2 mm. The slot antenna center frequency is around 2.25 GHz. The computed S_{11} parameters are presented in Figure 10.24. The antenna bandwidth is around 57% for VSWR better than 2:1. The antenna bandwidth is around 90% for VSWR better than 3:1. A varactor is connected to the slot feed line. The varactor bias voltage can be varied automatically to set the antenna resonant frequency at different locations and environments. The S_{11} parameters for varactor capacitances ranging from 0.1pF to 1pF are presented in Figure 10.25.

10.9 WEARABLE ACTIVE SLOT ANTENNAS FOR WIRELESS COMMUNICATION SYSTEMS

A wideband active wearable receiving slot antenna is shown in Figure 10.26. Active slot antennas are devices combining a radiating element with active components such

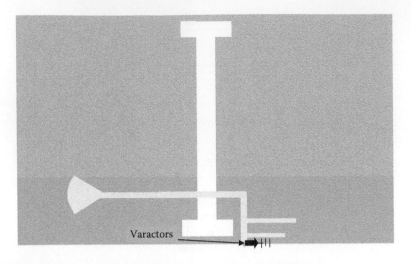

FIGURE 10.23   A wideband tunable wearable T-shape slot antenna.

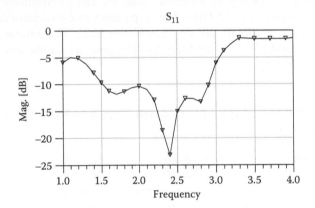

FIGURE 10.24 S_{11} of a wideband wearable T-shape slot antenna without a varactor.

as amplifiers and diodes. The radiating element is designed to provide the optimal load to the active elements. The slot antenna is printed on RT-DUROID 5880 dielectric substrate that is 1.2 mm thick with a dielectric constant of 2.2. The antenna electrical parameters were calculated and optimized using ADS software. The dimensions of the slot antenna shown in Figure 10.26 are 66 × 60 × 1.2 mm. An E PHEMT low noise amplifier (LNA) was connected to a slot antenna. The radiating element is connected to the LNA via an input matching network. An output matching network connects the amplifier port to the receiver. A DC bias network supplies the required voltages to the amplifiers. The amplifier specifications are listed in Table 9.1. The amplifier complex S parameters are listed are Table 9.2. The amplifier

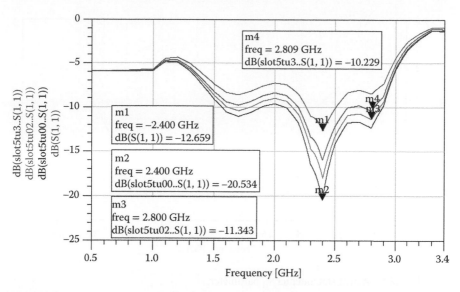

FIGURE 10.25 S_{11} of a wideband tunable wearable T-shape slot antenna.

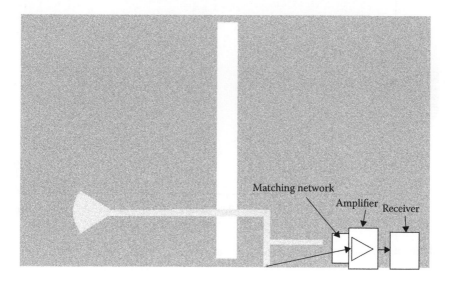

FIGURE 10.26 A wideband active receiving wearable slot antenna.

noise parameters are listed in Table 9.3. The active slot antenna S_{11} parameter is presented in Figure 10.27. The active slot antenna S_{22} parameter is presented in Figure 10.28. The antenna bandwidth is around 40% for VSWR better than 3:1. The active slot antenna S_{21} parameter, gain, is presented in Figure 10.29. The active antenna gain is 18±2.5 dB for frequencies ranging from 200 MHz to 580 MHz. The active antenna

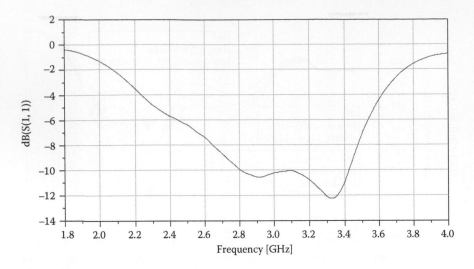

FIGURE 10.27   Active slot antenna S_{11} parameter.

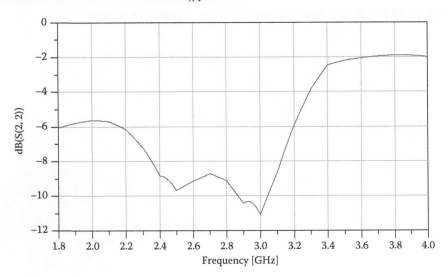

FIGURE 10.28   Active slot antenna S_{22} parameter.

gain is 12±2 dB for frequencies ranging from 1.3 GHz to 3.3 GHz. The active slot antenna noise figure is presented in Figure 10.30. The active slot antenna noise figure is 0.5±0.3 dB for frequencies ranging from 200 MHz to 3.3 GHz.

10.10   WEARABLE ACTIVE T-SHAPE SLOT ANTENNAS FOR WIRELESS COMMUNICATION SYSTEMS

A wideband active wearable receiving T-shape slot antenna is shown in Figure 10.31. The radiating element is designed to provide the optimal load to the active elements. The

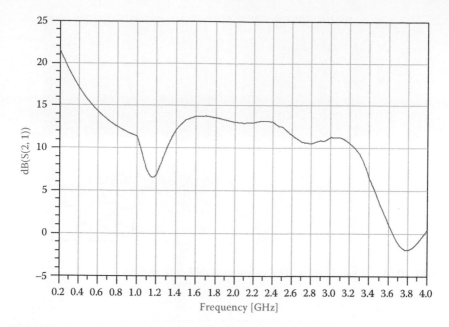

FIGURE 10.29 Active slot antenna S_{21} parameter, gain.

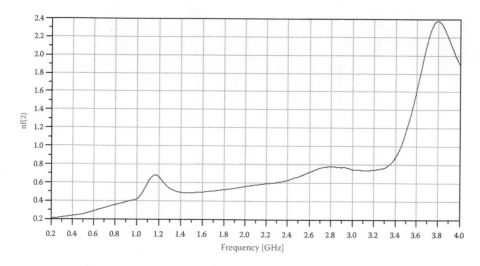

FIGURE 10.30 Active slot antenna noise figure.

slot antenna is printed on RT-DUROID 5880 dielectric substrate that is 1.2 mm thick with a dielectric constant of 2.2. The antenna electrical parameters were calculated and optimized using ADS software. The dimensions of the slot antenna shown in Figure 10.31 are $66 \times 60 \times 1.2$ mm. An E PHEMT LNA was connected to a slot antenna. The radiating element is connected to the LNA via an input matching network. An output

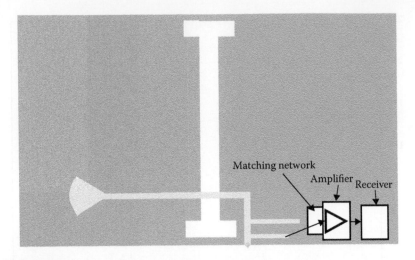

FIGURE 10.31   A wideband active receiving wearable slot antenna.

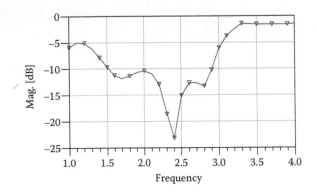

FIGURE 10.32   Active T-shape slot antenna S_{11} parameter.

matching network connects the amplifier port to the receiver. A DC bias network supplies the required voltages to the amplifiers. The amplifier specifications are listed in Table 9.1. The amplifier complex S parameters are listed in Table 9.2. The amplifier noise parameters are listed in Table 9.3. The active slot antenna S_{11} parameter is presented in Figure 10.32. The antenna bandwidth is around 40% for VSWR better than 2:1. The active slot antenna S_{21} parameter, gain, is presented in Figure 10.33. The active antenna gain is 18±2.5 dB for frequencies ranging from 200 MHz to 580 MHz. The active antenna gain is 12.5±2.5 dB for frequencies ranging from 1 GHz to 3 GHz. The active slot antenna noise figure is presented in Figure 10.34. The active slot antenna noise figure is 0.5±0.3 dB for frequencies ranging from 300 MHz to 3.2 GHz. The active slot antenna S_{22} parameter is presented in Figure 10.35.

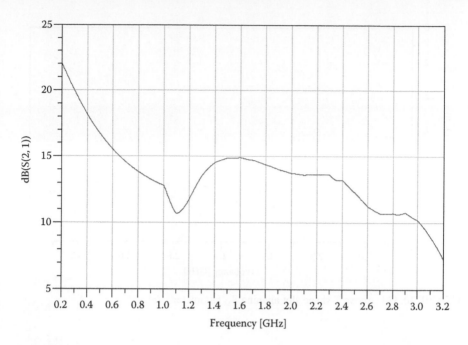

FIGURE 10.33 Active T-shape slot antenna S$_{21}$ parameter.

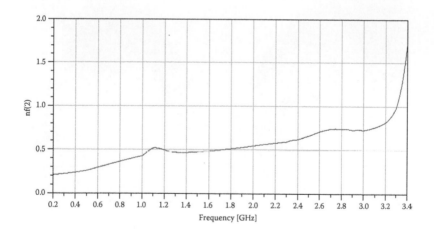

FIGURE 10.34 Active slot antenna noise figure.

10.11 NEW FRACTAL COMPACT ULTRA-WIDEBAND NOTCH ANTENNA, 1 GHZ–6 GHZ

A wideband notch antenna with a fractal structure has been designed. The antenna is printed on RT-DUROID 5880 dielectric substrate that is 1.2 mm thick with a

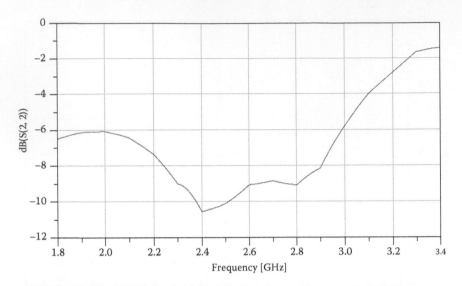

FIGURE 10.35   Active T-shape slot antenna S_{22} parameter.

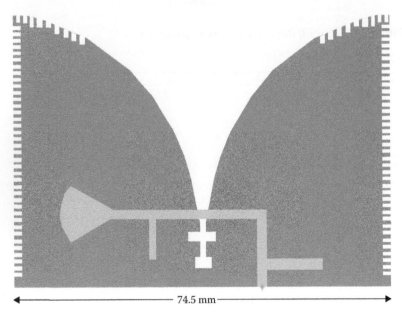

FIGURE 10.36   A wideband notch antenna with fractal structure.

dielectric constant of 2.2. The notch antenna is shown in Figure 10.36. Its dimensions are 74.5 × 57.1 mm. The antenna center frequency is 2.75 GHz. The antenna bandwidth is around 200% for S_{11} lower than −6.5 dB, as presented in Figure 10.37. The

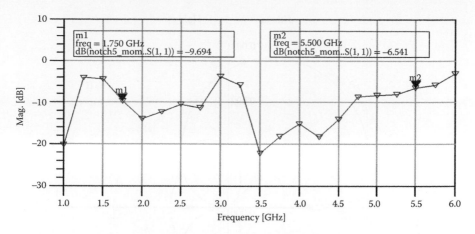

FIGURE 10.37 Computed S₁₁ for a wideband notch antenna with a fractal structure.

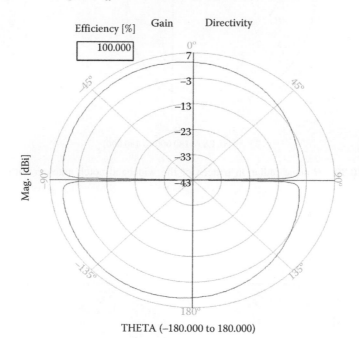

THETA (−180.000 to 180.000)

FIGURE 10.38 *E*-plane radiation pattern of the wideband notch antenna with a fractal structure.

notch antenna VSWR is better than 3:1 for frequencies from 1 GHz to 5.5 GHz. The antenna beam width is around 84°. The antenna gain is around 3.5 dBi as presented in Figure 10.38. *The H-plane* radiation pattern of the wideband notch antenna with a fractal structure is presented in Figure 10.39.

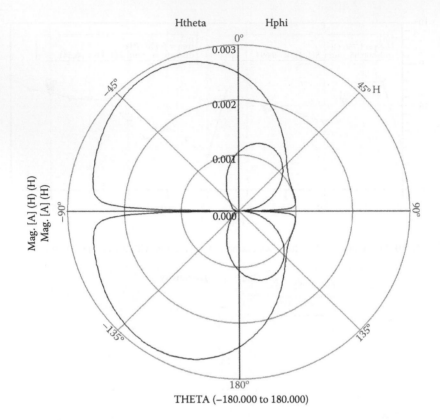

FIGURE 10.39 *H*-plane radiation pattern of the wideband notch antenna with a fractal structure.

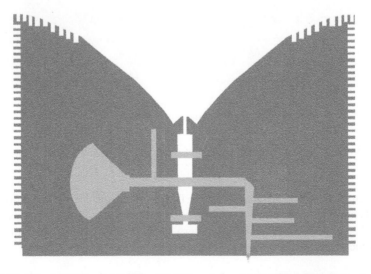

FIGURE 10.40 A wideband 1.3 GHz–3.9 GHz notch antenna with a fractal structure.

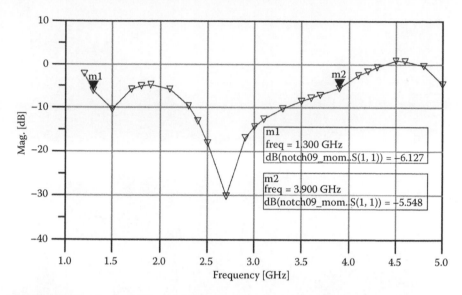

FIGURE 10.41 S_{11} results for a wideband 1.3 GHz–3.9 GHz notch antenna with a fractal structure.

10.12 NEW COMPACT ULTRA-WIDEBAND NOTCH ANTENNA, 1.3 GHZ–3.9 GHZ

A wideband notch antenna with a fractal structure has been designed. The antenna is printed on RT-DUROID 5880 dielectric substrate that is 1.2 mm thick with a dielectric constant of 2.2. The notch antenna is shown in Figure 10.40. Its dimensions are 52.2 × 36.8 mm. The antenna center frequency is 2.7 GHz. The antenna bandwidth is around 100% for S_{11} lower than −6.5 dB, as presented in Figure 10.41. The notch antenna VSWR is better than 3:1 for frequencies from 1.3 GHz to 3.9 GHz. The antenna beam width is around 84°. The antenna gain is around 3.5 dBi.

By using a fractal structure the notch antenna length and width was reduced by around 50%.

10.13 NEW COMPACT ULTRA-WIDEBAND NOTCH ANTENNA, 5.8 GHZ–18 GHZ

A wideband notch antenna with a fractal structure has been designed. The antenna is printed on RT-DUROID 5880 dielectric substrate that is 1.2 mm thick with a dielectric constant of 2.2. The notch antenna is shown in Figure 10.42. Its dimensions are 11 × 7.7 mm. The antenna center frequency is 12 GHz. The antenna bandwidth is around 100% for S_{11} lower than −5 dB, as presented in Figure 10.43. The notch antenna VSWR is better than 3:1 for more than 90% of the frequency range from 5.8 GHz to 18 GHz. The antenna beam width is around 84°. The antenna gain is around 3.5 dBi. Figure 10.44 Presents the radiation pattern of the wideband notch antenna with a fractal structure at 8 GHz.

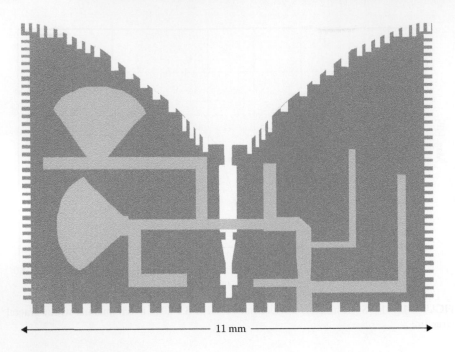

←	11 mm

FIGURE 10.42 A wideband 5.8 GHz–18 GHz notch antenna with a fractal structure.

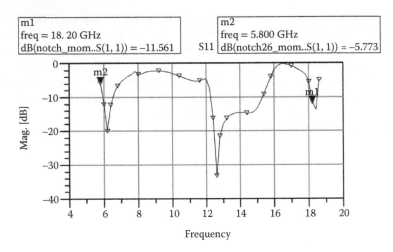

m1		m2
freq = 18. 20 GHz		freq = 5.800 GHz
dB(notch_mom..S(1, 1)) = −11.561	S11	dB(notch26_mom..S(1, 1)) = −5.773

FIGURE 10.43 S_{11} results for a wideband 5.8 GHz–18 GHz notch antenna with fractal structure.

The antenna matching network was optimized to get better S_{11} results at 16 GHz–18 GHz. The length and width of the stubs were tuned to get better S_{11} results at 16 GHz–18 GHz.

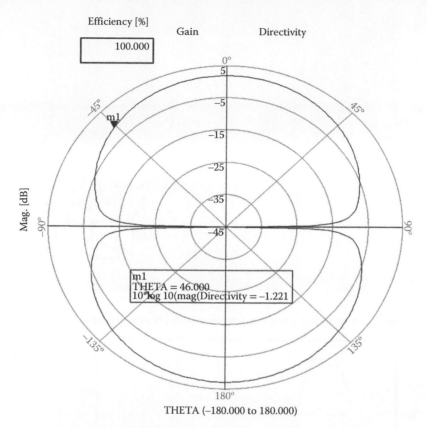

FIGURE 10.44 Radiation pattern of the wideband notch antenna with a fractal structure at 8 GHz.

10.14 NEW FRACTAL ACTIVE COMPACT ULTRA-WIDEBAND NOTCH ANTENNA, 0.5 GHZ–3 GHZ

A wideband active notch antenna with a fractal structure has been designed. The antenna is printed on RT-DUROID 5880 dielectric substrate that is 1.2 mm thick with a dielectric constant of 2.2. The active notch antenna is shown in Figure 10.45. Its dimensions are 74.5 × 57.1 mm. The antenna center frequency is 1.75 GHz. The active antenna bandwidth is around 200% for S_{11} lower than –5 dB. The active notch antenna VSWR is better than 3:1 for frequencies from 0.5 GHz to 3 GHz. The antenna beam width is around 84°.

An E PHEMT LNA was connected to a slot antenna. The radiating element is connected to the LNA via an input matching network. An output matching network connects the amplifier port to the receiver. A DC bias network supplies the required voltages to the amplifiers. The amplifier specifications are listed in Table 9.1. The amplifier complex S parameters are listed in Table 9.2. The amplifier noise parameters are listed in Table 9.3. The active notch antenna S_{21} parameter, gain, is presented in Figure 10.46. The active antenna gain is 22±2.5 dB for frequencies ranging from

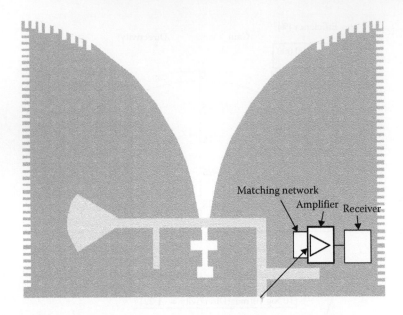

FIGURE 10.45 A wideband active notch antenna with a fractal structure.

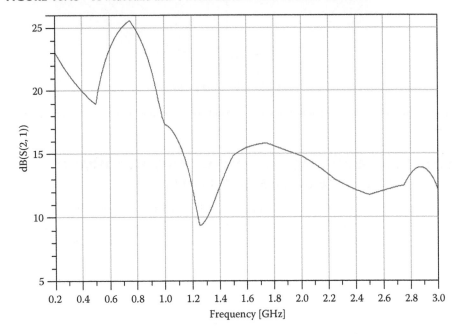

FIGURE 10.46 Active notch antenna S_{21} parameter.

200 MHz to 900 MHz. The active antenna gain is 12.5±2.5 dB for frequencies ranging from 1 GHz to 3 GHz. The active notch antenna noise figure is presented in Figure 10.47. The active notch antenna noise figure is 0.5±0.3 dB for frequencies ranging from 300 MHz to 3.0 GHz. The active notch antenna S_{22} parameter is lower than −5 dB for frequencies from 0.5 GHz to 3 GHz.

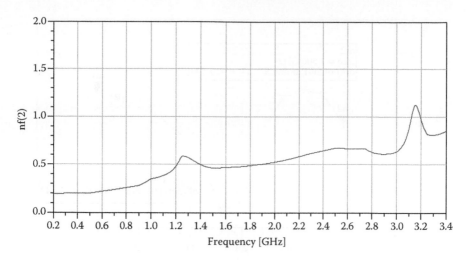

FIGURE 10.47 Active notch antenna noise figure.

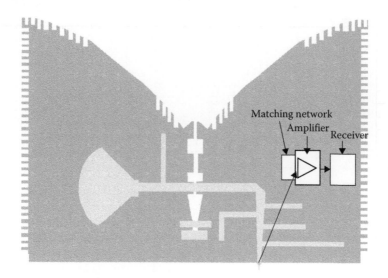

FIGURE 10.48 A wideband fractal active notch antenna with a fractal structure.

10.15 NEW COMPACT ULTRA-WIDEBAND ACTIVE NOTCH ANTENNA, 0.4 GHZ–3 GHZ

A wideband notch antenna with a fractal structure has been designed. The antenna is printed on RT-DUROID 5880 dielectric substrate that is 1.2 mm thick with a dielectric constant of 2.2. The notch antenna is shown in Figure 10.48. Its dimensions are 52.2 × 36.8 mm. The antenna center frequency is 1.7 GHz. The antenna bandwidth is around 100% for S_{11} lower than –5 dB as shown in Figure 10.49. The notch antenna

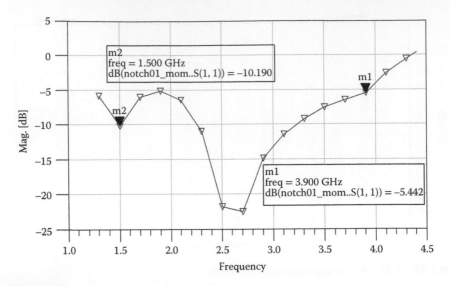

FIGURE 10.49   Fractal active notch antenna S_{11} parameter.

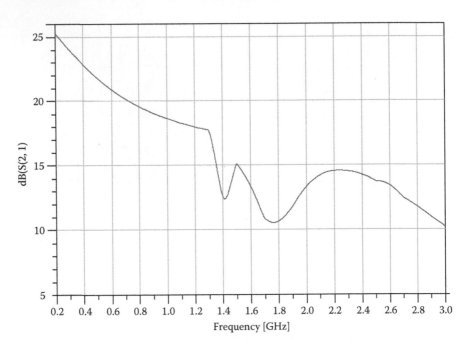

FIGURE 10.50   Fractal active notch antenna S_{21} parameter.

VSWR is better than 3:1 for frequencies from 0.4 GHz to 3 GHz. The antenna beam width is around 84°. An E PHEMT LNA was connected to a slot antenna. The radiating element is connected to the LNA via an input matching network. An output match-

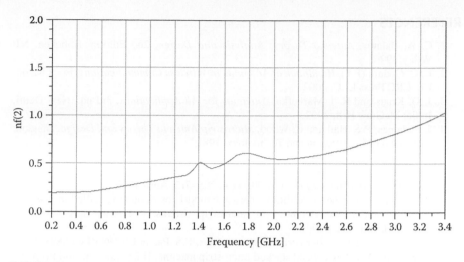

FIGURE 10.51 Active fractal notch antenna noise figure.

ing network connects the amplifier port to the receiver. A DC bias network supplies the required voltages to the amplifiers. The amplifier specifications are listed in Table 9.1. The amplifier complex S parameters are listed in Table 9.2. The amplifier noise parameters are listed in Table 9.3. The active notch antenna S_{21} parameter, gain, is presented in Figure 10.50. The active antenna gain is 20±2.5 dB for frequencies ranging from 400 MHz to 1.3 GHz. The active antenna gain is 12.5±2.5 dB for frequencies ranging from 1.3 GHz to 3 GHz. The active notch antenna noise figure is presented in Figure 10.51. The active notch antenna noise figure is 0.5±0.3 dB for frequencies ranging from 300 MHz to 3.0 GHz. The active notch antenna S_{22} parameter is lower than −5 dB for frequencies from 0.5 GHz to 3 GHz.

10.16 CONCLUSIONS

This chapter presents new compact ultra-wideband slot and notch antennas in frequencies ranging from 1 GHz to 18 GHz. The slot and notch antennas were analyzed by using 3D full-wave software. The antenna bandwidth is from 50% to 100% with VSWR better than 3:1. The antenna gain is around 3 dBi with efficiency higher than 90%. The antenna electrical parameters were computed in the vicinity of the human body. A compact new ultra-wideband notch antenna, 1 GHz–6 GHz, and a wideband notch antenna, 5.8 GHz–18, GHz are presented. The space-filling technique and Hilbert curves were employed to design the fractal notch antennas. The fractal notch antennas were analyzed using 3D full-wave software. The antenna bandwidth is around 100% with VSWR better than 3:1. The antenna gain is around 3.5 dBi with efficiency higher than 90%. By using a fractal structure the notch antenna length and width can be reduced by up to 50%. The chapter presents new compact ultra-wideband active slot and notch antennas in frequencies ranging from 1 GHz to 6 GHz.

REFERENCES

1. C. A. Balanis, *Antenna Theory: Analysis and Design*, 2nd Edition, Hoboken, NJ: Wiley, 1996.
2. L. C. Godara (Ed.), *Handbook of Antennas in Wireless Communications*, Boca Raton, FL: CRC Press LLC, 2002.
3. J. D. Kraus and R. J. Marhefka, *Antennas for All Applications*, 3rd ed., New Delhi, India: McGraw Hill, 2002.
4. J. R. James, P. S. Hall and C. Wood, *Microstrip Antenna Theory and Design*, London: Institution of Engineering and Technology, 1981.
5. A. Sabban and K. C. Gupta, Characterization of radiation loss from microstrip discontinuities using a multiport network modeling approach, *IEEE Transactions on Microwave Theory and Techniques*, vol. 39, no. 4, 705–712, April 1991.
6. A. Sabban, PhD Thesis, Multiport network model for evaluating radiation loss and coupling among discontinuities in microstrip circuits, University of Colorado at Boulder, CO, January 1991.
7. A. Sabban, Inventor, *Microstrip antenna arrays*, U.S. Patent US 1986/4,623,893, 1986.
8. A. Sabban, A new wideband stacked microstrip antenna, IEEE Antenna and Propagation Symposium, Houston, TX, June 1983.
9. A. Sabban, *Low Visibility Antennas for Communication Systems*, New York: Taylor & Francis Group, 2015.
10. A. Sabban, Wideband microstrip antenna arrays, IEEE Antenna and Propagation Symposium MELCOM, Tel-Aviv, Israel, June 1981.
11. A. Sabban, *RF Engineering, Microwave and Antennas*, Israel: Saar Publications, 2014.
12. K. Fujimoto and J. R. James, Editors, *Mobile Antenna Systems Handbook*, Boston, MA: Artech House, 1994.
13. A. Sabban, New wideband notch antennas for communication systems, *Wireless Engineering and Technology*, 75–82, April 2016.
14. A. Sabban, Inventor, *Dual polarized dipole wearable antenna*, U.S Patent 8203497, June 19, 2012, USA.
15. A. Sabban, Wideband tunable printed antennas for medical applications. IEEE Antenna and Propagation Symposium, Chicago, IL, July 2012.
16. A. Sabban, New wideband printed antennas for medical applications, *IEEE Transactions on Antennas and Propagation*, vol. 61, no. 1, 84–91, January 2013.
17. A. Sabban, Comprehensive study of printed antennas on human body for medical applications, *International Journal of Advance in Medical Science (AMS)*, vol. 1, 1–10, February 2013.

11 Microwave Technologies for Wearable Communication Systems

11.1 INTRODUCTION

Compact wearable communication systems can be designed using modern microwave technologies such as monolithic microwave integrated circuits (MMIC), micro-electro-mechanical systems (MEMS), and low temperature co-fired ceramic (LTCC) technologies. The communication industry in microwave and mm wave frequencies is currently seeing continuous growth. Radio frequency modules such as front end filters, power amplifiers, printed antennas, passive components, and limiters are important modules in wearable communication devices, see [1–20]. The electrical performance of the modules determines if the system will meet the required specifications. Moreover, in several cases the module's performance limits system performance. Minimization of the size and weight of the RF modules is achieved by employing MMIC and MIC technology. However, integration of MIC and MMIC components and modules raise several technical challenges. Design parameters that can be neglected for modular communication systems cannot be ignored in the design of wid band integrated RF modules. Powerful RF design software, such as advanced design software (ADS) and high frequency structure simulator (HFSS), is required to achieve accurate design of RF modules in microwave frequencies. Accurate design of mm wave RF modules is crucial. It is an impossible mission to tune mm wave RF modules in the fabrication process.

Microwave technologies for wearable communication systems
- MIC
- MMIC
- MEMS
- LTCC

11.2 MICROWAVE INTEGRATED CIRCUITS (MICs)

Traditional microwave systems consist of connectorized components (such as amplifiers, filters, and mixers) connected by coaxial cables. These modules have large dimensions and suffer from high losses and weight. Dimensions and losses can be minimized by using microwave integrated circuits (MIC technology). There are three types of MIC circuits: HMIC, standard MIC, and miniature HMIC. HMIC is a hybrid MIC. Solid state and passive elements are bonded to the dielectric substrate. The passive elements are fabricated by using thick or thin film technology. A standard MIC uses a single-level metallization for conductors and transmission lines. A miniature HMIC uses a multilevel process in which passive elements such as capacitors and resistors are batch deposited on the substrate. Semiconductor devices such as amplifiers and diodes are bonded on the substrate. Figure 11.1 presents a MIC transceiver. Figure 11.2 presents the layout of the MIC receiving link. The receiving channel consists of a low noise amplifier, filters, dielectric resonant oscillators, and a diode mixer.

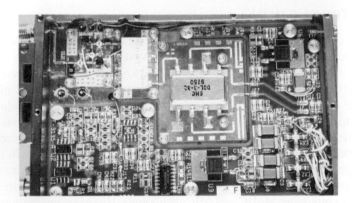

FIGURE 11.1   A MIC transceiver.

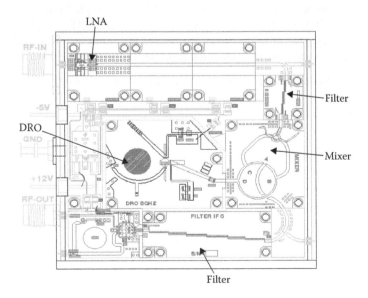

FIGURE 11.2   Layout of a MIC receiving link.

11.3 LOW NOISE K-BAND COMPACT RECEIVING CHANNEL FOR SATELLITE COMMUNICATION GROUND TERMINAL

In this section an example of a MIC receiving channel is presented.

11.3.1 INTRODUCTION

An increasing demand for wide bandwidth in communication links makes the K/Ka-band attractive for future commercial systems. The frequency allocations for the K/Ka-band VSAT system are 17.7–21.2 GHz for the receiving channel and 27.5–31 GHz for the transmitting channel. The communications industry is currently seeing continuous growth. In particular Very Small Aperture Terminal (VSAT) networks have gained wide use for business and private applications. Private organizations and banks are using VSAT networks to communicate between their various sites. VSAT applications cover a wide range such us telephony, message distribution, lottery, credit card approval, and inventory management. Commercial VSAT systems operate in the C-band and Ku-band, however there are many advantages to developing wideband K/Ka-band communication systems. However, only some commercial low-cost power amplifiers, low noise amplifiers, mixers, and DROs are published in commercial catalogs. Moreover, development of low-cost RF components is crucial the K/Ka-band satellite communication industry. This section describes the design and performance of a compact and low-cost K-band receiving channel.

11.3.2 RECEIVING CHANNEL DESIGN

The major objectives in the design of the receiving channel were electrical specifications and cost.
Receiving channel specifications
    The receiving channel specifications are listed in Table 11.1.

TABLE 11.1
Receiving Channel Specifications

Parameter	Specification
RF frequency range	18.8–19.3 GHz, 19.7–20.2 GHz
IF frequency range	0.95–1.45 GHz
Gain	50 dB
Noise figure	2 dB
Input VSWR	2:1
Output VSWR	2:1
Spurious level	-40 dBc
Frequency stability versus temperature	±2 MHz
Supply voltage	±5V
Connectors	K-connectors
Operating temperature	-40°C–60°C
Storage temperature	-50°C–80°C
Humidity	95%

11.3.3 Description of the Receiving Channel

A block diagram of the receiving channel is shown in Figure 11.3.

The receiving channel consists of a RF side coupled band-pass filter, low noise amplifier, mixer, DRO, IF filter, and MMC downconverter block. The noise figure, gain, and IP3 budget are given in Figure 11.4.

A receiving channel with improved NF (0.95 dB) and gain (77 dB) is obtained by adding a gain block after the LNA. However, for cost considerations we decided to realize the first configuration shown in Figure 11.4. The major objectives in the design of the receiving channel were specifications and cost.

11.3.4 Development of the Receiving Channel

A MIC and MMIC LNA were developed for K-band receiving links. The dimensions of the MMIC LNA are much smaller than the MIC LNA. However, the NF of the MIC LNA is around 1.2–1.5 dB and the NF of the MMIC LNA is around 1.7–2 dB.

Components of the receiving channel were printed on 10 mil thick RT-5880 Duroid substrate. Drawings of the MMIC LNA, and of the receiving channel, are shown in Figures 11.5 and 11.6. A photograph of the receiving channel with a MMIC LNA is shown in Figure 11.7.

11.3.5 Measured Test Results of the Receiving Channel

The measured test results of the receiving channel are summarized in Table 11.2.

11.4 MONOLITHIC MICROWAVE INTEGRATED CIRCUITS (MMICs)

Monolithic microwave integrated circuits (MMICs) are circuits in which active and passive elements are formed on the same dielectric substrate, as presented in Figure 11.8, by using such deposition schemes as epitaxy, ion implantation, sputtering, evaporation, and diffusion. In Figure 11.8 the MMIC chip consists of passive elements such as resistors, capacitors, inductors, and a field effect transistor (FET).

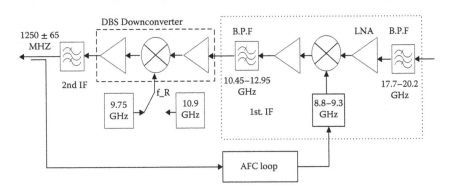

FIGURE 11.3   Block diagram of the receiving channel.

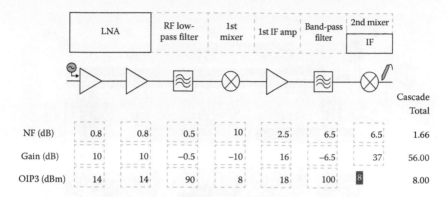

	LNA	RF low-pass filter	1st mixer	1st IF amp	Band-pass filter	2nd mixer IF	Cascade Total
NF (dB)	0.8	0.8	0.5	10	2.5	6.5	6.5	1.66
Gain (dB)	10	10	−0.5	−10	16	−6.5	37	56.00
OIP3 (dBm)	14	14	90	8	18	100	8	8.00

FIGURE 11.4 Noise figure, gain, IP3 budget.

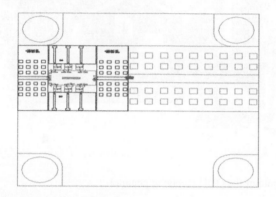

FIGURE 11.5 MMIC LNA on carrier.

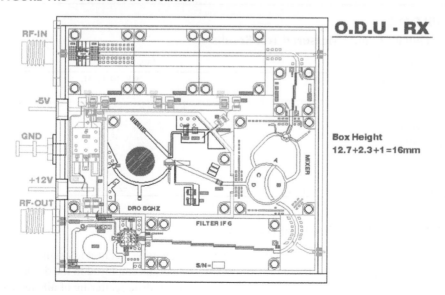

FIGURE 11.6 ODU receiving channel.

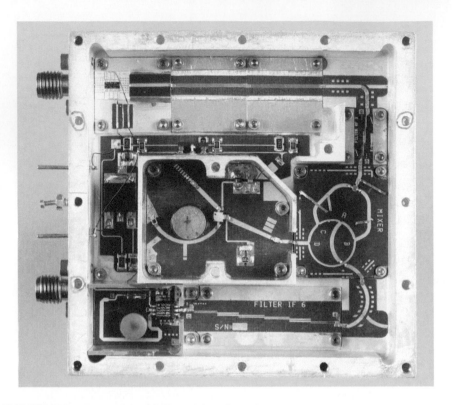

FIGURE 11.7   Photo of the ODU receiving channel.

TABLE 11.2
Receiving Channel Measured Test Results

Parameter	Measured Results
RF frequency range	18.8–19.3 GHz
IF frequency range	0.95–2 GHz
Gain	50 dB
Noise figure	2 dB
Input VSWR	2:1
Output VSWR	2:1
Spurious level	-40 dBc
Frequency stability versus temperature	±2 MHz

11.4.1   MMIC Technology Features

Accurate design is crucial in the design of MMIC circuits. Accurate design can be achieved by using 3D electromagnetic software. Materials employed in the design of MMIC circuits are GaAs, InP, GaN, and SiGe. Large statistic scattering of all electrical parameters causes sensitivity of the design.

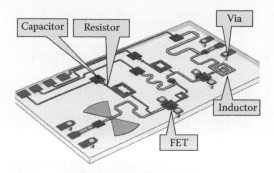

FIGURE 11.8 MMIC basic components.

FAB runs are expensive, around $200,000 per run. Miniaturization of components yields lower cost of the MMIC circuits. Figure 11.9 presents MMIC design flow.

The designer's goal is to comply with customer specifications in one design iteration. MMIC components can't be tuned.

- 0.25 micron GaAs PHEMT for power applications to Ku band.
- 0.15 micron GaAs PHEMT for applications to high Ka band.
- GaAs PIN process for low loss power switching applications.
- Future new processes: InP HBT, SiGe, GaN, RFCMOS, RFMEMS

Figure 11.10 presents a GaAs wafer layout. The wafer size can be 3″, 5″, or 6″.

11.4.2 MMIC COMPONENTS

Several microwave components are fabricated using MMIC technology.

- Mixers: balanced, star, sub-harmonic
- Amplifiers: LNA, general, power amplifiers, wideband power amplifiers, distributed TWA
- Switches: PIN, PHEMT, T/R matrix
- Frequency multipliers: active, passive
- Modulators: QPSK, QAM (PIN, PHEMT)
- Multifunction: RX chip, TX chip, switched amp chip, LO chain

FET: field effect Transistor
BJT: bipolar junction transistor
HEMT: high electron mobility transistor
PHEMT: pseudo-morphic HEMT
MHEMT: metamorphic HEMT
D-HBT: double hetero-structure bipolar transistor
CMOS: complementary metal-oxide semi-conductor

Table 11.3 presents types of devices fabricated using MMIC technology.

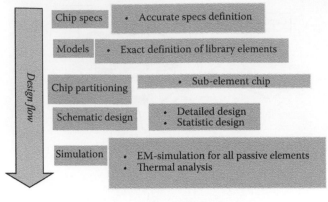

FIGURE 11.9   MMIC design flow.

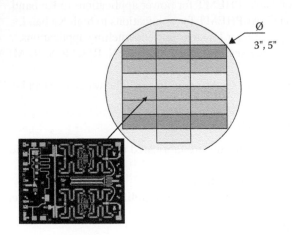

FIGURE 11.10   GaAs wafer layout.

TABLE 11.3
MMIC Technology

Material	FET	BJT	Diode
III–V-based	PHEMT GaAs	HBT GaAs	Schotky GaAs
	HEMT InP	D-HBT InP	
	MHEMT GaAs		
	HEMT GaN		
Silicon	CMOS	HBT SiGe	–

11.4.3 ADVANTAGES OF GaAs VERSUS SILICON

MMICs were originally fabricated by using gallium arsenide (GaAs), a III-V compound semiconductor. MMICs are dimensionally small (from around 1 mm² to 10 mm²) and can be mass-produced. GaAs has some electronic properties which are better than those of silicon. It has a higher saturated electron velocity and higher electron mobility, allowing transistors made from GaAs to function at frequencies higher than 250 GHz. Unlike silicon junctions, GaAs devices are relatively insensitive to heat due to their higher bandgap. Also, GaAs devices tend to have less noise than silicon devices especially at high frequencies, which is a result of higher carrier mobility and lower resistive device parasitic. These properties recommend GaAs circuitry in mobile phones, satellite communications, microwave point-to-point links, and higher frequency radar systems. It is used in the fabrication of Gunn diodes to generate microwaves. GaAs has a direct band gap, which means that it can be used to emit light efficiently. Silicon has an indirect bandgap and so is very poor at emitting light. Nonetheless, recent advances make silicon LEDs and lasers possible. Due to its lower bandgap though, Si LEDs cannot emit visible light and rather work in the IR range while GaAs LEDs function in visible red light. As a wide direct band gap material with the resulting resistance to radiation damage, GaAs is an excellent material for space electronics and optical windows in high power applications.

Silicon has three major advantages over GaAs for integrated circuit manufacturers. First, silicon is a cheap material. In addition, a Si crystal has an extremely stable structure mechanically; it can be grown to very large diameter boules and can be processed with very high yields. It is also a decent thermal conductor, thus enabling very dense packing of transistors, all very attractive for design and manufacturing of very large ICs. The second major advantage of Si is the existence of silicon dioxide—one of the best insulators. Silicon dioxide can easily be incorporated onto silicon circuits, and such layers are adherent to the underlying Si. GaAs does not easily form such a stable adherent insulating layer and does not have a stable oxide either. The third, and perhaps most important, advantage of silicon is that it possesses a much higher hole mobility. This high mobility allows the fabrication of higher-speed P-channel field effect transistors, which are required for CMOS logic. Because they lack a fast CMOS structure, GaAs logic circuits have much higher power consumption, which has made them unable to compete with silicon logic circuits. The primary advantage of Si technology is its lower fabrication cost compared with GaAs. Silicon wafer diameters are larger, typically 8″ or 12″ compared with 4″ or 6″ for GaAs. Si wafer costs are much lower than GaAs wafer costs, contributing to a less expensive Si IC.

Other III–V technologies, such as indium phosphide (InP), offer better performance than GaAs in terms of gain, higher cutoff frequency, and low noise. However they are more expensive due to smaller wafer sizes and greater material fragility.

Silicon germanium (SiGe) is a Si-based compound semiconductor technology offering higher speed transistors than conventional Si devices but with similar cost advantages.

Gallium nitride (GaN) is also an option for MMICs. Because GaN transistors can operate at much higher temperatures and work at much higher voltages than GaAs transistors, they make ideal power amplifiers at microwave frequencies. In Table 11.4 the properties of materials used in MMIC technology are compared.

11.4.4 SEMICONDUCTOR TECHNOLOGY

The cutoff frequency of Si CMOS MMIC devices is lower than 200 GHz. Si CMOS MMIC devices are usually low power and low cost devices. The cutoff frequency of SiGe MMIC devices is lower than 200 GHz. SiGe MMIC devices are used as medium power high gain devices. The cutoff frequency of InP HBT devices is lower than 400 GHz. InP HBT devices are used as medium power high gain devices. The cutoff frequency of InP HEMT devices is lower than 600 GHz. InP HEMT devices are used as medium power high gain devices. In Table 11.5 the properties of MMIC technologies are compared. Figure 11.11 presents a 0.15 micron PHEMT on GaAs substrate.

TABLE 11.4
Comparison of Material Properties

Property	Si	Si or Sapphire	GaAs	InP
Dielectric constant	11.7	11.6	12.9	14
Resistivity (Ω/cm)	10^3–10^5	$>10^{14}$	10^7–10^9	10^7
Mobility (cm^2/v-s)	700	700	4300	3000
Density (gr/cm^3)	2.3	3.9	5.3	4.8
Saturation velocity (cm/s)	9×10^6	9×10^6	1.3×10^7	1.9×10^7

TABLE 11.5
Summary of Semiconductor Technology

–	Si CMOS	SiGe HBT	InP HBT	InP HEMT	GaN HEMT
Cutoff frequency	>200 GHz	>200 GHz	>400 GHz	>600 GHz	>200 GHz
Published MMICs	170 GHz	245 GHz	325 GHz	670 GHz	200 GHz
Output power	Low	Medium	Medium	Medium	High
Gain	Low	High	High	Low	Low
RF noise	High	High	High	Low	Low
Yield	High	High	Medium	Low	Low
Mixed signal	Yes	Yes	Yes	No	No
1/f noise	High	Low	Low	High	High
Breakdown voltage	-1 V	-2 V	-4 V	-2 V	>20 V

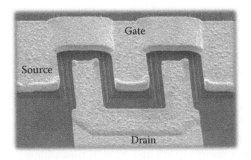

FIGURE 11.11   0.15 micron PHEMT on GaAs substrate.

11.4.5 MMIC Fabrication Process

The MMIC fabrication process consists of several controlled processes in a semiconductor FAB. The process is listed in the following list. In Figure 11.12 an MESFET cross section on GaAs substrate is shown.

MMIC fabrication process list

Wafer fabrication: Preparing the wafer for fabrication.

Wet cleans: Wafer cleaning by wet process.

Ion implantation: Dopants are embedded to create regions of increased or decreased conductivity. Selectively implant impurities. Create p or n type semiconductor regions.

Dry etching: Selectively remove materials.

Wet etching: Selectively remove materials using a chemical process.

Plasma etching: Selectively remove materials.

Thermal treatment: High temperature process to remove stress.

Rapid thermal anneal: High temperature process to remove stress.

Furnace anneal: After ion implantation, thermal annealing is required. Furnace annealing can take minutes and causes too much diffusion of dopants for some applications.

Oxidation: Substrate oxidation, for example: dry oxidation- $Si + O_2 \rightarrow SiO_2$. Wet oxidation $Si + 2H_2O \rightarrow SiO_2 + 2H_2$.

Chemical Vapor Deposition (CVD): Chemical vapor deposited on the wafer. Pattern defined by photoresist.

Physical Vapor Deposition (PVD): Vapor produced by evaporation or sputtering deposited on the wafer. Pattern defined by photoresist.

Molecular Beam Epitaxy (MBE): A beam of atoms or molecules produced in high vacuum. Selectively grow layers of materials. Pattern defined by photoresist.

Electroplating: Electromechanical process used to add metal.

Chemical mechanical polish (CMP)

Wafer testing: Electrical test of the wafer.

Wafer back-grinding

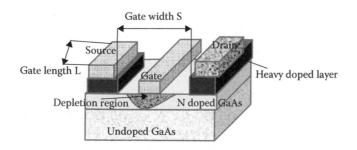

FIGURE 11.12 MESFET cross section on GaAs substrate.

> **Die preparation**
> **Wafer mounting**
> **Die cutting**

Lithography: Lithography is the process of transferring a pattern onto the wafer by selectively exposing and developing photoreists. Photolithography consists of four steps; the order depends on whether we are etching or lifting off the unwanted material.

Contact lithography: A glass plate is used that contains the pattern for the entire wafer. It is literally led against the wafer during exposure of the photoresist. In this case the entire wafer is patterned in one shot.

Electron-beam lithography is a form of direct-write lithography. Using E-beam lithography you can write directly to the wafer without a mask. Because an electron beam is used, rather than light, much smaller features can be resolved.

Exposure can be done with light, UV light, or electron beam, depending on the accuracy needed. An E beam provides much higher resolution than light, because the particles are bigger (greater momentum), and the wavelength is shorter.

Etching versus lift-off removal processes

There are two principal means of removing material, etching and lift-off.
The steps for an etch-off process are:

1. Deposit material
2. Deposit photoresist
3. Pattern (expose and develop)
4. Remove material where it is not wanted by etching

Etching can be isotropic (etching wherever we can find the material we like to etch) or anisotropic (directional, etching only where the mask allows). Etches can be dry (reactive ion etching or RIE) or wet (chemical). Etches can be very selective (only etching what we intend to etch) or non-selective (attacking a mask to the substrate).

In a lift-off process, the photoresist *forms a mold*, into which the desired material is deposited. The desired features are completed when photoresist B under unwanted areas is dissolved, and unwanted material is "lifted off."

The steps of a lift-off process are:

1. Deposit photo-resist
2. Pattern
3. Deposit material conductor or insulator
4. Remove material where it is not wanted by *lifting off*

In Figure 11.13, a MESFET cross section on GaAs substrate is shown. In Figure 11.14 a MMIC resistor cross section is shown. In Figure 11.15 a MMIC capacitor cross section is shown.

Figure 11.16 presents the ion implantation process. Figure 11.17 presents the ion etch process. Figure 11.18 presents the wet etch process.

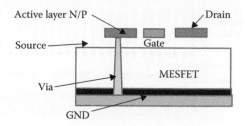

FIGURE 11.13 MESFET cross section.

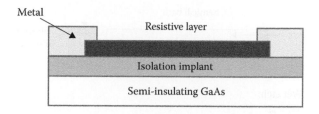

FIGURE 11.14 Resistor cross section.

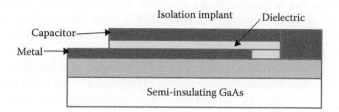

FIGURE 11.15 Capacitor cross section.

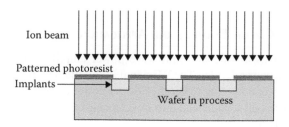

FIGURE 11.16 Ion implantation.

11.4.6 Generation of Microwave Signals in Microwave and mm Wave

Microwaves signals can be generated by solid state devices and vacuum-tube based devices. Solid state microwave devices are based on semiconductors such as silicon or gallium arsenide, and include field-effect transistors (FETs), bipolar junction transistors (BJTs), Gunn diodes, and IMPATT diodes. Microwave variations of BJTs

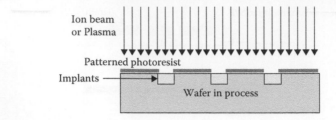

FIGURE 11.17   Ion etch.

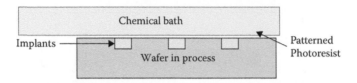

FIGURE 11.18   Wet etch.

include the hetero-junction bipolar transistor (HBT), and microwave variants of FETs include the MESFET, the HEMT (also known as HFET), and LDMOS transistor. Microwaves can be generated and processed using integrated circuits known as monolithic microwave integrated circuits (MMIC). They are usually manufactured using gallium arsenide (GaAs) wafers, though silicon germanium (SiGe) and heavy-dope silicon are increasingly used. Vacuum-tube-based devices operate on the ballistic motion of electrons in a vacuum under the influence of controlling electric or magnetic fields, and include the magnetron, klystron, traveling wave tube (TWT), and gyrotron. These devices work in the density modulated mode, rather than the current modulated mode. This means that they work on the basis of clumps of electrons flying ballistically through them, rather than using a continuous stream.

11.4.7   MMIC Circuit Examples and Applications

Figure 11.19 presents a wideband mm wave power amplifier. The input power is divided by using a power divider. The RF signal is amplified by power amplifiers and combined by a power combiner to get the desired power at the device output.

Figure 11.20 presents a wideband mm wave upconverter. The MMIC process cost is listed in Table 11.6.

MMIC applications

- Ka-band satellite communication
- 60 GHz wireless communication
- Automotive radars
- Imaging in security
- Gbit WLAN

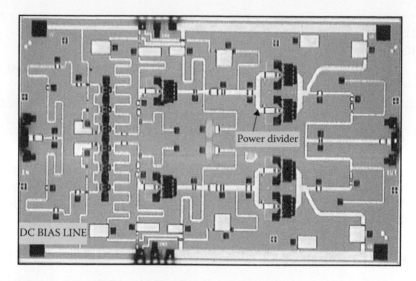

FIGURE 11.19 Wideband power amplifier.

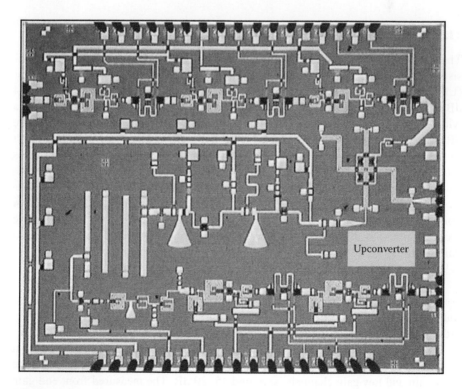

FIGURE 11.20 Ka-band upconverter.

TABLE 11.6
MMIC Cost

	Si CMOS	SiGe HBT	GaAs HEMT	InP HEMT
Chip cost ($/mm²)	0.01	0.1–0.5	1–2	10
Mask cost (M$/mask set)	1.35	0.135	0.0135	0.0135

11.5 18 TO 40 GHZ FRONT END

Development and design considerations of a compact wideband 18–40 GHz front end are described in this section. The RF modules and the system was designed using ADS system software and momentum RF software. There is good agreement between computed and measured results.

11.5.1 18 TO 40 GHz FRONT END REQUIREMENTS

The front end electrical specifications are listed in Table 11.7. The front end design presented in this section meet the frontend electrical specifications. Physical characteristics, interfaces, and connectors are listed in Table 11.8.

11.5.2 FRONT END DESIGN

The front end block diagram is shown in Figure 11.21. The front end module consists of a limiter and a wideband 18–40 GHz Filtronic low noise amplifier (LMA406). The LMA406's gain is around 12 dB with a 4.5 dB noise figure and 14 dBm saturated output power. The LNA dimensions are 1.44 × 1.1 mm. We used a wideband PHEMT MMIC SPDT manufactured by Agilent, AMMC-2008. The SPDT insertion loss is lower than 2 dB. The isolation between the SPDT input port to the output ports is better than 25 dB. The SPDT 1 dBc compression point is around 14 dBm. The SPDT dimensions are 1 × 0.7 × 0.1 mm. The front end electrical characteristics were evaluated using ADS Agilent software and SYSCAL software. Figure 11.22 presents the front end module noise figure and gain for LNA noise figure of 6 dB. The overall computed module noise figure is 9.46 dB. The module gain is 21 dB. Figure 11.23 presents the front end module noise figure and gain for the LNA noise figure of 5.5 dB. The overall computed module noise figure is 9.25 dB. The module gain is 21 dB.

The MMIC amplifiers and the SPDT are glued to the surface of the mechanical box. The MMIC chips are assembled on a Covar carrier. During development it was found that the spacing between the front end carriers should be less than 0.03 mm in order to achieve flatness requirements and VSWR better than 2:1.

The front end voltage and current consumption are listed in Table 11.9. The front end module has high gain and low gain channels. The gain difference between the high gain and low gain channels is around 15–20 dB. The measured front end gain is presented in Figure 11.24. The front end gain is around 20±4 dB for the 18–40 GHz frequency range.

TABLE 11.7
Front end Electrical Specifications

Parameter	Requirements	Performance
Frequency range	18–40 GHz	Comply
Gain	24/3 dB typical, switched by external control (-40 dB or lower for off state)	Comply
Gain flatness	±0.5 dB max for any 0.5 GHz BW in 18–40 GHz. ±2 dB max for any 4 GHz BW in 18–40 GHz. ±3 dB max for the whole range 18–40 GHz.	Comply
Noise figure (high gain)	10 dB max for 40°C baseplate temperature 11 dB over temperature	Comply
Inputs power range	-60 dBm–10 dBm	Comply
Output power range	-39 dBm–11 dBm not saturated, 13 dBm saturated	Comply
Linearity	Output 1 dB compression point at 12 dBm min. Third intercept point (Ip3) at 21 dBm. Single tone. Second harmonic power -25 dBc max for 10 dBm output.	Comply
VSWR	2:1	Comply
Power input protection	No damage at +30 dBm CW and +47 dBm Pulses (for average power higher then 30 dBm) input power at 0.1–40 GHz. Test for pulses: PW = 1 usec, PRF = 1 KHz	Comply
Power Supply voltages	±5 V, ±15 V	Comply
Control logic	LVTTL standard "0" = 0–0.8 V; "1" = 2.0–3.3 V	Comply
Switching time	Less then 100 nsec	Comply
Non-harmonic spurious (output)	-50 dBm max (when it isn't correlative with the input signals)	Comply
Video leakage	Video leakage signals will be below the RF output level for terminated input.	Comply
Dimensions	60 × 40 × 20 mm	Comply

TABLE 11.8
Physical Characteristics: Interface Connectors

Interface	Type
RF input	Waveguide WRD180 (Double Ridge)
RF output	K connector
DC supply	D type
Dimensions	60 × 40 × 20 mm
Control	D type

11.5.3 HIGH GAIN FRONT END MODULE

To achieve a high gain front end module a medium power Hittite MMIC amplifier, HMC283, was added to the front end module presented in Figure 11.25. The HMC283 gain is around 21 dB with a 10 dB noise figure and 21 dBm saturated output power.

FRONT END BLOCK DIAGRAM

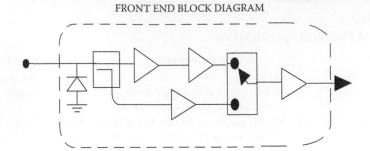

FIGURE 11.21   Frontend block diagram.

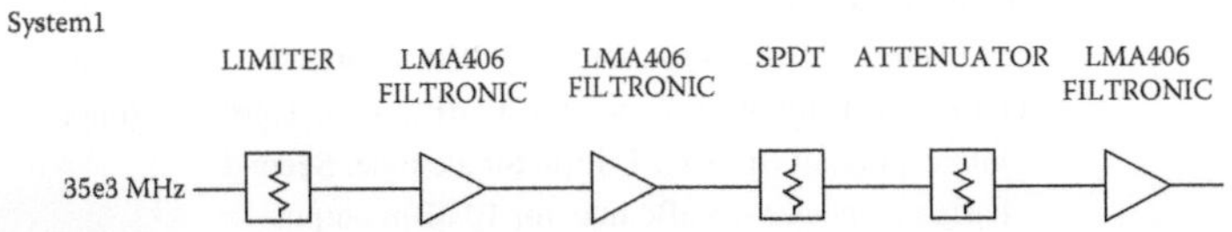

System1

	LIMITER	LMA406 FILTRONIC	LMA406 FILTRONIC	SPDT	ATTENUATOR	LMA406 FILTRONIC	Total
35e3 MHz							
NF (dB)	3.00	6.00	6.00	3.00	3.00	6.00	9.46
Gain (dB)	–3.00	10.00	10.00	–3.00	–3.00	10.00	21.00
OIP3 (dBm)	30.00	25.00	25.00	30.00	30.00	25.00	23.14

Input Pwr (dBm)	–60.00	System Temp (K)	290.00	IM Offset (MHz)	.025
OIP2 (dBm)	23.14	OIP3 (dBm)	23.14	Output P1dB (dBm)	11.37
IIP2 (dBm)	2.14	IIP3 (dBm)	2.14	Input P1dB (dBm)	–8.63
OIM2 (dBm)	–101.14	OIM3 (dBm)	–163.28	Compressed (dB)	0.00
ORR2 (dB)	62.14	ORR3 (dB)	124.28	Gain, Actual (dB)	21.00
IRR2 (dB)	31.07	IRR3 (dB)	41.43		
SFDR2 (dB)	61.34	SFDR3 (dB)	81.79	Gain, Linear (dB)	21.00
AGC Controlled Range:		Min Input (dBm)	N/A	Max Input (dBm)	N/A

FIGURE 11.22   Front end module design for LNA NF = 6 dB.

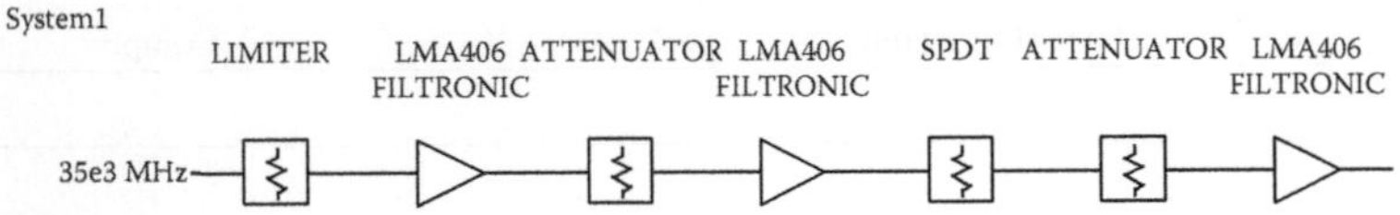

System1

	LIMITER	LMA406 FILTRONIC	ATTENUATOR	LMA406 FILTRONIC	SPDT	ATTENUATOR	LMA406 FILTRONIC	Total
35e3 MHz								
NF (dB)	3.00	5.50	3.00	5.50	3.00	1.00	5.50	9.25
Gain (dB)	–3.00	10.50	–3.00	10.50	–3.00	–1.00	10.00	21.00
OIP3 (dBm)	30.00	25.00	30.00	25.00	30.00	30.00	25.00	23.61

Input Pwr (dBm)	–60.00	System Temp (K)	290.00	IM Offset (MHz)	.025
OIP2 (dBm)	24.04	OIP3 (dBm)	23.61	Output P1dB (dBm)	11.74
IIP2 (dBm)	3.04	IIP3 (dBm)	2.61	Input P1dB (dBm)	–8.26
OIM2 (dBm)	–102.04	OIM3 (dBm)	–164.23	Compressed (dB)	0.00
ORR2 (dB)	63.04	ORR3 (dB)	125.23	Gain, Actual (dB)	21.00
IRR2 (dB)	31.52	IRR3 (dB)	41.74		
SFDR2 (dB)	61.90	SFDR3 (dB)	82.24	Gain, Linear (dB)	21.00
AGC Controlled Range:		Min Input (dBm)	N/A	Max Input (dBm)	N/A

FIGURE 11.23   Front end module design for LNA NF = 6 dB.

The amplifier dimensions are 1.72 × 0.9 mm. The high gain front end module block diagram is shown in Figures 11.25 and 11.26. The front end module has high gain and low gain channels. The gain difference between the high gain and low gain

TABLE 11.9
Front End Module Voltage and Current Consumption

Voltage (V)	3	5	-12	-5	5 Digital
Current (A)	0.25	0.15	0.1	0.1	0.1

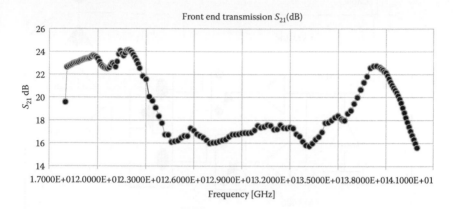

FIGURE 11.24 Measured front end gain.

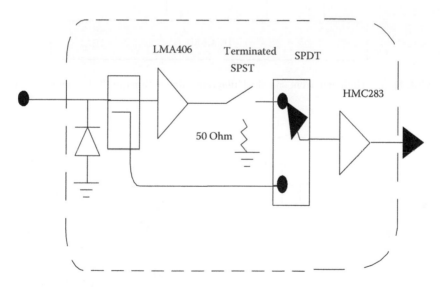

FIGURE 11.25 High gain front end block diagram.

channels presented in Figure 11.26 is around 15–20 dB. The gain difference between the high gain and low gain channels presented in Figure 11.27 is around 10–15 dB. A detailed block diagram of the high gain module is shown in Figure 11.28.

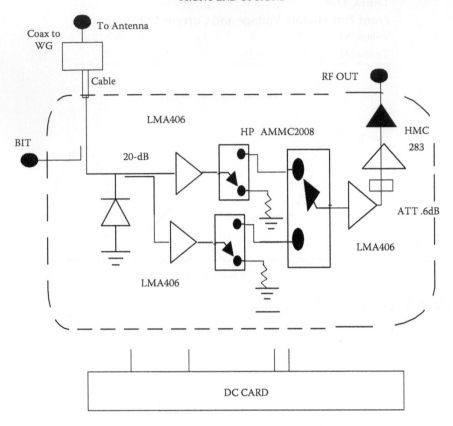

FIGURE 11.26   High gain front end block diagram with amplifier in the low gain channel.

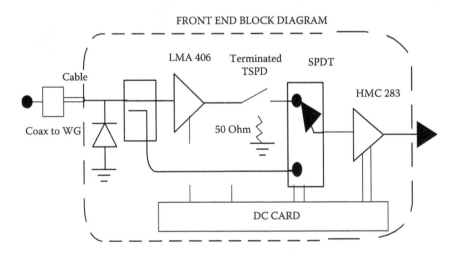

FIGURE 11.27   Detailed block diagram for high gain front end.

11.5.4 HIGH GAIN FRONT END DESIGN

The high front end electrical characteristics were evaluated using ADS Agilent software and SYSCAL software. Figure 11.28 presents the front end module noise figure and gain for an LNA noise figure of 9.5 dB. The overall computed module noise figure is 13.3 dB. The module gain is 32.48 dB. Figure 11.29 presents the front end module noise figure and gain for an LNA noise figure of 5 dB. The overall computed module noise figure is 10 dB. The module gain is 29.5 dB.

Measured results for front end modules are listed in Table 11.10. An HMC283 assembly is shown in Figure 11.30. A photo of the front end is shown in Figure 11.31. There is a good agreement between computed and measured results.

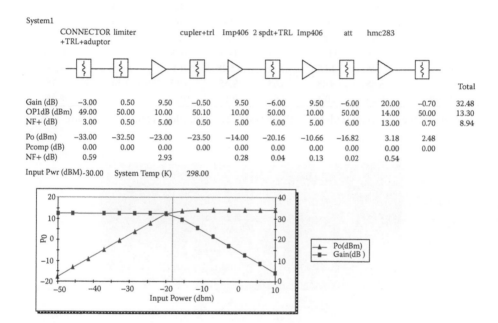

FIGURE 11.28 Front end module design for LNA NF = 9.5 dB.

						Total
NF (dB)	3.50	5.00	5.00	5.00	6.00	9.00	10.02
Gain (dB)	−3.50	11.00	−5.00	11.00	−6.00	22.00	29.50
OIP3 (dBm)		20.00		20.00		20.00	19.87
NF+ (dB)		2.85		0.56		0.57	
Po (dBm)	−63.50	−52.50	−57.50	−46.50	−52.50	−30.50	
Input pwr (dBm)	−60.00	System temp (K)		290.00			

FIGURE 11.29 Front end module design for LNA NF = 5 dB.

TABLE 11.10

Measured Results of Front End Modules

Parameter	DF6	DF4	DF3	DF2	DF1	OMNI02	OMNI01
High gain max	31	32	32.5	32.5	31	31.5	32
High gain min	26	26	27.5	27	26	28.5	28
High gain avg	29	29	29	29	29	30	30
Amp. nal.	5	6	5	5	4	3	4
S_{11}(dB)	4.5	5	5	5	5	5	4
S_{22}(dB)	7.5	6	5	6	5	7	6
Isolation(dB)	9	9	10	10	6.5	21.5	22.5
Low gain max	19	18	17	17	17	16.5	18
Low gain min	13	10	7.5	12	12	10.5	11
Low gain avg	15	14	12	14	14	13.5	14.5
Amp. nal.	6	8	9.5	5	5	6	7
P1 dB 30 GHz	11.6	11.93	11.7	11.4	10.9	14	15.96
P1 dB 40 GHz	13.96	14.5	15.58	15.28	14	14.48	16.8
NF 30 GHz	8.68	9.48	8.65	8.45	10.5	8.14	8.75
NF 40 GHz	9.28	10.1	8.64	9.17	10.24	–	8.75

A photo of the compact wideband 18–40 GHz RF modules is shown in Figure 11.32.

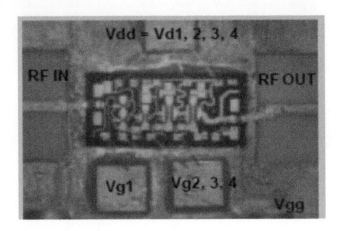

FIGURE 11.30   HMC283 assembly.

11.6   MEMS TECHNOLOGY

A micro-electro-mechanical system (MEMS) is the integration of mechanical elements, sensors, actuators, and electronics on a common silicon substrate through micro-fabrication technology. These devices replace bulky actuators and sensors with micron-scale equivalents that can produced in large quantities by using the fabrication process used for integrated circuits in photolithography. They reduce cost, bulk, weight, and power consumption while increasing performance, production volume, and functionality by orders of magnitude.

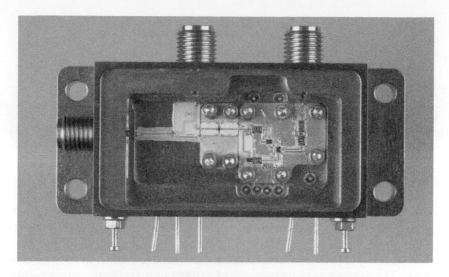

FIGURE 11.31   18–40 GHz front end module.

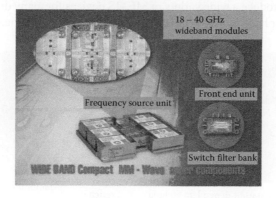

FIGURE 11.32   Photo of 18–40 GHz compact modules.

The electronics are fabricated using integrated circuit (IC) process sequences (e.g., CMOS, bipolar, or BICMOS processes); the micromechanical components are fabricated using compatible "micromachining" processes that selectively etch away parts of the silicon wafer or add new structural layers to form the mechanical and electromechanical devices.

11.6.1   MEMS Technology Advantages

- Low insertion loss, <0.1 dB
- High isolation, >50 dB
- Low distortion
- High linearity
- Very high Q
- Size reduction, system-on-a-chip

- High power handling, ~40 dBm
- Low power consumption (~mW and no LNA)
- Low-cost, high-volume fabrication

11.6.2 MEMS Technology Process

Bulk micromachining fabricates mechanical structures in the substrate by using orientation-dependent etching. Bulk micro-machined substrate is shown in Figure 11.33.

Surface micromachining fabricates mechanical structures above the substrate surface by using a sacrificial layer. Surface micro-machined substrate is presented in Figure 11.34.

In the bulk micromachining process silicon is machined using various etching processes. Surface micromachining uses layers deposited on the surface of a substrate as the structural materials, rather than using the substrate itself. The surface micromachining technique is relatively independent of the substrate used, and therefore can be easily mixed with other fabrication techniques which modify the substrate first. An example is the fabrication of MEMS on a substrate with embedded control circuitry, in which MEMS technology is integrated with IC technology. This is being used to produce a wide variety of MEMS devices for many different applications. On the other hand, bulk micromachining is a subtractive fabrication technique,

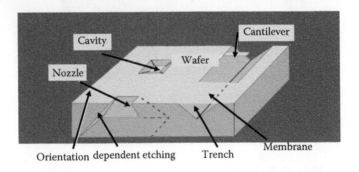

FIGURE 11.33 Bulk micromachining.

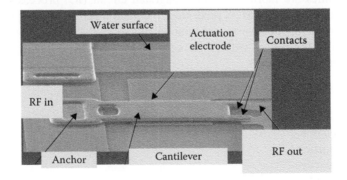

FIGURE 11.34 Surface micromachining.

which converts the substrate, typically a single-crystal silicon, into the mechanical parts of the MEMS device. A MEMS device is first designed with a computer-aided design (CAD) tool. The design outcome is a layout and masks that are used to fabricate the MEMS device. In Figure 11.35, the MEMS fabrication process is presented. A summary of MEMS fabrication technology is listed in Table 11.11. In Figure 11.36, the block diagram of a MEMS bolometer coupled antenna array is presented.

Packaging of the device tends to be more difficult, but structures with increased heights are easier to fabricate when compared to surface micromachining. This is

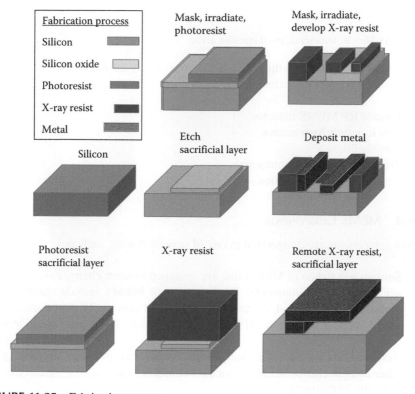

FIGURE 11.35   Fabrication process.

TABLE 11.11
Fabrication Technology

Fabrication Technology	Process
Surface micromachining	Release and drying systems to realize free-standing microstructures.
Bulk micromachining	Dry etching systems to produce deep 2D free-form geometries with vertical sidewalls in substrates. Anisotropic wet etching systems with protection for wafer front sides during etching. Bonding and aligning systems to join wafers and perform photolithography on the stacked substrates.

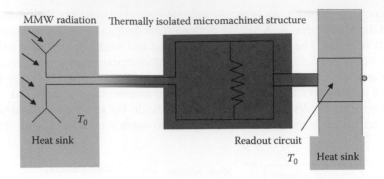

FIGURE 11.36   Bolometer coupled antenna array.

because the substrates can be thicker, resulting in relatively thick unsupported devices. Applications of RF MEMS technology include:

- Tunable RF MEMS inductor
- Low loss switching matrix
- Tunable filters
- Bolometer coupled antenna array
- Low cost W-band detection array

11.6.3   MEMS COMPONENTS

MEMS components are categorized in one of several classes, such as:

1. **Sensors** are a class of MEMS that are designed to sense changes and inter-act with their environments. These classes of MEMS include chemical, motion, inertia, thermal, RF sensors, and optical sensors. Microsensors are useful because of their small physical size, which allows them to be less invasive.
2. **Actuators** are a group of devices designed to provide power or stimulus to other components or MEMS devices. MEMS actuators are either electro-statically or thermally driven.
3. **RF MEMS** are a class of devices used to switch or transmit high frequency RF signals. Typical devices include metal contact switches, shunt switches, tunable capacitors, antennas, etc.
4. **Optical MEMS** are devices designed to direct, reflect, filter, and/or amplify light. These components include optical switches and reflectors.
5. **Microfluidic MEMS** are devices designed to interact with fluid-based environments. Devices such as pumps and valves have been designed to move, eject, and mix small volumes of fluid.
6. **Bio MEMS** are devices that, much like microfluidic MEMS, are designed to interact specifically with biological samples. Devices such as these are designed to interact with proteins, biological cells, medical reagents, etc. and can be used for drug delivery or other in-situ medical analysis.

11.7   W BAND MEMS DETECTION ARRAY

In this section we present the development of a millimeter wave radiation detection array. The detection array can employ around 256–1024 patch antennas. These patches are coupled to a resistor. Optimization of the antenna structure, feed network dimensions, and resistor structure allow us to maximize the power rate dissipated on the resistor. Design considerations of the detection antenna array are given in this section. Several imaging approaches are presented in the literature [10–14]. The common approach is based on an array of radiators (antennas) that receives radiation from a specific direction by using a combination of electronic and mechanical scanning. Another approach is based on a steering array of radiation sensors at the focal plane of a lens of reflector. The sensor can be an antenna coupled to a resistor.

11.7.1   DETECTION ARRAY CONCEPT

Losses in the microstrip feed network are very high in the W band frequency range. In W band frequencies we can design a detection array. The array concept is based on an antenna coupled to a resistor. A direct antenna-coupling surface to a micromachined micro-bridge resistor is used for heating and sensing. The feed network determines the antenna efficiency. The insertion loss of a gold microstrip line with width of 1 μm and 188 μm length is 4.4 dB at 95 GHz. The insertion loss of a gold microstrip line with width of 10 μm and 188 μm length is 3.6 dB at 95 GHz. The insertion loss of a gold microstrip line with width of 20 μm and 188 μm length is 3.2 dB at 95 GHz. To minimize losses the feed line dimensions were selected as 60 × 10 × 1 μm. An analog CMOS readout circuit can be employed as a sensing channel per pixel. Figure 11.37 presents a pixel block diagram.

11.7.2   THE ARRAY PRINCIPLE OF OPERATION

The antenna receives effective mm wave radiation. The radiation power is transmitted to a thermally isolated resistor coupled to a Ti resistor. The electrical power raises the structure temperature with a short response time. The same resistor changes its temperature and therefore its electrical resistance. Figure 11.38 shows a single array pixel. The pixel consists of a patch antenna, a matching network, a printed resistor, and DC pads. The printed resistor consist of titanium lines, and a titanium resistor coupled to an isolated resistor.

The operating frequency range of 92–100 GHz is the best choice. In the frequency range of 30–150 GHz there is a proven contrast between land, sky, and high transmittance of clothes. Size and resolution considerations promote higher frequencies above 100 GHz. Typical penetration of clothing at 100 GHz is 1 dB and 5–10 dB at 1 THz. Characterization and measurement considerations promote lower frequencies. The frequency range of 100 GHz allows sufficient bandwidth when working with illumination, and is the best compromise. Figure 11.39 presents the array concept. Several types of printed antennas can be used as the array element such as bowtie dipole, patch antenna, and ring resonant slot.

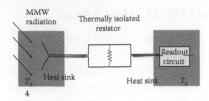

FIGURE 11.37   Antenna coupled to a resistor.

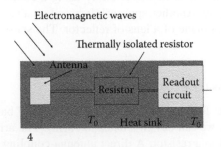

FIGURE 11.38   A single array pixel.

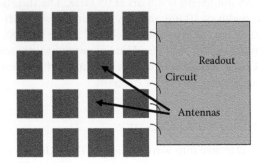

FIGURE 11.39   Array concept.

11.7.3   W Band Antenna Design

The bowtie dipole and a patch antenna have been considered as the array element. Computed results shows that the directivity of the bowtie dipole is around 5.3 dBi and the directivity of a patch antenna is around 4.8 dBi. However the length of the bowtie dipole is around 1.5 mm while the size of the patch antenna is around 700 × 700 μm. We used a quartz substrate with thickness of 250 μm. The bandwidth of the bowtie dipole is wider than that of a patch antenna. However, the patch antenna bandwidth meets the detection array electrical specifications. We chose the patch antenna as the array element since the patch size is significantly smaller than that of the bowtie dipole. This feature allows us to design an array with a higher number of radiating elements. The resolution of the detection array with a higher number of radiating elements is improved. We also realized that the matching network between the antenna and the resistor has a smaller size for a patch antenna than that for a bowtie dipole. The matching network between the antenna and the resistor consists of microstrip open stubs. Figure 11.40 shows the 3D radiation pattern of the bowtie dipole. Figure 11.41 presents the S_{11} parameter of the patch antenna. The electrical performance of the bowtie dipole and the patch antenna was compared. The VSWR of the patch antenna is better than 2:1 for 10% bandwidth. Figure 11.42 presents the 3D radiation pattern of the patch antenna at 95 GHz.

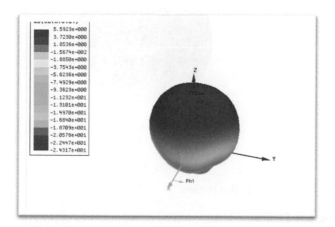

FIGURE 11.40 Dipole 3D radiation pattern.

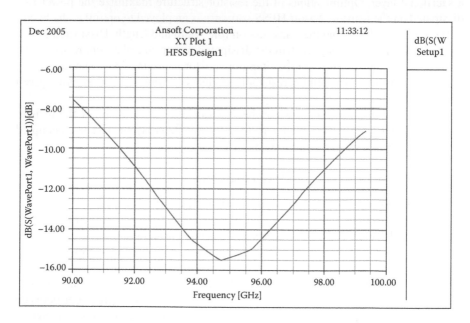

FIGURE 11.41 Patch S_{11} computed results.

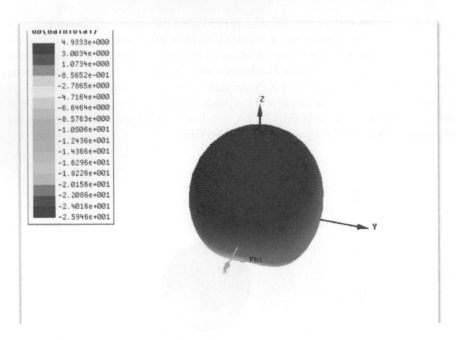

FIGURE 11.42 Patch 3D radiation pattern.

11.7.4 Resistor Design

As described in [6], the resistor is thermally isolated from the patch antenna by using a sacrificial layer. Optimizations of the resistor structure maximize the power rate dissipated on the resistor. Ansoft HFSS software is employed to optimize the height of the sacrificial layer, and the transmission line width and length. Dissipated power on a titanium resistor is higher than the dissipated power on a platinum resistor. The rate of the dissipated power on the titanium resistor is around 25%. The rate of the dissipated power on the platinum resistor is around 4%. Material properties are given in Table 11.12.

The sacrificial layer thickness can be 2–3 μm. Figure 11.43 shows the resistor configuration. Figure 11.44 presents the MEMS bolometer layout. The patch coupled to a bolometer is shown in Figure 11.45.

11.7.5 Array Fabrication and Measurement

Nine masks are used to fabricate the detection array. The mask process and layer thickness are listed in Table 11.13. Layer thickness has been determined as the best compromise between technology limits and design consideration.

Dimensions of detection array elements have been measured in several array pixels as part of a visual test of the array after its fabrication; some of the measured results are listed in Table 11.14. From results listed in Table 11.14 we can conclude that the fabrication process is very accurate. There is a good agreement between computed and measured results of the array electrical and mechanical parameters.

TABLE 11.12

Material Properties

Property	Units	siNi	Ti
Conductivity (K)	W/m/K	1.6	7
Capacity (C)	J/Kg/K	770	520
Density (ρ)	Gr/cm³	2.85	4.5
Resistance	Ω/□	>1e8	90
Thickness	μm	0.1	0.1

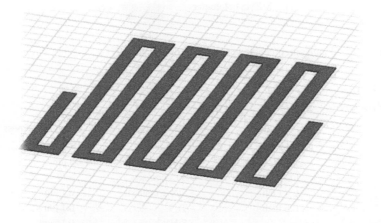

FIGURE 11.43 Resistor configuration.

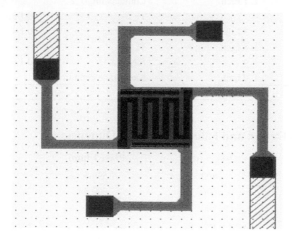

FIGURE 11.44 MEMS bolometer layout.

Figure 11.46 presents how we measure the bolometer output voltage. V_{ref} is the bolometer output voltage when no radiated power is received by the detection array. The voltage difference between the bolometer voltage and V_{ref} is amplified by a low

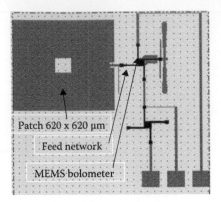

FIGURE 11.45   Patch antenna coupled to bolometer.

TABLE 11.13
Mask Process

Mask	Layer	Process	Layer thickness
1	L 1 Lift or Etch	Gold reflector Au	1 μm
2	L 2 Etch	Streets open S.L.	3 μm
3	L 3 Etch	S.L. contacts	–
4	L 4 Etch	SiN + contacts	0.1 μm
5	L 5 Etch	Ti_1	0.1 μm
–	–	SiN	0.15 μm
6	L 6 Etch	VOx	0.1 μm
7	L 7 Etch	Contacts for Ti_2	
–	–	Ti_2	0.1 μm
–	L 3 Lift	Metal cap	0.1–0.5 μm
8	L 8 Etch	Ti_2	–
–	–	SiN	0.1 μm
9	L 9 Etch	Membrane definition	

TABLE 11.14
Comparison of Design and Fabricated Array Dimensions

Element	Design (μm)	Pixel 1 (μm)	Pixel 2 (μm)
Patch width	600	599.5	600.5
Patch length	600	600.3	600.5
Hole width	100	99.8	100
Hole length	100	100	99.8
Feed line	10	10	10
Feed line	10	9.8	10
Stub width	2	2	1.8
Tapered line	15	15.2	14.8
Stub width	2	1.8	2
Tapered line	25	25.3	25.2

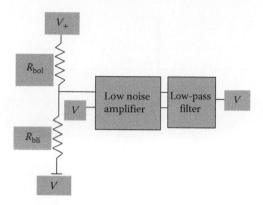

FIGURE 11.46   Measurements of bolometer voltage.

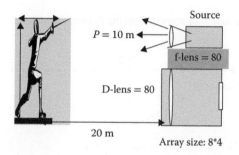

FIGURE 11.47   Detection array.

noise differential amplifier. The rate of the dissipated power on the titanium resistor is around 25%–30%.

Figure 11.47 presents the operational concept of the detection array.

11.7.6   MUTUAL COUPLING EFFECTS BETWEEN PIXELS

HFSS software has been used to compute mutual coupling effects between pixels in the detection array as shown in Figure 11.48. Computation results indicate that the power dissipated on the centered pixels in the array is higher by 1%–2% than the pixels located at the corners of the array.

11.8   MEMS BOWTIE DIPOLE WITH BOLOMETER

A bowtie dipole with bolometer printed on quartz substrate is shown in Figure 11.49. The length of the bowtie dipole is around 1.5 mm. The bolometer length is 0.6 mm. The bolometer line width is 5 µm. Figure 11.50 presents the $S11$ parameter of the bowtie dipole. Figure 11.51 shows the 3D radiation pattern of the bowtie dipole.

Computed results shows that the directivity of the bowtie dipole is around 5.3 dBi.

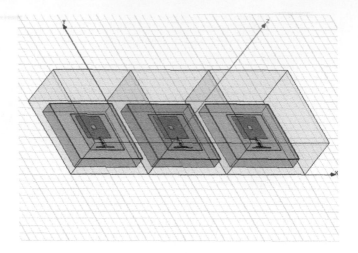

FIGURE 11.48 Computation of mutual coupling between pixels.

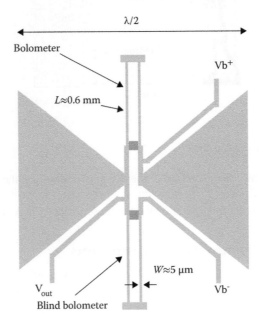

FIGURE 11.49 MEMS bowtie dipole with bolometer.

11.9 LTCC AND HTCC TECHNOLOGY

Co-fired ceramic devices are monolithic, ceramic microelectronic devices where the entire ceramic support structure and any conductive, resistive, and dielectric materials are fired in a kiln at the same time. Typical devices include capacitors, inductors, resistors, transformers, and hybrid circuits. The technology is also used

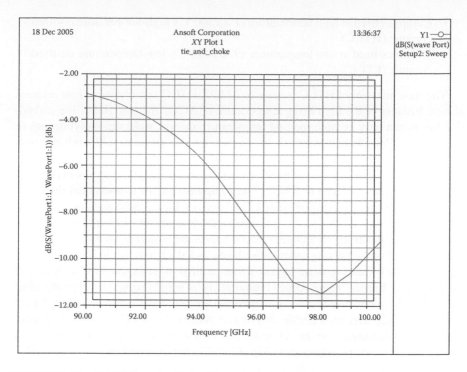

FIGURE 11.50   MEMS bowtie dipole $S11$ computed results.

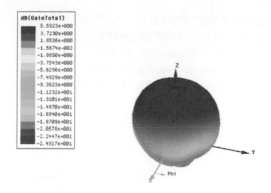

FIGURE 11.51   Bowtie dipole 3D radiation pattern.

for multilayer packaging for the electronics industry, such as for military electronics. Co-fired ceramic devices are made by processing a number of layers independently and assembling them into a device as a final step. Co-firing can be divided into low temperature (LTCC) and high temperature (HTCC) applications: low temperature means that the sintering temperature is below 1,000°C (1,830°F), while high temperature is around 1,600°C (2,910°F). There are two types of raw ceramics to manufacture multilayer ceramic (MLC) substrate:

- Ceramics fired at high temperature ($T \geq 1500°C$): high-temperature co-fired ceramic (HTCC)
- Ceramics fired at low temperature ($T \leq 1000°C$): low-temperature co-fired ceramic (LTCC).

The base material of HTCC is usually Al2O3. HTCC substrates are row ceramic sheets. Because of the high firing temperature of Al2O3 the material of the embedded layers can only be high melting temperature metals: wolfram, molybdenum or manganese. The substrate is unsuitable to bury passive elements, although it is possible to produce thick-film networks and circuits on the surface of HTCC substrates.

The breakthrough for LTCC fabrication came when the firing temperature of ceramic-glass substrate was reduced to 850°C. The equipment for the conventional thick-film process could then be used to fabricate LTCC devices. LTCC technology evolved from HTCC technology combined the advantageous features of thick-film technology. Because of the low firing temperature (850°C), the same materials are used for producing buried and surface wiring and resistive layers as a thick-film hybrid IC (i.e., Au, Ag, Cu wiring RuO_2-based resistive layers). It can be fired in an oxygen-rich environment unlike HTCC boards, where reduced atmosphere is used. During co-firing the glass melts, and the conductive and ceramic particles are sintered. On the surface of LTCC substrates hybrid integrated circuits can be realized, as shown in Figure 11.52. Passive elements can be buried into the substrate, and we can place semiconductor chips in a cavity. The dielectric properties at 9 GHz of LTCC substrates are listed in Table 11.15.

11.9.1   LTCC and HTCC Technology Process

- Low Temperature   LTCC 875°C
- High Temperature   HTCC 1400°C–1600°C
- Co-fired   Co-firing of (di)electric pastes
    LTCC: precious metals (Au, Ag, Pd, Cu)
        HTCC: refractory metals (W, Mo, MoMn)
- Ceramic   Mix of: alumina Al_2O_3
        Glasses SiO_2 - B_2O_3 - CaO - MgO
        Organic binders
        HTTC: essentially Al_2O_3

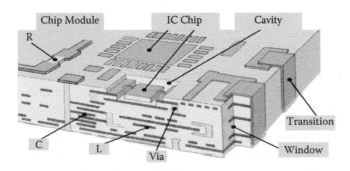

FIGURE 11.52   LTCC module.

TABLE 11.15
Dielectric Properties at 9 GHz of LTCC Substrates

Material	ε_r	Tan $\delta \times 10^{-3}$
99.5% AL	9.98	0.1
LTCC1	7.33	3.0
LTCC2	6.27	0.4
LTCC3	7.2	0.6
LTCC4	7.44	1.2
LTCC5	6.84	1.3
LTCC6	8.89	1.4

Advantages of LTCC

- Low permittivity tolerance
- Good thermal conductivity
- Low TCE (adapted to silicon and GaAs)
- Excellently suited for multilayer modules
- Integration of cavities and passive elements such as R, L, and C components
- Very robust against mechanical and thermal stress (hermetically sealed)
- Composable with fluidic, chemical, thermal, and mechanical functionalities
- Low material costs for silver conductor paths
- Low production costs for medium and large quantities

Advantages for high frequency applications

- Parallel processing (high yield, fast turnaround, lower cost)
- Precisely defined parameters
- High performance conductors
- Potential for multilayer structures
- High interconnect density

In Table 11.16, the LTCC process steps are listed. LTCC raw material comes as sheets or rolls. Material manufacturers are DuPont, ESL, Ferro, and Heraeus. In Table 11.17 several electrical, thermal, and mechanical characteristics of several LTCC materials are listed. In Figure 11.53, the LTCC process block diagram is presented.

In Table 11.18, the LTCC line loss at 2 GHz is listed for several LTCC materials. For LTTC1, material losses are 0.004 dB/mm.

11.9.2 Design of High-Pass LTCC Filters

The trend in the wireless industry toward miniaturization, cost reduction, and improved performance drives microwave designers to develop microwave compo-

TABLE 11.16
LTCC Process List

Tape casting
Sheet cutting
Laser punching
Printing
Cavity punching
Stacking
Bottom side printing
Pressing
Side hole formation
Side hole printing
Snap line formation
Pallet firing
Plating Ni-Au

TABLE 11.17
LTCC Material Characteristics

Material	LTCC DP951	Al2O3 96%	BeO	AIN 98%
Electrical Characteristics at 10 MHz				
Dielectric constant, ε_r	7.8	9.6	6.5	8.6
Dissipation factor, $\tan\delta$	0.00015	0.0003	0.0002	0.0005
Thermal Characteristics				
Thermal expansion, $10^{-6}/°C$	5.8	7.1	7.5	4.6
Thermal conductivity, W/mk 25°C–300°C	3	20.9	251	180
Mechanical Characteristics				
Density	3.1	3.8	2.8	3.3
Flexural strength, MPa	320	274	241	340
Young's modulus, GPa	120	314	343	340

nents using LTCC technology. A significant reduction in the size and the cost of microwave components can be achieved by using LTCC technology. When using LTCC technology discrete surface-mounted components such as capacitors and inductors are replaced by integrated printed components. LTCC technology allows the designer to use multilayer design if needed to reduce the size and cost of the circuit. However, multilayer design results in more losses due to via connections and to parasitic coupling between different parts of the circuit. To improve filter performance all filter parmeters have been optimized. Package effects were taken into account in the design.

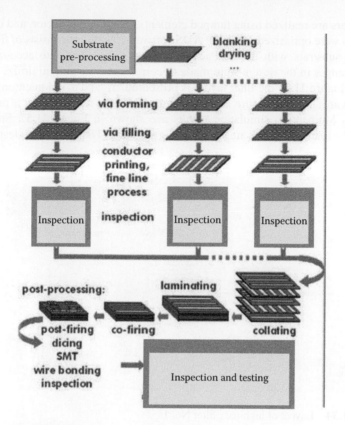

FIGURE 11.53 LTCC process.

TABLE 11.18
LTCC Line Loss

Material	Dissipation Factor, $\tan\delta \times 10^{-3}$	Line Loss, dB/mm, at 2 GHz
LTTC1	3.8	0.004
LTTC2	2.0	0.0035
LTTC6-CT2000	1.7	0.0033
Alumina 99.5%	0.65	0.003

High-pass filter specification

Frequency 1.5–2.5 GHz
Insertion loss 1.1 Fo – 1 dB
Rejection 0.9 Fo – 3 dB
Rejection 0.75 Fo – 20 dB
Rejection 0.5 Fo – 40 dB
VSWR - 2:1
Case dimensions - 700 × 300 × 25.5 mil inch

The filters are realized using lumped elements. The filter, inductor, and capacitor parameters were optimized using HP ADS software. The filter consists of five layers of 5.1 mil substrate with ε_r=7.8. Package effects were taken into account in the design. Changes in the design were made to compensate for and minimize package effects. In Figure 11.54 the filter layout is presented. S_{11} and S_{12} Momentum simulation results are shown in Figure 11.55. In Figure 11.56 the filter 2 layout is presented. S_{11} and S_{12} Momentum simulation results are shown in Figure 11.57. Simulation results of the tolerance check are shown in Figure 11.58. The parameters tested in the

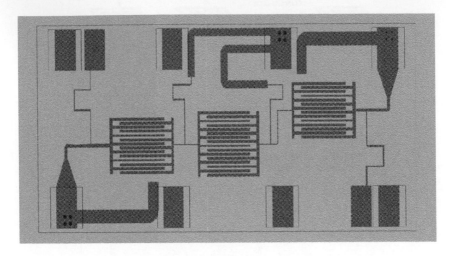

FIGURE 11.54　Layout of high-pass filter No. 1.

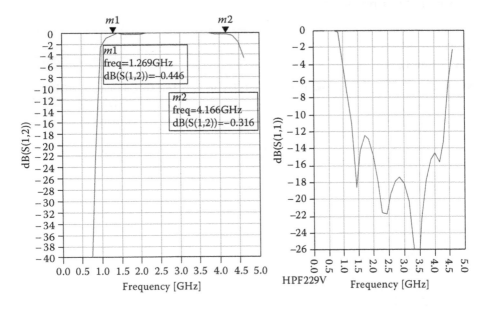

FIGURE 11.55　S_{12} and S_{11} results of high-pass filter no. 1.

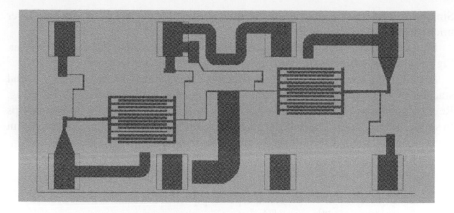

FIGURE 11.56 Layout of high-pass filter no. 2.

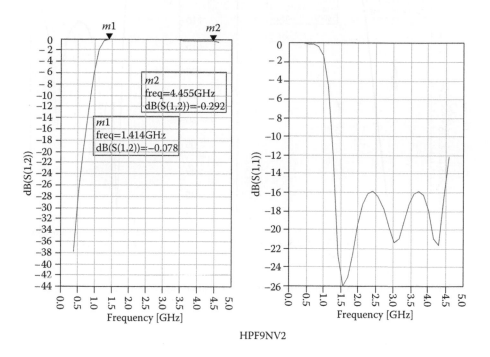

HPF9NV2

FIGURE 11.57 S_{12} and S_{11} results of high-pass filter no. 2.

tolerance check are inductor and capacitor line width and length and spacing between capacitor fingers.

11.9.3 COMPARISON OF SINGLE-LAYER AND MULTILAYER MICROSTRIP CIRCUITS

In a single-layer microstrip circuit all conductors are in a single layer. Coupling between conductors is achieved through edge or end proximity (across narrow gaps).

Single-layer microstrip circuits are cheap to produce. In Figure 11.59, a single-layer microstrip edge-coupled filter is shown.

Figure 11.60 presents the layout of a single-layer microstrip directional coupler. Figure 11.61 presents the structure of a multilayer microstrip coupler.

In multilayer microwave circuits conductors are separated by dielectric layers and stacked on different layers. This structure allows for (strong) broadside coupling. Registration between layers is not difficult to achieve as narrow gaps between strips in single-layer circuits. The multilayer structure technique is well-suited to thick-film print technology and also suitable for LTCC technology.

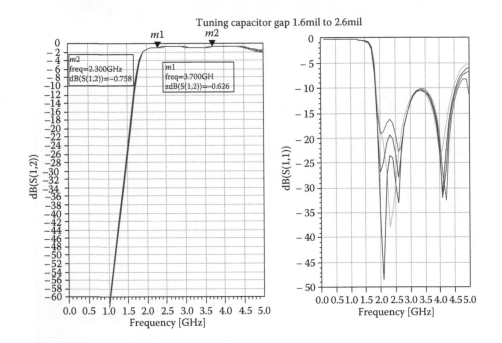

FIGURE 11.58   Tolerance simulation for spacing between capacitor fingers.

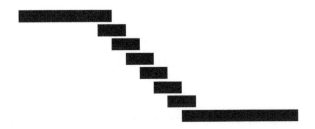

FIGURE 11.59   Edge-coupled filter.

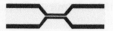

FIGURE 11.60 Single-layer microstrip directional coupler.

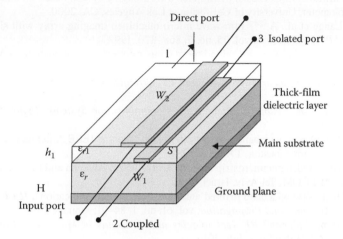

FIGURE 11.61 Multilayer microstrip coupler.

11.10 CONCLUSIONS

The dimensions and losses of microwave systems are minimized using monolithic microwave integrated circuit (MMIC) technology, MEMS, and LTCC technology, as well as the multi-layer structure technique. The multilayer structure technique is well-suited to thick-film print technology and LTCC technology. LTCC technology allows integration of cavities and passive elements such as R, L, and C components as part of the LTCC circuits. Sensors, actuators, and RF switches can be manufactured using MEMS technology. Losses in MEMS components are considerably lower than in MIC and MMIC RF components. MMICs are circuits in which active and passive elements are formed on the same dielectric substrate. MMICs are dimensionally small (from around 1 mm² to 10 mm²) and can be mass-produced. MMIC components can't be tuned. Accurate design is crucial in the design of MMIC circuits. The goal of MMIC, MEMS, and LTCC designers is to comply with customer specifications in one design iteration.

REFERENCES

1. J._Rogers and C. Plett, *Radio Frequency Integrated Circuit Design*, Norwood, MA: Artech House, 2003.
2. N. Maluf and K. Williams, *An Introduction to Microelectromechanical System Engineering*, Norwood, MA: Artech House, 2004.
3. A. Sabban, Microstrip antenna arrays, in *Microstrip Antennas*, N. Nasimuddin (Ed.), ISBN: 978-953-307-247-0, Croatia: InTech, pp. 361–384, 2011.

4. A. Sabban, Applications of MM wave microstrip antenna arrays, ISSSE 2007 Conference, Montreal, Canada, August 2007.
5. G. P. Gauthier et al., 94 GHz micro-machined aperture-coupled microstrip antenna, *IEEE Transactions on Antenna and Propagation*, vol. 47, no. 12, 1761–1766, December 1999.
6. M. M. Milkov, MSc. Thesis, Millimeter-wave imaging system based on antenna-coupled bolometer, University of California at Los Angeles, CA, 2000.
7. G. de Lange et al., A 3*3 mm-wave micro machined imaging array with sis mixers, *Applied Physical Letters*, vol. 75, no. 6, 868–870, 1999.
8. A. Rahman et al., Micro-machined room temperature micro bolometers for MM-wave detection, *Applied Physical Letters*, vol. 68, no. 14, 2020–2022, 1996.
9. S. A. Mass, *Nonlinear Microwave and RF Circuits*, Norwood, MA: Artech House, 1997.
10. A. Sabban, *Low Visibility Antennas for Communication Systems*, Taylor & Francis Group, 2015.
11. A. Sabban, A new wideband stacked microstrip antenna, IEEE Antenna and Propagation Symposium, Houston, TX, June 1983.
12. A. Sabban, Wideband microstrip antenna arrays, IEEE Antenna and Propagation Symposium MELCOM, Tel-Aviv, Israel, 1981.
13. A. Sabban, New wideband printed antennas for medical applications, *IEEE Transactions on Antennas and Propagation*, vol. 61, no. 1, 84–91, January 2013.
14. A. Sabban, *Wideband RF Technologies and Antennas in Microwave Frequencies*, Hoboken, NJ: Wiley Sons, July 2016.
15. A. Sabban, Small wearable meta materials antennas for medical systems, *Applied Computational Electromagnetics Society*, vol. 31, no. 4, April 2016.
16. A. Sabban, Ultra-wideband RF modules for communication systems, PARIPEX, *Indian Journal of Research*, vol. 5, no. 1, 91–95, January 2016.
17. A. Sabban, New compact wearable meta-material antennas, *Global Journal For Research and Analysis*, vol. 4, 268–271, August 2015.
18. A. Sabban, New wideband meta materials printed antennas for medical applications, *Journal of Advance in Medical Science (AMS)*, vol. 3, 1–10, April 2015. Invited paper.
19. A. Sabban, Wideband RF modules and antennas at microwave and MM wave frequencies for communication applications, *Journal of Modern Communication Technologies & Research*, vol. 3, 89–97. March 2015.
20. A. Sabban, Wideband MEMS detection arrays, *Journal of Modern Communication Technologies & Research*, vol. 2, 9–13, December 2014.

12 Body Area Networks (BANs)

The personal communication and biomedical industry has witnessed continuous growth in the last few years. Due to the huge progress in the development of communication systems in the last decade, development of low-cost wearable communication systems is not risky. However, development of compact efficient wearable antennas is one of the major challenges in the development of wearable communication and medical systems. Low profile compact antennas and transceivers are crucial in the development of wearable human communication and biomedical systems. Development of wearable antennas and compact transceivers for communication and biomedical systems is described in this chapter as well as design considerations, computational results, and measured results of wearable compact transceivers. The main goal of wireless BANs, WBANs, is to continuously provide medical data to the physician.

12.1   INTRODUCTION

Wearable systems have several applications in personal communication devices and medical devices as presented in [1–8]. Several medical devices and systems have been developed to monitor patient health as presented in several books and papers [1–44]. Wearable technology provides a powerful new tool to medical and surgical rehabilitation services. Wireless body area networks, WBANs, can record electrocardiograms, measure body temperature and blood pressure, and measure heartbeat rate, electro-dermal activity, and other healthcare parameters. The recorded and collected data can be stored and analyzed by employing cloud storage and cloud computing services.

12.2   CLOUD STORAGE AND COMPUTING SERVICES

Cloud storage is a service package in which data is stored, managed, backed up remotely, and made available to users over a network and internet services. Cloud storage is based on a virtualized infrastructure with accessible interfaces. Cloud-based data is stored in servers located in data centers managed by a cloud provider. A file and its associated metadata are stored in the server by using an object storage protocol. The server assigns an identification number (ID) to each stored file. When a file needs to be retrieved, the user presents the ID to the system and the content is assembled with all its metadata, authentication, and security. The most common uses of cloud services are cloud backup, disaster recovery, and archiving infrequently accessed data. Cloud storage providers are responsible for keeping the data available and accessible, and the physical environment protected and running. People and organizations buy or lease storage capacity from the providers to store and archive data files. Cloud storage services can be accessed via cloud computers and web services that use application programming interfaces (API) such as cloud desktop storage and cloud storage gateways.

Advantages of cloud storage

- Cloud storage can provide the benefits of greater accessibility, reliability, rapid deployment, and strong protection for data backup, archival, and disaster recovery purposes.
- Cloud storage is used as a natural disaster-proof backup. Usually there are at least two backup servers located in different places around the world.
- Cloud storage can be used for copying virtual machine images from the cloud to a desired location or to import a virtual machine image from any designated location to the cloud image library. Cloud storage can also be used to move virtual machine images between user accounts or between data centers.
- Cloud storage provides users with immediate access to a broad range of resources and applications hosted in the infrastructure of another organization via a web service interface.
- By using cloud storage companies can cut computing expenses such as storage maintenance task and purchasing additional storage capacity, and cut their energy consumption as well.
- Storage availability and data protection are provided by cloud storage services. So depending on the application, the additional technology efforts and cost to ensure availability and protection of data storage can be eliminated.

Disadvantages of cloud storage

- Increase in the risk of unauthorized physical access to the data.
- In a cloud-based architecture, data is replicated and moved frequently so the risk of unauthorized data recovery increases dramatically.
- Decrease in the security level of the stored data.
- It increases the number of networks over which the data travels. Instead of just a local area network (LAN) or storage area network, data stored on a cloud requires a wide area network to connect them both.
- A cloud storage company has many customers and thousands of servers. Therefore there is a larger team of technical staff with physical and electronic access to almost all of the data at the entire facility. Encryption keys that are kept by the service user, as opposed to the service provider, limit the access to data by service provider employees. A large number of keys has to be distributed to users via secure channels for decryption. The keys have to be securely stored and managed by the users in their devices. Storing these keys requires expensive secure storage.

- Cloud storage companies are not permanent and the services and products they provide can change.
- Cloud storage companies can be purchased by other larger foreign companies, or can go bankrupt and suffer from an irrecoverable disaster.
- Cloud storage is a rich resource for both hackers and national security agencies. The cloud stores data from many different users and organizations. Hackers see it as a very valuable target.
- Cloud storage sites have faced lawsuits from the owners of the intellectual property uploaded and shared in the site. Piracy and copyright problems can be enabled by sites that permit file sharing.

There are three main cloud-based storage architecture models: public, private and hybrid.

Public cloud storage services provide a multi-customer storage environment that is most suited for data storage. Data is stored in global data centers with storage data spread across multiple regions or continents.

Private cloud storage provides local storage services to a dedicated environment protected behind an organization's firewall. Private clouds are appropriate for users who need customization and more control over their data.

Hybrid cloud storage is a mix of private cloud and third-party public cloud services with synchronization between the platforms. The model offers businesses flexibility and more data deployment options. An organization might, for example, store actively used and structured data in a local cloud, and unstructured and archival data in a public cloud. In recent years, a greater number of customers have adopted the hybrid cloud model. Despite its benefits, a hybrid cloud presents technical, business, and management challenges. For example, private workloads must access and interact with public cloud storage providers, so compatibility and solid network connectivity are very important factors.

Cloud computing

Cloud computing is a type of Internet computing service that provides shared computer processing resources and data to computers and other devices on demand. Cloud computing enables on-demand access to a shared pool of configurable computing resources such as computer networks, servers, storage, applications, and services. It relies on sharing of computing resources. Cloud computing services can be rapidly provisioned and released with minimal management effort. Cloud computing and storage solutions provide users and enterprises with various capabilities to store and process their data in privately owned data centers. It allows companies to avoid high infrastructure costs such as servers and expensive software, and allows organizations to focus on their core businesses instead of spending time and money on computer networks. Cloud computing also allows companies to get their applications up and running faster, with improved manageability and less maintenance costs. Information technology teams can rapidly adjust resources to meet unpredictable business demands. Cloud computing applies high-performance computing power to perform tens of trillions of computations per second.

12.3 WIRELESS BODY AREA NETWORKS (WBANs)

The main goal of WBANs is to continuously provide biofeedback data. WBANs can record electrocardiograms, and measure body temperature and blood pressure, heartbeat rate, electro-dermal activity, and other healthcare parameters in an efficient way. For example, accelerometers can be used to sense heartbeat rate, movement, or even muscular activity. Body area networks (BANs) include the applications and communication devices using wearable and implantable wireless networks. A sensor network that senses health parameters is called a body sensor network (BSN). A wireless body area network (WBAN) is a special purpose wireless sensor network that incorporates different networks and wireless devices to enable remote monitoring in various environments.

An application of WBANs is in medical centers where the conditions of a large number of patients are constantly being monitored. Wireless monitoring of physiological signals of a large number of patients is needed in order to deploy a complete WSN in healthcare centers. Human health monitoring is emerging as a significant application of embedded sensor networks. A WBAN can monitor vital signs, providing real-time feedback to allow many patient diagnostic procedures using continuous monitoring of chronic conditions, or to monitor progress of recovery from an illness. Recent technological advances in wireless networking promise a new generation of wireless sensor networks suitable for human body wearable network systems.

Data acquisition in WBAN devices can be point-to-point or multipoint-to-point, depending on specific applications. Detection of an athlete's health condition would require point-to-point data sharing across various on-body sensors. Human body monitoring of vital signs will require routing data from several wearable sensors, multipoint-to-point, to a sink node, which in turn can relay the information wirelessly to an out-of-body computer. Data can be transferred in real-time mode or non-real-time. Human body monitoring applications require real-time data transfer. An athlete's physiological data can be collected offline for processing and analysis purposes.

A typical wireless body area network consists of a number of compact low-power sensing devices, a control unit, and wireless transceivers. The power supply for these components should be compact, lightweight, and long lasting as well. WBANs consist of small devices that allow fewer opportunities for redundancy and cover less space. To improve the efficiency of a WBAN it is important to minimize the number of nodes in the network. Adding more devices and path redundancy for solving node failure and network problems cannot be a practical option in WBAN systems. WBANs receive and transmit a large amount of data constantly. Data processing must be hierarchical and efficient to deal with asymmetry of several resources, to maintain system efficiency, and to ensure the availability of data. WBANs in a medical area consist of wearable and implantable sensor nodes that can sense biological information from the human body and transmit it over a short distance wirelessly to a control device worn on the body or placed in an accessible location. The sensor electronics must be miniaturized, low-power, and able to detect medical signals such

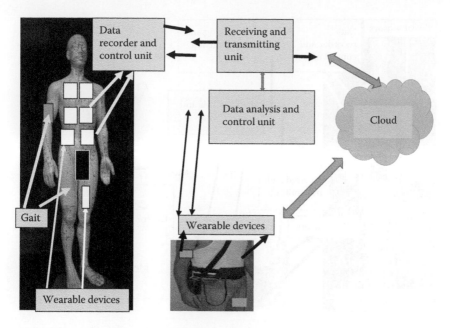

FIGURE 12.1 Wearable devices for various medical applications.

as electrocardiograms, electroencephalography, pulse rate, pressure, and temperature. The gathered data from the control devices are then transmitted to remote destinations in a wireless body area network for diagnostic and therapeutic purposes by including other wireless networks for long-range transmission. A wireless body area network with various wearable devices for medical applications is presented in Figure 12.1.

A wireless control unit is used to collect information from sensors through wires and transmits it to a remote station for monitoring. The recorded and collected data can be stored and analyzed by employing cloud storage and cloud computing services. A wireless wearable body area network (WWBAN) with various wearable devices for medical applications is presented in Figure 12.2. A WBAN health monitoring system is presented in Figure 12.3. The recorded and monitoring data can be stored and analyzed by employing cloud storage and cloud computing services.

12.4 WEARABLE WIRELESS BODY AREA NETWORKS (WWBANs)

Wireless communication systems offer a wide range of benefits to medical centers, patients, physicians, and sport centers through continuous measuring and monitoring of medical information, early detection of abnormal conditions, supervised rehabilitation, and potential discovery of knowledge through data analysis of the collected information. Wearable health monitoring systems allow the person to closely follow changes in important health parameters and provide feedback for maintaining optimal health status. If the WWBAN is part of the telemedicine system, the medical system can alert medical personnel when life-threatening events occur. In addition,

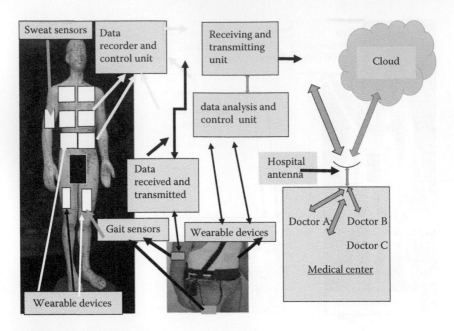

FIGURE 12.2   Wearable body area network (WBAN) for various medical applications.

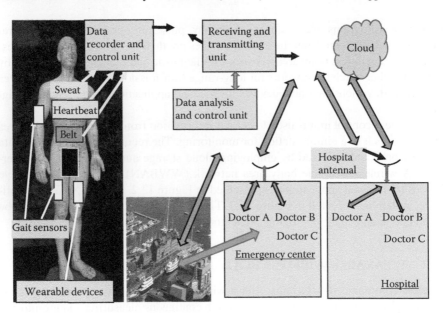

FIGURE 12.3   Wearable body area network (WBAN) health monitoring system.

patients can benefit from continuous long-term monitoring as a part of a diagnostic procedure. We can achieve optimal maintenance of a chronic condition, or can monitor the recovery period after an acute event or surgical procedure. The collected medical data can be a very good indicator of cardiac recovery of patients after heart

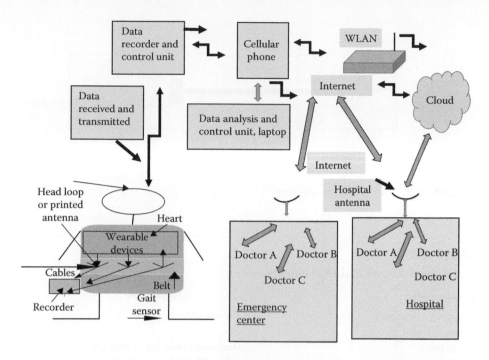

FIGURE 12.4 Wireless wearable body area network (WWBAN) health monitoring system.

surgery. Long-term monitoring can also confirm adherence to treatment guidelines or help monitor the effects of drug therapy. Health monitors can be used to monitor physical rehabilitation of patients during stroke rehabilitation or brain trauma reha-bilitation and after hip or knee surgeries. Many people use WBAN devices such as wearable heart rate monitors, respiration rate monitors, and pedometers for medical reasons or as part of fitness regimes. WBANs can be attached to cotton shirts to mea-sure respiratory activity, electrocardiograms, electromyograms, and body posture.

The recorded patient data can be stored and analyzed by employing cloud storage and cloud computing services. A wireless wearable body area network (WWBAN) health monitoring system is presented in Figure 12.4.

12.5 434 MHZ RECEIVING CHANNEL FOR COMMUNICATION AND MEDICAL SYSTEMS

A medical system can be implanted or inserted into the human body as a swal-lowed capsule. The medical device then transmits medical data to a recorder. The medical data can be analyzed by the medical stuff online or stored as medical data about the patient. The receiving channel is part of the recorder and consists of receiving wearable antennas, an RF head, and a signal processing unit. A block diagram of the receiver is shown in Figure 12.5. The receiving channel main spec-ifications are listed in Table 12.1.

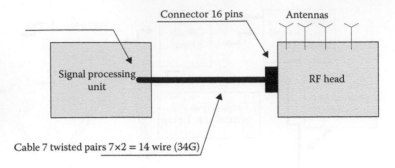

FIGURE 12.5   Recorder block diagram.

TABLE 12.1
Receiving Channel Main Specifications

Requirement	Specification
Frequency range uplink	430–440 MHz
Return loss (dB)	–9
Group delay	Maximum 50 nsec for 12 MHz BW
Input power	–30 to –60 dBm
SNR	>20 dB
Current consumption (mA)	50
Dimensions (cm)	12 × 12 × 5
Frequency range downlink	13.56 MHz
Received power downlink	–8 dBm ± 1 dB
Current consumption (mA)	100–110

A block diagram of the receiving channel is shown in Figure 12.6. The receiving channel consists of an uplink channel at 434 MHz and a downlink at 13.56 MHz.

The uplink channel consists of a switching matrix, low noise amplifier, and filter. The switching matrix losses are around 2 dB. The LNA noise figure is around 1 dB with 21 dB gain. The downlink channel consists of a transmitting antenna, antenna matching network, and differential amplifier. The downlink channel transmits commands to the medical system. The receiving channel gain and noise figure budget is shown in Figure 12.7. The receiving channel noise figure is around 3.5 dB.

A receiving channel with lower noise figure values is shown in Figure 12.8. The LNA amplifier is connected to the receiving antenna. The receiving channel gain and noise figure budget is shown in Figure 12.9. The receiving channel noise figure is around 3.5 dB.

Four folded dipole or loop antennas can be assembled in a belt and attached to the patient's stomach as shown in Figure 12.10a and b. The cable from each antenna is connected to a recorder. The received signal is routed to a switching matrix. The signal with the highest level is selected during the medical test. The antennas receive

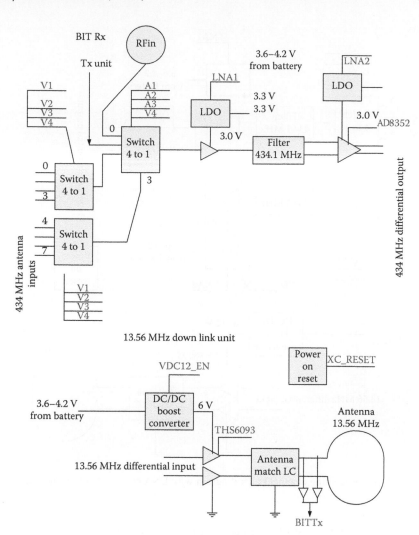

FIGURE 12.6 Receiving channel block diagram.

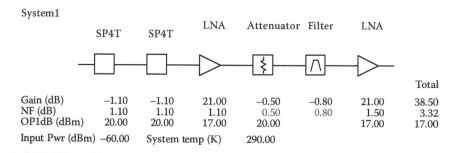

System1

	SP4T	SP4T	LNA	Attenuator	Filter	LNA	Total
Gain (dB)	−1.10	−1.10	21.00	−0.50	−0.80	21.00	38.50
NF (dB)	1.10	1.10	1.10	0.50	0.80	1.50	3.32
OP1dB (dBm)	20.00	20.00	17.00	20.00		17.00	17.00
Input Pwr (dBm)	−60.00	System temp (K)	290.00				

FIGURE 12.7 Receiving channel gain and noise figure budget.

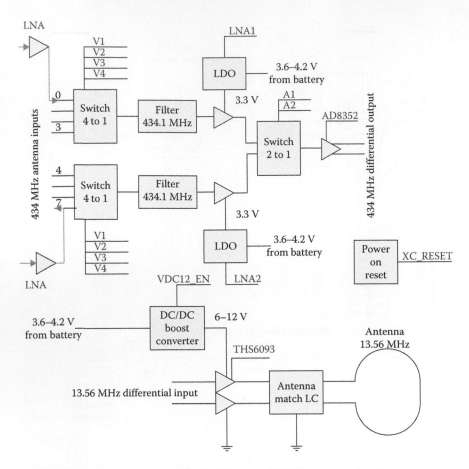

FIGURE 12.8 Receiving channel block diagram with LNA connected to the antennas.

	LNA	SP4T	Filter	SP2T	LNA	Attenuator	LNA	Total
Gain (dB)	21.00	−1.20	−0.80	−1.00	17.00	−1.00	15.50	49.50
NF (dB)	1.10	1.20	0.80	2.00	1.10	1.00	2.00	1.16
OP1dB (dBm)	17.00	20.00		20.00	17.00	20.00	17.00	17.00

Input Pwr (dBm) −60.00   System temp (K) 290.00

FIGURE 12.9 Receiving channel with LNA connected to the antennas: gain and noise figure budget.

a signal that is transmitted from various positions in the human body. Wearable antennas can be also attached on the patient's back in order to improve the level of the received signal from different locations in the human body.

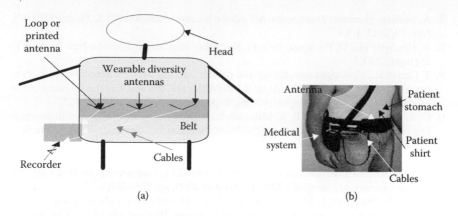

FIGURE 12.10 (a) Wearable medical system. (b) Medical system on patient.

12.6 CONCLUSIONS

Wearable technology provides a powerful new tool to medical and surgical rehabilitation services. The wearable body area network (WBAN) is emerging as an important option for medical centers and patients. Wearable technology provides a convenient platform that can quantify the long-term context and physiological response of individuals. Wearable technology will support the development of individualized treatment systems with real-time feedback to help promote patient health. Wearable medical systems and sensors can perform gait analysis, and measure body temperature, heartbeat, blood pressure, sweat rate, and other physiological parameters of the person wearing the medical device. Gait analysis is a useful tool both in clinical practice and biomechanical research. Gait analysis using wearable sensors provides quantitative and repeatable results over extended time periods with low cost and good portability, showing better prospects and making great progress in recent years. At present, commercialized wearable sensors have been adopted in various applications of gait analysis.

REFERENCES

1. S. C. Mukhopadhyay, (Ed.), *Wearable Electronics Sensors*, Switzerland: Springer, 2015.
2. A. Sabban, *Wideband RF Technologies and Antennas in Microwave Frequencies*, Hoboken, NJ: Wiley Sons, July 2016.
3. A. Sabban, *Low Visibility Antennas for Communication Systems*, Taylor & Francis Group, 2015.
4. A. Sabban, Small wearable meta materials antennas for medical systems, *Applied Computational Electromagnetics Society*, vol. 31, no. 4, April 2016.
5. A. Sabban, Microstrip antenna arrays, in *Microstrip Antennas*, N. Nasimuddin (Ed.), ISBN: 978-953-307-247-0, Croatia: InTech, pp. 361–384, 2011, Available from: http://www.intechopen.com/articles/show/title/microstrip-antenna-arrays.
6. A. Sabban, New wideband printed antennas for medical applications, *IEEE Transactions on Antennas and Propagation*, vol. 61, no. 1, 84–91, January 2013.

7. A. Sabban, Inventor, *Dual polarized dipole wearable antenna*, U.S. Patent 8203497, June 19, 2012, USA.
8. A. Bonfiglio and D. De Rossi, Editors, *Wearable Monitoring Systems*, New York, NY: Springer, 2011.
9. T. Gao et al., Vital signs monitoring and patient tracking over a wireless network, Proceedings of IEEE-EMBS 27th Annual International Conference of the Engineering in Medicine and Biology, Shanghai, China, September 1–5, 2005, pp. 102–105.
10. C. A. Otto, E. Jovanov and E. A. Milenkovic, WBAN-based system for health monitoring at home, Proceedings of IEEE/EMBS International Summer School, Medical Devices and Biosensors, Boston, MA, September 4–6, 2006, pp. 20–23.
11. G. H. Zhang et al., A biometric method to secure telemedicine systems, Proceedings of the 31st Annual International Conference of the IEEE Engineering in Medicine and Biology Society, Minneapolis, MN, September 2009, pp. 701–704.
12. S. Bao, Y. Zhang and L. Shen, Physiological signal based entity authentication for body area sensor networks and mobile healthcare systems, Proceedings of the 27th Annual International Conference of the IEEE EMBS, Shanghai, China, September 1–4, 2005, pp. 2455–2458.
13. V. Ikonen and E. Kaasinen, Ethical assessment in the design of ambient assisted living, Proceedings of Assisted Living Systems—Models, Architectures and Engineering Approaches, Schloss Dagstuhl, Germany, November 2008, pp. 14–17.
14. V. Srinivasan, J. Stankovic and K. Whitehouse, Protecting your daily in home activity information from a wireless snooping attack, Proceedings of the 10th International Conference on Ubiquitous Computing, Seoul, Korea, September 21–24, 2008, pp. 202–211.
15. R. Casas et al., User modelling in ambient intelligence for elderly and disabled people, Proceedings of the 11th International Conference on Computers Helping People with Special Needs, Linz, Austria, July 2008, pp. 114–122.
16. Y. Jasemian, Elderly comfort and compliance to modern telemedicine system at home, Proceedings of the Second International Conference on Pervasive Computing Technologies for Healthcare, Tampere, Finland, 30 January–1 February 2008, pp. 60–63.
17. L. Atallah et al., Wirelessly accessible sensor populations (WASP) for elderly care monitoring, Proceedings of the Second International Conference on Pervasive Computing Technologies for Healthcare, Tampere, Finland, 30 January–1 February 2008, pp. 2–7.
18. T. Hori et al., SELF-Network: Design and implementation of network for distributed embedded sensors, Proceedings of IEEE/RSJ International Conference on Intelligent Robots and Systems, Takamatsu, Japan, 30 October–5 November 2000, pp. 1373–1378.
19. Y. Mori, M. Yamauchi and K. Kaneko, Design and implementation of the Vital Sign Box for home healthcare, Proceedings of IEEE EMBS International Conference on Information Technology Applications in Biomedicine, Arlington, VA, November 2000, pp. 104–109.
20. C. Lauterbach et al., Smart clothes self-powered by body heat, Proceedings of Avantex Symposium, Frankfurt, Germany, Can 2002, pp. 5259–5263.
21. S. Marinkovic and E. Popovici, Network coding for efficient error recovery in wireless sensor networks for medical applications, Proceedings of International Conference on Emerging Network Intelligence, Sliema, Malta, October 11–16, 2009, pp. 15–20.
22. T. Schoellhammer et al., Lightweight temporal compression of microclimate datasets, Proceedings of the 29th Annual IEEE International Conference on Local Computer Networks, Tampa, FL, November 16–18, 2004, pp. 516–524.
23. A. T. Barth et al., Tempo 3.1: A body area sensor network platform for continuous movement assessment, Proceedings of the 6th International Workshop on Wearable and Implantable Body Sensor Networks, Berkeley, CA, June 2009, pp. 71–76.

24. M. Gietzelt., Automatic self-calibration of body worn triaxial-accelerometers for application in healthcare, Proceedings of the Second International Conference on Pervasive Computing Technologies for Healthcare, Tampere, Finland, January 2008, pp. 177–180.

25. T. Gao et al., Vital signs monitoring and patient tracking over a wireless network, Proceedings of the 27th Annual International Conference of the *IEEE EMBS*, Shanghai, China, September 1–4, 2005, pp. 102–105.

26. A. Purwar, D. U. Jeong and W. Y. Chung, Activity monitoring from realtime triaxial accelerometer data using sensor network, Proceedings of International Conference on Control, Automation and Systems, Hong Kong, March 21–23, 2007, pp. 2402–2406.

27. C. Baker et al., Wireless sensor networks for home health care, Proceedings of the 21st International Conference on Advanced Information Networking and Applications Workshops, Niagara Falls, Canada, Can 21–23, 2007, pp. 832–837.

28. L. Schwiebert, S. K. S. Gupta and J. Weinmann, Research challenges in wireless networks of biomedical sensors, Proceedings of the 7th annual International Conference on Mobile Computing and Networking, Rome, Italy, July 16–21, 2001, pp. 151–165.

29. O. Aziz et al., Pervasive body sensor network: An approach to monitoring the postoperative surgical patient, Proceedings of International Workshop on Wearable and implantable Body Sensor Networks *(BSN 2006)*, Cambridge, MA, 2006, pp. 13–18.

30. J. M. Kahn, R. H. Katz, K. S. J. Pister, Next century challenges: Mobile networking for smart dust, Proceedings of the ACM MobiCom'99, Washington, DC, August 1999, pp. 271–278.

31. N. Noury et al., Monitoring behavior in home using a smart fall sensor, Proceedings of IEEE-EMBS Special Topic Conference on Micro-technologies in Medicine and Biology, Lyon, France, October 12–14, 2000, pp. 607–610.

32. D. Y. Kwon and M. Gross, Combining body sensors and visual sensors for motion training, Proceedings of the 2005 ACM SIGCHI International Conference on Advances in Computer Entertainment Technology, Valencia, Spain, June 15–17, 2005, pp. 94–101.

33. N. K. Boulgouris, D. Hatzinakos and K.N. Plataniotis, Gait recognition: A challenging signal processing technology for biometric identification, *IEEE Signal Processing Magazine,* vol. 22, 78–90, 2005.

34. S. Kimmeskamp and E. M. Hennig, Heel to toe motion characteristics in parkinson patients during free walking, *Clinical Biomechanics*, 16, 806–812, 2001.

35. K. Turcot et al., New accelerometric method to discriminate between asymptomatic subjects and patients with medial knee osteoarthritis during 3-D gait, *IEEE Transactions on Biomedical Engineering*, 55, 1415–1422, 2008.

36. H. Furnée, Real-time motion capture systems, in *Three-Dimensional Analysis of Human Locomotion*, P. Allard et al. (Eds.), Chichester: John Wiley & Sons, pp. 85–108, 1997.

37. S. J. M. Bamberg et al., Gait analysis using a shoe-integrated wireless sensor system, *IEEE Transactions on Information Technology in Biomedicine*, 12, 413–423, 2008.

38. J. H. Choi et al., An efficient gait phase detection device based on magnetic sensor array, Proceedings of the 4th Kuala Lumpur International Conference on Biomedical Engineering, Kuala Lumpur, Malaysia, vol. 21, June 25–28, 2008, pp. 778–781.

39. J. Hidler, Robotic-assessment of walking in individuals with gait disorders, Proceedings of the 26th Annual International Conference of the IEEE Engineering in Medicine and Biology Society, San Francisco, CA, vol. 7, September 1–5, 2004, pp. 4829–4831.

40. Y. Wahab and N. A. Bakar, Gait analysis measurement for sport application based on ultrasonic system, Proceedings of the 2011 IEEE 15th International Symposium on Consumer Electronics, Singapore, June 14–17, 2011, pp. 20–24.

41. B. De Silva et al., A real-time feedback utility with body sensor networks, Proceedings of the 5th International Workshop on Wearable and Implantable Body Sensor Networks (BSN 08), Hong Kong, June 1–3, 2008, pp. 49–53.

42. A. Salarian et al., Gait assessment in Parkinson's disease: Toward an ambulatory system for long-term monitoring, *IEEE Transactions on Biomedical Engineering*, 51, 1434–1443, 2004.
43. L. Atallah et al., Observing recovery from knee-replacement surgery by using wearable sensors, Proceedings of the 2011 International Conference on Body Sensor Networks, Dallas, TX, Can 23–25, 2011, pp. 29–34.
44. M. El Sayed et al., Ambient and wearable sensing for gait classification in pervasive healthcare environments, Proceedings of the 12th IEEE International Conference on e-Health Networking Applications and Services (Healthcom), Lyon, France, July 1–3, 2010, pp. 240–245.

13 Measurements of Wearable Systems and Antennas

13.1 INTRODUCTION

This chapter describes electromagnetics, microwave engineering, wearable systems, and antenna measurements. Measurement techniques of wearable antennas and RF medical systems in the vicinity of the human body are presented in Sections 13.2 through 13.5. Basic radio frequency (RF) measurement theory is presented in Sections 13.6 and 13.7, see [1–5]. S parameter measurements are the first stage in electromagnetics, microwave engineering, and antenna measurements. Setups for microwave engineering measurements are also presented in this chapter, as well as maximum input and output measurements of communication systems, intermodulation measurements, IP2 and IP3, and antenna measurements. It is most convenient to measure antennas in receiving mode. If the antenna measured is reciprocal the antenna radiation characteristics are identical for receiving and transmitting modes. Active antennas, however, are not reciprocal. Radiation characteristics of antennas are usually measured in the far field. Far field antenna measurements suffer from some disadvantages. A long free-space area is needed. Reflections from the ground and from walls affect measured results and add errors to measured results. It is difficult, indeed almost impossible, to measure the antenna in the antenna's operating environment, such as an airplane or satellite. Antenna measurement facilities are expensive. Some of these drawbacks can be solved by near field and indoor measurements. Near field measurements are presented in [1]. Small communication companies do not own antenna measurement facilities. However, several companies around the world provide antenna measurement services, both near field and far field measurements. One day of near field measurements may cost as much as 5,000USD. One day of far field measurements may cost as much as 2,000USD.

13.2 WEARABLE ANTENNA MEASUREMENTS IN THE VICINITY OF THE HUMAN BODY

This section presents measurement techniques for wearable antennas and RF medical systems in the vicinity of the human body. Measurement results of wearable antennas and radio frequency (RF) medical systems in the vicinity of the human body are presented in [5–23]. Wearable antenna and RF medical system radiation characteristics on the human body can be measured by using a phantom. The phantom's electrical characteristics represent the human body's electrical characteristics. The phantom has a cylindrical shape with a 40 cm diameter and a length of 1.5 m.

The wearable antenna under test is placed on the phantom during the measurements of the antenna's radiation characteristics. The phantom is employed to compare the electrical performance of several new wearable antennas and to measure the electrical performance of several antenna belts in the vicinity of the human body.

13.3   PHANTOM CONFIGURATION

The phantom represents human body tissues. It contains a mix of water, sugar, and salt. The relative concentration of water, sugar, and salt determines the electrical characteristics of the phantom environment. A mixture of 55% water, 44% sugar, and 1% salt presents the electrical characteristics of stomach tissues. The phantom can be used to measure electromagnetic radiation from inside or outside the phantom. It is a fiberglass cylinder with 1.5 m height and 0.4 m diameter as shown in Figure 13.1. The cylinder surface is around 2.5 mm thick. The phantom contains a plastic rod 5 mm thick. The position of the plastic rod inside the phantom can be adjusted. The plastic rod can be rotated as shown in Figure 13.2. A small transmitting antenna can be attached to the plastic rod at different heights. The antenna can be rotated in the x–y plane.

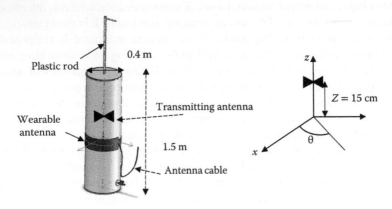

FIGURE 13.1   Phantom configuration.

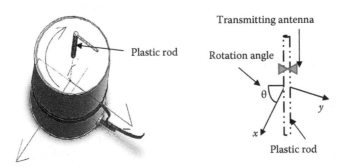

FIGURE 13.2   Transmitting antenna rotation.

13.4   MEASUREMENTS OF WEARABLE ANTENNAS USING A PHANTOM

The electrical characteristics of several wearable antennas were measured using the phantom. The position of the transmitting antennas along the z axis and x axis varied as listed in tables ($Z = 0$, $Z = -15$ cm, and $Z = 15$ cm). The angular angle of the transmitting antenna varied from 0° to 270°. Signal reception levels and immunity to noise were measured for several types of wearable antenna. The antennas' electrical performance was compared and the best antenna was chosen according to the system electrical requirements.

13.4.1   TEST PROCEDURE AND PROCESS

The test procedure and process is described below.

13.4.1.1   Test Procedure

The test checks two parameters of the antenna array:

- Signal reception levels
- Immunity to noise

13.4.1.2   Measured Antennas

The test checks the following antenna arrays:

- Four-sensor antenna array in a belt, antennas in orientations of +45°, +45°, +45°, −45°
- Sensor belt with four loop antennas in orientations of +45°, +45°, +45°, −45°
- Sensor belt with four antennas in orientations of +45°, −45°, +45°, −45°
- Thin belt with four-sensor array in orientations of +45°, −45°, +45°, −45°
- Four loop antenna array in a sleeve

13.4.1.3   Test Process

- Place the antenna array on the phantom as shown in Figure 13.2 and connect to the recorder.

Signal reception levels:

- Place the transmitter in the phantom in the following coordinates, 5 minutes per each location:
  - **Z values**: from −15 cm to +15 cm in 15 cm increments, 0 being the level of the antenna center.
  - **X values**: from −5 cm to −20 cm in 15 cm increments, 0 being the container wall where the antennas are attached.
  - **θ values**: from 0° to 270° in 90° increments, 0° being perpendicular to the middle of the antenna set.

13.4.1.4 Immunity to noise:
- Place the transmitter outside the phantom in the following coordinates, 5 minutes per location:
  - **Z values**: from −40 cm to +40 cm in 10 cm increments, 0 being the level of the antenna center.
  - **X values**: 100 cm from container wall θ values: from 0° to 270° in 90° increments, 0° being perpendicular to the middle of the antenna set.

13.5 MEASUREMENT RESULTS OF WEARABLE ANTENNAS

Measurements of five antenna array configurations were taken. For all the configurations the lowest measured signal level was when the transmitting antenna was located at $z = 15$ cm and $x = -5$ cm. For all the configurations the highest measured signal level was when the transmitting antenna was located at $z = 0$ cm and $x = -5$ cm.

13.5.1 MEASUREMENTS OF ANTENNA ARRAY 1

The measured antenna consists of four loop antennas with a tuning capacitor as shown in Figure 13.3. The loop antenna are printed on FR4 substrate with dielectric constant of 4.8 and 0.25 mm thickness. The loop radiator orientations are +45°, −45°, −45°, −45°. The antennas were inserted in a thin belt. The measurement results of antenna number 1 are listed in Table 13.1.

13.5.2 MEASUREMENTS OF ANTENNA ARRAY 2

The measured antenna consists of four loop antennas without a tuning capacitor as shown in Figure 13.4. The loop radiator orientations are +45°, −45°, −45°, −45°. The antennas was inserted in a thin belt. The measurement results of antenna number 2 are listed in Table 13.2.

13.5.3 MEASUREMENTS OF ANTENNA ARRAY 3

The measured antenna consists of four tuned loop antennas with a tuning capacitor as shown in Figure 13.5. The loop radiator orientations are +45°, −45°, +45°, −45°. The antenna was inserted in a belt. The measurement results of antenna number 3 are listed in Table 13.3.

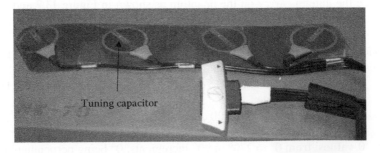

FIGURE 13.3 Sensor belt with four antennas in orientations of +45°, +45°, +45°, −45°.

TABLE 13.1

Measurements of Antenna 1

Antenna 1 (X cm , Z cm)	Angle θ			
	0°	90°	180°	270°
$Z = 0$ cm	0°	90°	180°	270°
Signal level (dB) $X = -5$, $Z=0$	−60	−63	−81	−65
Signal level (dB) $X = -20$, $Z = 0$	−78	−70	−65	−74
$Z = 15$ cm	−	−	−	−
Signal level (dB) $X = -5$, $Z=15$	−81	−89	−83	−82
Signal level (dB) $X = -20$, $Z = 15$	−86	−89	−81	−85
$Z = -15$ cm	−	−	−	−
Signal level (dB) $X = -5$, $Z = -15$	−70	−76	−81	−68
Signal level (dB) $X = -20$, $Z = -15$	−79	−64	−74	−81
Noise test	Angle θ			
$Z = 0$ cm	0°	90°	180°	270°
Signal level (dB)	−72	−74	−74	−74
Noise level (dB)	−95	−95	−95	−95
$Z = 40$ cm	−			
Signal level (dB)	−72	−74	−74	−74
Noise level (dB)	−88	−88	−88	−88
$Z = -40$ cm	−			
Signal level (dB)	−72	−74	−74	−74
Noise level (dB)	−94	−93	−94	−95

The highest signal level is at $Z = 0$ cm, $X = -5$ cm, $\theta = 0°$. At $\theta = 180°$ the signal level is lower by 21 dB. The lowest signal level is at $Z = \pm 15$ cm, $X = -5$ cm, $\theta = 90°$. The noise level is lower by 14–21 dB than the signal level.

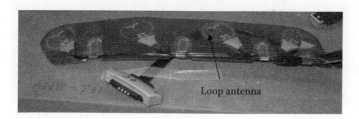

FIGURE 13.4 Sensor belt with four antennas in orientations of +45°, +45°, +45°, −45° without a tuning capacitor.

13.5.4 MEASUREMENTS OF ANTENNA ARRAY 4 IN A THINNER BELT

The measured antenna consists of four loop antennas with a tuning capacitor as shown in Figure 13.6. The loop radiator orientations are +45°, −45°, +45°, −45°. The antenna was inserted in a thinner belt. The measurement results of antenna number 4 are listed in Table 13.4.

TABLE 13.2
Measurements of Antenna 2

Antenna2 (X cm, Z cm)		Angle θ		
Z = 0 cm	0°	90°	180°	270°
Signal level (dB) X = −5, Z = 0	−63	−70	−82	−72
Signal level (dB) X = −20, Z = 0	−84	−66	−66	−79
Z = 15 cm	–	–	–	–
Signal level (dB) X = −5, Z = 15	−82	−93	−90	−84
Signal level (dB) X = −20, Z = 15	−88	−83	−79	−90
Z = −15 cm	–	–	–	–
Signal level (dB) X = −5, Z = −15	−74	−82	−85	−92
Signal level (dB) X = −20, Z = −15	−86	−70	−77	−81
Noise test		**Angle θ**		
Z = 0 cm	0°	90°	180°	270°
Signal level (dB)	−67	−69	−72	−68
Noise level (dB)	−85	−85	−86	−85
Z = 40 cm	–			
Signal level (dB)	−66	−69	−72	−68
Noise level (dB)	−80	−83	−86	−85
Z = −40 cm	–			
Signal level (dB)	−68	−69	−72	−69
Noise level (dB)	−84	−82	−83	−83

The highest signal level is at $Z = 0$ cm, $X = −5$ cm, $θ = 0°$. At $θ = 180°$ the signal level is lower by 19 dB. The lowest signal level is at $Z = 15$ cm, $X = −5$ cm, $θ = 90°$. The noise level is lower by 14–18 dB than the signal level.

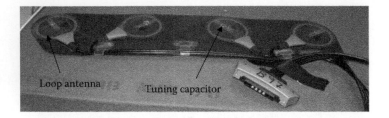

FIGURE 13.5   Sensor belt with four antennas in orientations of +45°, −45°, +45°, −45°.

13.5.5   MEASUREMENTS OF ANTENNA ARRAY 5

The measured antenna consists of four loop antennas without a tuning capacitor inserted in a sleeve, as shown in Figure 13.7. The sleeve improves the antenna VSWR from 4:1 to 2:1. The loop radiator orientations are 90°, 90°, 90°, 90°.

The antenna was inserted in a thin sleeve. The measurement results of antenna number 5 are listed in Table 13.5.

TABLE 13.3

Measurements of Antenna 3

Antenna3 (X cm, Z cm)		Angle θ		
Z = 0 cm	0°	90°	180°	270°
Signal level (dB) $X = -5, Z = 0$	−63	−63	−82	−69
Signal level (dB) $X = -20, Z = 0$	−83	−70	−68	−76
Z = 15 cm	−	−	−	−
Signal level (dB) $X = -5, Z = 15$	−85	−86	−85	−86
Signal level (dB) $X = -20, Z = 15$	−89	−88	−86	−85
Z = −15 cm	−	−	−	−
Signal level (dB) $X = -5, Z = -15$	−72	−79	−83	−74
Signal level (dB) $X = -20, Z = -15$	−85	−69	−77	−82
Noise test		**Angle θ**		
Z = 0 cm	0°	90°	180°	270°
Signal level (dB)	−68	−70	−76	−70
Noise level (dB)	−91	−91	−92	−92
Z = 40 cm	−			
Signal level (dB)	−68	−70	−76	−70
Noise level (dB)	−90	−88	−90	−88
Z = −40 cm	−			
Signal level (dB)	−68	−70	−76	−70
Noise level (dB)	−89	−87	−90	−87

The highest signal level is at Z = 0 cm, X = −5 cm, θ = 0°. At θ = 180° the signal level is lower by 19 dB. The lowest signal level is at Z = 15 cm, X = −20 cm, θ = 0°. The noise level is lower by 18–23 dB than the signal level.

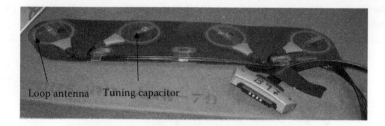

FIGURE 13.6 Four antennas in orientations of +45°, −45°, +45°, −45°, in a thinner belt.

13.6 REPRESENTATION OF WEARABLE SYSTEMS WITH N PORTS

Antenna systems and communication systems can be represented as multiport networks with N ports as shown in Figure 13.8. We can assume that only one mode propagates in each port. The electromagnetic fields in each port represents incident and reflected waves. The electromagnetic fields can be represented by equivalent voltages and currents as given in Equations 13.1 and 13.2, see [1–5].

$$V_n^- = Z_n I_n^-$$

$$V_n^+ = Z_n I_n^+$$

(13.1)

TABLE 13.4
Measurements of Antenna 4

Antenna4 (X cm, Z cm)	Angle θ			
Z = 0 cm	0°	90°	180°	270°
Signal level (dB) X = −5, Z = 0	−61	−62	−81	−63
Signal level (dB) X = −20, Z = 0	−79	−69	−67	−73
Z = 15 cm	−	−	−	−
Signal level (dB) X = −5, Z = 15	−86	−88	−88	−83
Signal level (dB) X = −20, Z = 15	−90	−84	−82	−86
Z = −15 cm	−	−	−	−
Signal level (dB) X = −5, Z = −15	−70	−81	−82	−67
Signal level (dB) X = −20, Z = −15	−80	−67	−74	−81
Noise test	**Angle θ**			
Z = 0 cm	0°	90°	180°	270°
Signal level (dB)	−70	−70	−76	−70
Noise level (dB)	−95	−95	−95	−95
Z = 40 cm	−			
Signal level (dB)	−70	−70	−76	−70
Noise level (dB)	−92	−92	−91	−92
Z = −40 cm	−			
Signal level (dB)	−70	−70	−76	−70
Noise level (dB)	−92	−92	−91	−92

The highest signal level is at Z = 0 cm, X = −5 cm, θ = 0°. At θ = 180° the signal level is lower by 20 dB. The lowest signal level is at Z = 15 cm, X = −20 cm, θ = 0°. The noise level is lower by 18–25 dB than the signal level.

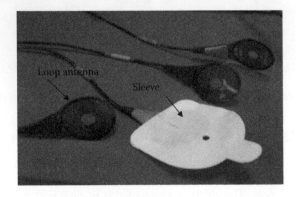

FIGURE 13.7   Four loop antennas in a sleeve; radiator orientations are 90°, 90°, 90°, 90°.

$$I_n^- = Y_n V_n^-$$

$$I_n^+ = Y_n V_n^+$$

(13.2)

TABLE 13.5
Measurements of Antenna 5

Antenna5 (X cm, Z cm)		Angle θ		
Z = 0 cm	0°	90°	180°	270°
Signal level (dB) X = −5, Z = 0	−67	−52	−58	−60
Signal level (dB) X = −20, Z = 0	−68	−70	−77	−78
Z = 15 cm	–	–	–	–
Signal level (dB) X = −5, Z = 15	−90	−86	−92	−90
Signal level (dB) X = −20, Z = 15	−84	−86	−90	−86
Z = −15 cm	–	–	–	–
Signal level (dB) X = −5, Z = −15	−85	−90	−85	−92
Signal level (dB) X = −20, Z = −15	−90	−85	−75	−78
Noise test		**Angle θ**		
Z = 0 cm	0°	90°	180°	270°
Signal level (dB)	−70	70	−70	−70
Noise level (dB)	−90	−90	−90	−90
Z = 40 cm	–			
Signal level (dB)	−72	−72	−72	−72
Noise level (dB)	−90	−90	−90	−90
Z = −40 cm	–			
Signal level (dB)	−73	−73	−73	−73
Noise level (dB)	−90	−90	−90	−90

The highest signal level is at Z = 0 cm, X = −5 cm, θ = 90°. At θ = 180° the signal level is lower by 6 dB. At θ = 270° the signal level is lower by 8 dB. The lowest signal level is at Z = 15 cm, X = −20 cm, θ = 180°. The noise level is lower by 18–22 dB than the signal level.

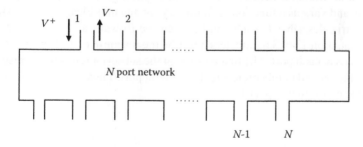

FIGURE 13.8 Multiport network with N ports.

The voltages and currents in each port are given in Equation 13.3.

$$I_n = I_n^+ - I_n^-$$
$$V_n = V_n^+ + V_n^-$$

(13.3)

The relations between the voltages and currents can be represented by the Z matrix as given in Equation 13.4. The relations between the currents and voltages can be represented by the Y matrix as given in Equation 13.5. The Y matrix is the inverse of the Z matrix.

$$
[V] = \begin{bmatrix} V_1 \\ V_2 \\ \\ V_N \end{bmatrix} = \begin{bmatrix} Z_{11} & Z_{12} & Z_{1N} \\ Z_{21} & Z_{22} & Z_{2N} \\ \\ Z_{N1} & Z_{N2} & Z_{NN} \end{bmatrix} \begin{bmatrix} I_1 \\ I_2 \\ \\ I_N \end{bmatrix} = [Z][I] \quad (13.4)
$$

$$
[I] = \begin{bmatrix} I_1 \\ I_2 \\ \\ I_N \end{bmatrix} = \begin{bmatrix} Y_{11} & Y_{12} & Y_{1N} \\ Y_{21} & Y_{22} & Y_{2N} \\ \\ Y_{N1} & Y_{N2} & Y_{NN} \end{bmatrix} \begin{bmatrix} V_1 \\ V_2 \\ \\ V_N \end{bmatrix} = [Y][V] \quad (13.5)
$$

13.7   SCATTERING MATRIX

We cannot measure voltages and currents in microwave networks. However, we can measure power, VSWR, and the location of the minimum field strength. We can calculate the reflection coefficient from these data. The scattering matrix is a mathematical presentation that describes how electromagnetic energy propagates through a multiport network. The S matrix allows us to accurately describe the properties of complicated networks. S parameters are defined for a given frequency and system impedance, and vary as a function of frequency for any non-ideal network. The scattering S matrix describes the relation between the forward and reflected waves as written in Equation 13.6. S parameters describe the response of an N-port network to voltage signals at each port. The first number in the subscript refers to the responding port, while the second number refers to the incident port. Thus S_{21} means the response at port 2 due to a signal at port 1.

$$
[V^-] = \begin{bmatrix} V_1^- \\ V_2^- \\ \\ V_2^+ \end{bmatrix} = \begin{bmatrix} S_{11} & S_{12} & S_{1N} \\ S_{21} & S_{22} & S_{2N} \\ \\ S_{N1} & S_{N2} & S_{NN} \end{bmatrix} \begin{bmatrix} V_1^+ \\ V_2^+ \\ \\ V_2^+ \end{bmatrix} = [S][V^+] \quad (13.6)
$$

The S_{nn} elements represent reflection coefficients. The S_{nm} elements represent transmission coefficients as written in Equation 13.7, where a_i represents the forward voltage in the i port.

$$S_{nn} = \frac{V_n^-}{V_n^+}\bigg|a_i = 0 \qquad i \neq n$$

$$\text{(13.7)}$$

$$S_{nm} = \frac{V_n^-}{V_m^+}\bigg|a_i = 0 \qquad i \neq m$$

By normalizing the S matrix we can represent the forward and reflected voltages as written in Equation 13.8. S parameters depend on the frequency and are given as a function of frequency. In a reciprocal microwave network $S_{nm} = S_{mn}$ and $[S]^t = [S]$.

$$I = I^+ - I^- = V^+ - V^-$$

$$V = V^+ + V^-$$

$$\text{(13.8)}$$

$$V^+ = \frac{1}{2}(V + I)$$

$$V^- = \frac{1}{2}(V - I)$$

The relation between the Z and S matrix is derived by using Equations 13.8 and 13.9 and is given in Equations 13.10 and 13.11.

$$I_n = I_n^+ - I_n^- = V_n^+ - V_n^-$$

$$\text{(13.9)}$$

$$V_n = V_n^+ + V_n^-$$

$$[V] = [V^+] + [V^-] = [Z][I] = [Z][V^+] - [Z][V^-]$$

$$([Z] + [U])[V^-] = ([Z] - [U])[V^+]$$

$$[V^-] = ([Z] + [U])^{-1}([Z] - [U])[V^+]$$

$$\text{(13.10)}$$

$$[V^-] = [S][V^+]$$

$$[S] = ([Z] + [U])^{-1}([Z] - [U])$$

$$[V^+] = \frac{1}{2}([V] + [I]) = \frac{1}{2}([Z] + [U])[I]$$

$$[V^-] = \frac{1}{2}([V] - [I]) = \frac{1}{2}([Z] - [U])[I]$$

$$\frac{1}{2}[I] = ([Z] + [U])^{-1}[V^+]$$

$$\text{(13.11)}$$

$$[V^-] = ([Z] - [U])([Z] + [U])^{-1}[V^+]$$

$$[S] = ([Z] - [U])([Z] + [U])^{-1}$$

A network analyzer is employed to measure S parameters, as shown in Figure 13.2a. A network analyzer can have 2 to 16 ports.

13.8   S PARAMETER MEASUREMENTS

Antenna S parameter measurement is usually a one-port measurement. First we calibrate the network analyzer to the desired frequency range. A one-port, S1P, calibration process consists of three steps.

- Short calibration
- Open calibration
- Load calibration

Connect the antenna to the network analyzer and measure the S_{11} parameter. Save and plot the S_{11} results. An antenna S parameter measured result is shown in Figure 13.9. A setup for S parameter measurement is shown in Figure 13.10a. S_{11} parameter measurement results are shown in Figure 13.10b. Two-port S parameter measurements setup is shown in Figure 13.11. The two-port, S2P, calibration process consists of four steps.

- Short calibration
- Open calibration
- Load calibration
- Through calibration

Measure S parameters S_{11}, S_{22}, S_{12}, and S_{21} for N channels. The RF head gain is given by the S_{21} parameter. Gain flatness and phase balance between channels is measured by comparing the S_{21} magnitude and phase measured values. RF head gain

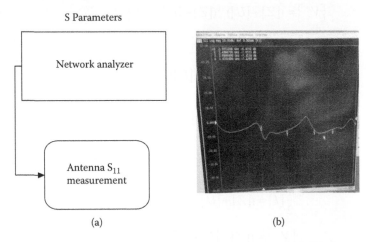

(a)   (b)

FIGURE 13.9   (a) Antenna S parameter measurements. (b) Measured antenna S_{11}.

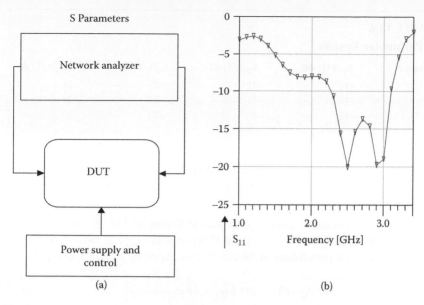

FIGURE 13.10   (a) Two-port S parameter measurements. (b) S_{11} parameter results.

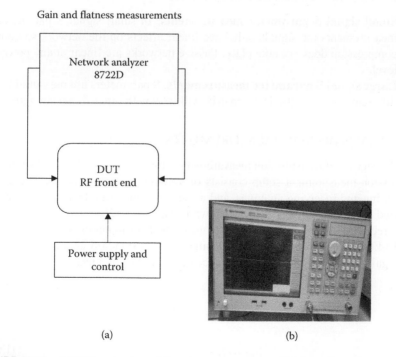

FIGURE 13.11   (a) RF head gain and flatness measurements. (b) Network analyzer.

TABLE 13.6

S Parameter Results

Channel	S_{11}(E/T) dB		S_{22}(E/T) dB		S_{12}(E/T) dB		S_{21}(E/T) dB	
1	−12	–	−11	–	−22	–	31	–
2	−10.5	–	−11	–	−23	–	29	–
3	−11	–	−10	–	−20	–	29	–
–	–	–	–	–	–	–	–	–
$n-1$	−10	–	−9	–	−20	–	29	–
n	−9	–	−10.5	–	−19	–	28	–

and flatness measurement setup is presented in Figure 13.11a. A two-port network analyzer is shown in Figure 13.11b. Table 13.6 presents a typical table of measured S parameter results. S parameters in dB can be calculated by using Equation 13.12.

$$S_{ij}(\text{dB}) = 20 * \log\left[S_{ij}(\text{magnitude})\right] \tag{13.12}$$

13.8.1 TYPES OF S PARAMETER MEASUREMENTS

Small signal S parameter measurements: In small signal S parameter measurements the signals only have linear effects on the network so gain compression does not take place. Passive networks are linear at any power level.

Large signal S parameter measurements: S parameters are measured for different power levels. The S matrix will vary with input signal strength.

13.9 TRANSMISSION MEASUREMENTS

A block diagram of transmission measurement setup is shown in Figure 13.12a. The transmission measurement setup consists of a sweep generator, device under test, transmitting and receiving antennas, and a spectrum analyser. Transmission results measured by a spectrum analyser are shown in Figure 13.12b.

The received power can be calculated using the Friis equation as given in Equations 13.13 and 13.14. The receiving antenna can be a standard gain antenna with a known gain where r represents the distance between the antennas.

$$P_R = P_T G_T G_R \left(\frac{\lambda}{4\pi r}\right)^2$$

$$\text{For} - G_T = G_R = G \tag{13.13}$$

$$G = \sqrt{\frac{P_R}{P_T}}\left(\frac{4\pi r}{\lambda}\right)$$

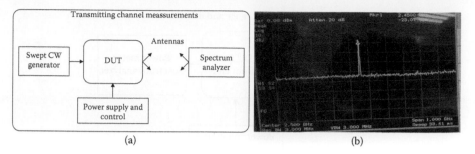

(a)   (b)

FIGURE 13.12   (a) Transmission measurement setup. (b) Measured transmission results.

TABLE 13.7
Transmission Measurement Results

Transmission Results for Antennas under Test (AUT) dBm

Antenna	F1 (MHz)	F2 (MHz)	F3 (MHz)	Remarks
1	10	9	8	–
2	9	8	7	–
3	9.5	8.5	7.5	–
4	10	9	8	–
5	9	8	7	–
6	10.5	9.5	8.5	–
7	9	8	7	–
8	11	10	9	–

$$P_R = P_T G_T G_R \left(\frac{\lambda}{4\pi r} \right)^2$$

$$\text{For} - G_T \neq G_R \tag{13.14}$$

$$G_T = \frac{1}{G_R} \frac{P_R}{P_T} \left(\frac{4\pi r}{\lambda} \right)^2$$

Transmission measurement results can be summarized as in Table 13.7.

13.10   OUTPUT POWER AND LINEARITY MEASUREMENTS

A block diagram of the output power and linearity measurement setup is shown in Figure 13.13. The output power and linearity measurement setup consists of a sweep generator, device under test, and a spectrum analyzer or power meter. In output power and linearity measurements we increase the synthesizer power in 1 dB steps and measure the output power level and linearity.

Output power range and linearity

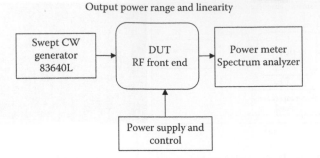

FIGURE 13.13   Output power and linearity measurements setup.

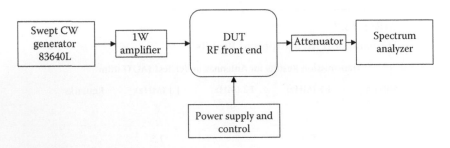

FIGURE 13.14   Power input protection measurement.

13.11   POWER INPUT PROTECTION MEASUREMENT

A block diagram of power input protection measurement setup is shown in Figure 13.14. The power input protection measurement setup consists of a sweep generator, power amplifier, device under test, attenuator and spectrum analyzer or power meter. In power input protection measurements we increase the synthesizer power in 1 dB steps from 0 dBm and measure the output power level and observe that the device under test (DUT) function with no damage.

13.12   NON-HARMONIC SPURIOUS MEASUREMENTS

A block diagram of a non-harmonic spurious measurement setup is shown in Figure 13.15a. The spectrum analyzer is shown in Figure 13.15b.

The non-harmonic spurious measurements setup consists of a sweep generator, device under test (DUT), and a spectrum analyser. In non-harmonic spurious measurements we increase the synthesizer power in 1 dB steps, up to 1 dBc point, and measure the spurious level.

13.13   SWITCHING TIME MEASUREMENTS

A block diagram of a switching time measurements setup is shown in Figure 13.16. The switching time measurement setup consists of a sweep generator, device under test (DUT), detector, pulse generator, and oscilloscope. In switching time measurements we transmit an RF signal through the DUT. We inject a pulse via the switch control port. The pulse envelope can be observed on the oscilloscope. Switching time can be measured using the oscilloscope.

13.14   IP2 MEASUREMENTS

The setup for IP2 and IP3 measurements is shown in Figure 13.17. Second-order intermodulation results are shown in Figure 13.17. IP2 can be computed by Equation 13.15.

$$IP_{2[dBm]} = P_{out[dBm]} + \Delta_{[dB]} \tag{13.15}$$

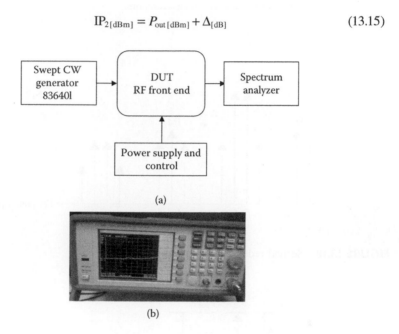

(a)

(b)

FIGURE 13.15   (a) Non-harmonic spurious measurements. (b) Spectrum analyzer.

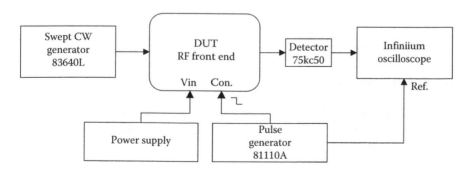

FIGURE 13.16   Switching time measurement setup.

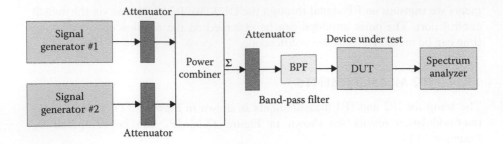

FIGURE 13.17 Setup for IP2 and IP3 measurements.

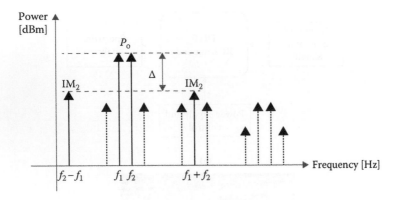

FIGURE 13.18 Second-order intermodulation results.

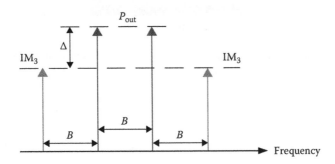

FIGURE 13.19 Third-order intermodulation results.

Second-order intermodulation results are shown in Figure 13.18.

Third-order intermodulation results are shown in Figure 13.19. IP3 can be computed by Equation 13.16.

$$\mathrm{IP}_{3[\mathrm{dBm}]} = P_{\mathrm{out}[\mathrm{dBm}]} + \frac{\Delta_{[\mathrm{dB}]}}{2} \tag{13.16}$$

13.15   IP3 MEASUREMENTS

A block diagram of output IP3 measurement setup is shown in Figure 13.20. IP3 setup consists of two sweep generators, a device under test (DUT), and a spectrum analyser. In an IP3 test we inject two signals the DUT and measure the intermodulation signals. The test results listed in Table 13.8 present IP3 measurements of a receiving channel. Input and output measured IP3 can be calculated by using Equations 13.16 through 13.18.

$$IP3_{out} = P_{F1} + \frac{\left(\left(\frac{P_{F1}+P_{F2}}{2}\right) - P_{IM1}\right)}{2} \tag{13.17}$$

$$IP3_{IN} = \frac{(P_{F1}+P_{F2})}{2} + \frac{\left(\frac{(P_{F1}+P_{F2})}{2} - P_{IM2}\right)}{2} - \left(\left(\frac{P_{F1}+P_{F2}}{2}\right) - P_{in}\right) \tag{13.18}$$

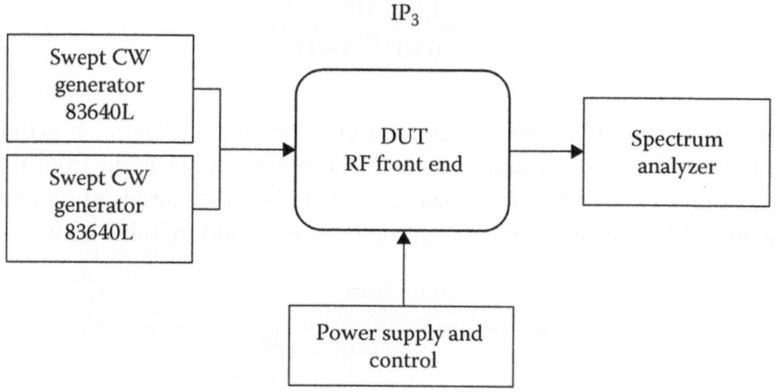

FIGURE 13.20   Two-tone measurements.

TABLE 13.8
IP3 Measurements

Pin (dBm)	19.999 (GHz) IM1	F1 = 20 (GHz)	F2 = 20.001 (GHz)	20.002 (GHz) IM2	IP3 OUT	IP3 INPUT
B	C (dBm)	D (dBm)	E (dBm)	F (dBm)	(dBm)	(dBm)
−17	−10.8	10	10	−13.8	20.4	−5.1
Pin (dBm)	29.999 (GHz) IM1	F1 = 30 (GHz)	F2 = 30.001 (GHz)	30.002 (GHz) IM2	IP3 OUT	IP3 INPUT
−14.50	−17	10	10	−18.8	23.5	−0.1
Pin (dBm)	39.998 (GHz) IM1	F1 = 39.999 (GHz)	F2 = 40 (GHz)	40.001 (GHz) IM2	IP3 OUT	IP3 INPUT
−14.5	−12	10	10	−11.2	21	−3.9

For example the first signal is at 20 GHz with a power level of 10 dBm. The second signal is at 20.001 GHz with a power level of 10 dBm. The first intermodulation signal is at 19.999 GHz with a power level of −10.8 dBm. The second intermodulation signal is at 20.001 GHz with a power level of −13.8 dBm. The power level of IP3 at the output is 20.4 dBm. The power level of IP3 at the input is −5.1 dBm.

13.16   NOISE FIGURE MEASUREMENTS

A block diagram of a noise figure measurement setup is shown in Figure 13.21. The noise figure measurement setup consists of a noise source, device under test (DUT), amplifier, and spectrum analyser. The noise level is measured without the DUT as a calibration level. We measure the difference, delta (Δ) value, between the noise figure when the noise source is on and the measured noise figure when the noise source is off.

$$NF = \frac{10LOG(10^{0.1*ENR})}{((10^{0.1*\Delta}) - 1)} \tag{13.19}$$

where ENR is listed on the noise source for a given frequency. Delta, Δ, is the difference in the noise figure measurement when the noise source is on from the noise figure measurement when the noise source is off. The measured NF is calculated using Equation 13.19. Noise figure measurements are listed in Table 13.9.

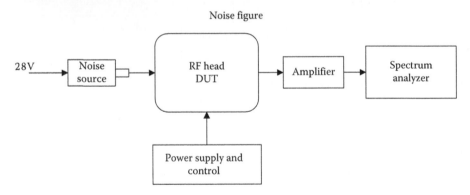

FIGURE 13.21   Noise figure measurement setup.

TABLE 13.9
Noise Figure Measurements

Parameter	Measurement 1	Measurement 2	Measurement 3
ENR	23.62	23.62	24
Delta (dB)	14	15	14
NF (dB)	9.777	8.740	10.159

13.17 ANTENNA MEASUREMENTS

Typical parameters of antennas are radiation pattern, gain, directivity, beam width, polarization, and impedance. During antenna measurements we ensure that the antenna meets the required specifications and we can characterize the antenna parameters.

13.17.1 RADIATION PATTERN MEASUREMENTS

A radiation pattern is the antenna radiated field as a function of its direction in space. The radiated field is measured at various angles at a constant distance from the antenna. The radiation pattern of an antenna is defined as the locus of all points where the emitted power per unit surface is the same. The radiated power per unit surface is proportional to the square of the electric field of the electromagnetic wave. The radiation pattern is the locus of points with the same electrical field strength. Usually the antenna radiation pattern is measured in a far field antenna range. The antenna under test is placed in the far-field distance from the transmitting antenna. Due to the size required to create a far-field range for large antennas near-field techniques are employed. Near-field techniques allow measurement of the fields on a surface close to the antenna (usually 3–10 wavelengths). The near-field measurements are transferred to far field by using a Fourier transform.

The far-field distance or Fraunhofer distance, R, is given in Equation 13.20.

$$R = \frac{2D^2}{\lambda} \tag{13.20}$$

where D is the maximum antenna dimension and λ is the antenna wavelength.

The radiation pattern graphs can be drawn using Cartesian (rectangular) coordinates as shown in Figure 13.22, see [1–5]. A polar radiation pattern plot is shown in Figure 13.23. The polar plot is useful to measure the beam width, which is the angle at the −3 dB points around the maximum gain. A 3D radiation pattern of a loop antenna is shown in Figure 13.24.

Main beam: The main beam is the region around the direction of maximum radiation, usually the region that is within 3 dB of the peak of the main lobe.

Beam width: The beam width is the angular range of the antenna pattern in which at least half of the maximum power is emitted. This angular range of the major lobe is defined as the points at which the field strength falls to around 3 dB with regard to the maximum field strength.

Side lobe level: Side lobes are smaller beams that are away from the main beam. Side lobes present radiation in undesired directions. The level is a parameter used to characterize the antenna radiation pattern. It is the maximum value of the side lobes away from the main beam and is expressed usually in decibels.

Radiated power: Total radiated power when the antenna is excited by a current or voltage of known intensity.

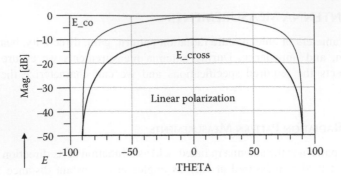

FIGURE 13.22   Radiation pattern of folded dipole dual polarized antenna.

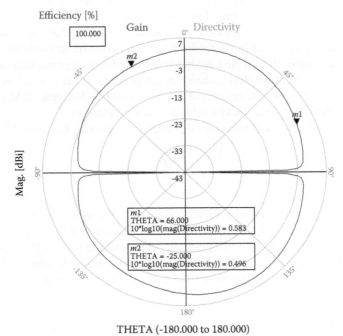

THETA (-180.000 to 180.000)

FIGURE 13.23   Radiation pattern of a wideband wearable printed slot antenna at 2 GHz.

13.17.2   DIRECTIVITY AND ANTENNA EFFECTIVE AREA

Antenna directivity is the ratio between the amounts of energy propagating in a certain direction compared to the average energy radiated to all directions over a sphere as given in Equation 13.21, see [1–4].

$$D = \frac{P(\theta,\phi)\ \text{maximal}}{P(\theta,\phi)\ \text{average}} = 4\pi \frac{P(\theta,\phi)\ \text{maximal}}{P\ \text{rad}} \qquad (13.21)$$

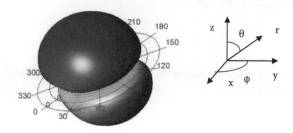

FIGURE 13.24 Loop antenna 3D radiation pattern.

where $P(\theta, \phi)$ average $= \dfrac{1}{4\pi} \displaystyle\iint P(\theta, \phi)\sin\theta \, d\theta = \dfrac{P \, \text{rad}}{4\pi}$. An approximation used to calculate antenna directivity is given in Equation 13.22.

$$D \sim \frac{4\pi}{\theta E \times \theta H} \tag{13.22}$$

θE – Measured beam widh in radians in EL plane

θH – Measured beam widh in AZ plane

Measuring the beam width radians in the AZ plane and in the EL plane allows us to calculate antenna directivity.

Antenna effective area (A_{eff}): The antenna area which contributes to the antenna directivity is given in Equation 13.23.

$$A_{\text{eff}} = \frac{D\lambda^2}{4\pi} \sim \frac{\lambda^2}{\theta E \times \theta H} \tag{13.23}$$

13.17.3 Radiation Efficiency (α)

Radiation efficiency is the ratio of power radiated to the total input power, $\alpha = \dfrac{G}{D}$. The efficiency of an antenna takes into account losses, and is equal to the total radiated power divided by the radiated power of an ideal lossless antenna. Efficiency is equal to the radiation resistance divided by total resistance (real part) of the feedpoint impedance. Efficiency is defined as the ratio of the power that is radiated to the total power used by the antenna as given in Equation 13.24. Total power equal to power radiated plus power loss.

$$\alpha = \frac{P_r}{P_r + P_l} \tag{13.24}$$

The E- and H-plane radiation pattern of a wire loop antenna in free space is shown in Figure 13.25.

13.17.4 TYPICAL ANTENNA RADIATION PATTERN

A typical antenna radiation pattern is shown in Figure 13.26. The antenna main beam is measured between the points that the maximum relative field intensity E decays to $0.707E$. Half of the radiated power is concentrated in the antenna main beam. The antenna main beam is called the 3 dB beam width. Radiation to undesired directions is concentrated in the antenna side lobes.

The antenna radiation pattern is usually measured in free space ranges. An elevated free space range is shown in Figure 13.27. An anechoic chamber is shown in Figure 13.28.

13.17.5 GAIN MEASUREMENTS

Antenna gain (G): The ratio between the amounts of energy propagating in a certain direction compared to the energy that would be propagating in the same direction if the antenna were not directional is known as its gain.

Figure 13.27 presents the antenna far field range for radiation pattern measurements. Antenna gain is measured by comparing the field strength measured by the antenna under test to the field strength measured by a standard gain horn as shown in Figure 13.27. The gain as a function of frequency of the standard gain horn is supplied by the standard gain horn manufacturer. Figure 13.28 presents an anechoic chamber used to indoor antenna measurements. The chamber metallic walls are covered with absorbing materials.

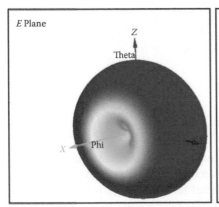
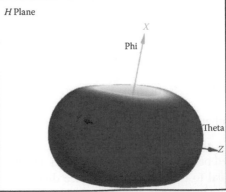

FIGURE 13.25 E- and H-plane radiation pattern of loop antenna in free space.

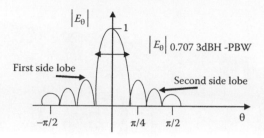

FIGURE 13.26 Antenna typical radiation pattern.

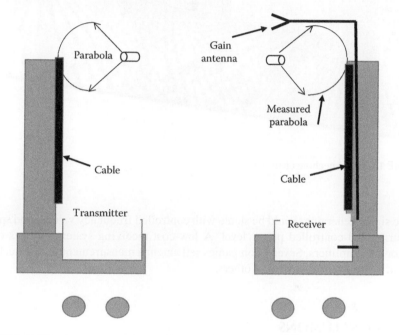

FIGURE 13.27 Antenna range for radiation pattern measurements.

13.18 ANTENNA RANGE SETUP

Antenna range setup consists of the following instruments:

- Transmitting system that consists of a wideband signal generator and transmitting antenna
- Measured receiving antenna
- Receiver
- Positioning system
- Recorder and plotter
- Computer and data processing system

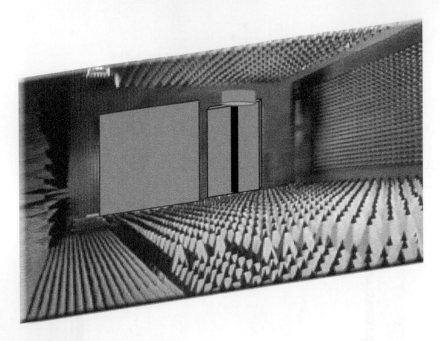

FIGURE 13.28   Anechoic chamber.

The signal generator should be stable with controlled frequency value, good spectral purity, and controlled power level. A low-cost receiving system consists of a detector and amplifiers. Several companies sell antenna measurement setups, such as Agilent, Tektronix, Antritsu, and others.

13.19   CONCLUSIONS

In this chapter electromagnetic, microwave engineering, wearable systems, and antenna measurements are presented. The wearable antenna's radiation characteristics on the human body can be measured by using a phantom. This low-cost measurement technique is used to compare several wearable antennas. The best results are achieved with the first antenna with tuning capacitor antennas in orientations of $+45°, +45°, +45°, -45°$. The results of antenna number 4 with a thinner belt are better than the results of the same antenna array with a thicker belt. For all the configurations, the highest measured signal level was when the transmitting antenna was located at $z = 0$ cm and $x = -5$ cm. For all the configurations the lowest measured signal level was when the transmitting antenna was located at $z = 15$ cm and $x = -5$ cm. The noise level is lower by 18–22 dB than the signal level.

The effect of the antenna location on the human body should be considered in the antenna design process.

REFERENCES

1. C. A. Balanis, *Antenna Theory: Analysis and Design*, 2nd Edition. Hoboken, NJ: Wiley, 1996.
2. L. C. Godara,)Ed.), *Handbook of Antennas in Wireless Communications*, Boca Raton, FL: CRC Press, 2002.
3. J. D. Kraus and R. J. Marhefka, *Antennas for All Applications*, 3rd edition, McGraw Hill, 2002.
4. A. Sabban, *RF Engineering, Microwave and Antennas*, Tel Aviv: Saar Publication, 2014.
5. A. Sabban, *Low Visibility Antennas for Communication Systems*, Taylor < Francis Group, 2015.
6. A. Sabban, *Wideband RF Technologies and Antenna in Microwave Frequencies*, Hoboken, NJ: Wiley Sons, July 2016.
7. A. Sabban, Small wearable meta materials antennas for medical systems, *Applied Computational Electromagnetics Society*, vol. 31, no. 4, pp. 434-443, April 2016.
8. A. Sabban, New compact wearable meta-material antennas, *Global Journal for Research and Analysis*, vol. 4, 268–271, August 2015.
9. A. Sabban, New wideband meta materials printed antennas for medical applications, *Journal of Advance in Medical Science (AMS)*, vol. 3, 1–10, April 2015. Invited paper.
10. A. Sabban, New wideband printed antennas for medical applications, *IEEE Transactions on Antennas and Propagation*, vol. 61, no. 1, 84–91, January 2013.
11. A. Sabban, Comprehensive study of printed antennas on human body for medical applications, *Journal of Advance in Medical Science (AMS)*, vol. 1, 1–10, February 2013.
12. A. Sabban, Wearable Antennas in Advancements in Microstrip and Printed Antennas, A. Kishk (Ed.), ISBN 980-953-307-543-8, 2013. Croatia: Intech, 2013, Available from: http://www.intechopen.com/books/show/title/advancement-in-microstrip-antennas-with-recent-applications.
13. A. Sabban, *Microstrip Antenna Arrays, in Microstrip Antennas*, N. Nasimuddin (Ed.), ISBN: 978-953-307-247-0, Croatia: InTech, 2011, Available from: http://www.intechopen .com/articles/show/title/microstrip-antenna-arrays.
14. A. Sabban, Dually polarized tunable printed antennas for medical applications, IEEE European Antennas and Propagation Conference (EUCAP), 2015, Lisbon, Portugal, April 2015.
15. A. Sabban, New microstrip meta materials antennas, *IEEE Antennas and Propagation*, Memphis, TN, July 2014.
16. A. Sabban, Wearable antennas for medical applications, *in IEEE BodyNet 2013*, Boston, MA, October 2013, pp. 1–7.
17. A. Sabban, New meta materials antennas, *IEEE Antennas and Propagation*, Orlando, FL, July 2013.
18. A. Sabban, Meta materials antennas, New Tech Magazine, Tel Aviv, Israel, pp. 16–19, June 2013.
19. A. Sabban, Wideband tunable printed antennas for medical applications. *IEEE APS/ URSI Conference*, Chicago, IL, July 2012, pp. 1–2.
20. A. Sabban, MM wave microstrip antenna arrays, New Tech Magazine, Tel Aviv, Israel, June 2012, pp. 16–21.
21. A. Sabban, New compact wideband printed antennas for medical applications. *IEEE APS/URSI Conference*, Spokane, WA, July 2011, pp. 251–254.
22. A. Sabban, Interaction between new printed antennas and human body in medical applications, *Asia Pacific Symposium*, Japan, December 2010, pp. 187–190.
23. A. Sabban, Wideband printed antennas for medical applications *APMC 2009 Conference*, Singapore, December 2009, pp. 393–396 .

Index

Printed and bound by CPI Group (UK) Ltd, Croydon, CR0 4YY

01/11/2024

01782619-0015